T0142318

# Advances in Intelligent Systems and Computing

Volume 779

**Series editor**

Janusz Kacprzyk, Polish Academy of Sciences, Warsaw, Poland
e-mail: kacprzyk@ibspan.waw.pl

The series "Advances in Intelligent Systems and Computing" contains publications on theory, applications, and design methods of Intelligent Systems and Intelligent Computing. Virtually all disciplines such as engineering, natural sciences, computer and information science, ICT, economics, business, e-commerce, environment, healthcare, life science are covered. The list of topics spans all the areas of modern intelligent systems and computing such as: computational intelligence, soft computing including neural networks, fuzzy systems, evolutionary computing and the fusion of these paradigms, social intelligence, ambient intelligence, computational neuroscience, artificial life, virtual worlds and society, cognitive science and systems, Perception and Vision, DNA and immune based systems, self-organizing and adaptive systems, e-Learning and teaching, human-centered and human-centric computing, recommender systems, intelligent control, robotics and mechatronics including human-machine teaming, knowledge-based paradigms, learning paradigms, machine ethics, intelligent data analysis, knowledge management, intelligent agents, intelligent decision making and support, intelligent network security, trust management, interactive entertainment, Web intelligence and multimedia.

The publications within "Advances in Intelligent Systems and Computing" are primarily proceedings of important conferences, symposia and congresses. They cover significant recent developments in the field, both of a foundational and applicable character. An important characteristic feature of the series is the short publication time and world-wide distribution. This permits a rapid and broad dissemination of research results.

More information about this series at http://www.springer.com/series/11156

Nancy J. Lightner
Editor

# Advances in Human Factors and Ergonomics in Healthcare and Medical Devices

Proceedings of the AHFE 2018 International
Conference on Human Factors and Ergonomics
in Healthcare and Medical Devices, July 21–25,
2018, Loews Sapphire Falls Resort at Universal Studios,
Orlando, Florida, USA

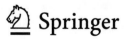 Springer

*Editor*
Nancy J. Lightner
Veterans Affairs - Center for Applied
Systems Engineering
Indianapolis, IN, USA

ISSN 2194-5357          ISSN 2194-5365  (electronic)
Advances in Intelligent Systems and Computing
ISBN 978-3-319-94372-5          ISBN 978-3-319-94373-2   (eBook)
https://doi.org/10.1007/978-3-319-94373-2

Library of Congress Control Number: 2018947355

Printed on acid-free paper

This Springer imprint is published by the registered company Springer International Publishing AG
part of Springer Nature
The registered company address is: Gewerbestrasse 11, 6330 Cham, Switzerland

# Advances in Human Factors and Ergonomics 2018

**AHFE 2018 Series Editors**

*Tareq Z. Ahram, Florida, USA*
*Waldemar Karwowski, Florida, USA*

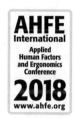

**9th International Conference on Applied Human Factors and Ergonomics and the Affiliated Conferences**

**Proceedings of the AHFE 2018 International Conference on Healthcare and Medical Devices, held on July 21–25, 2018, in Loews Sapphire Falls Resort at Universal Studios, Orlando, Florida, USA**

| | |
|---|---|
| *Advances in Affective and Pleasurable Design* | *Shuichi Fukuda* |
| *Advances in Neuroergonomics and Cognitive Engineering* | *Hasan Ayaz and Lukasz Mazur* |
| *Advances in Design for Inclusion* | *Giuseppe Di Bucchianico* |
| *Advances in Ergonomics in Design* | *Francisco Rebelo and Marcelo M. Soares* |
| *Advances in Human Error, Reliability, Resilience, and Performance* | *Ronald L. Boring* |
| *Advances in Human Factors and Ergonomics in Healthcare and Medical Devices* | *Nancy J. Lightner* |
| *Advances in Human Factors in Simulation and Modeling* | *Daniel N. Cassenti* |
| *Advances in Human Factors and Systems Interaction* | *Isabel L. Nunes* |
| *Advances in Human Factors in Cybersecurity* | *Tareq Z. Ahram and Denise Nicholson* |
| *Advances in Human Factors, Business Management and Society* | *Jussi Ilari Kantola, Salman Nazir and Tibor Barath* |
| *Advances in Human Factors in Robots and Unmanned Systems* | *Jessie Chen* |
| *Advances in Human Factors in Training, Education, and Learning Sciences* | *Salman Nazir, Anna-Maria Teperi and Aleksandra Polak-Sopińska* |
| *Advances in Human Aspects of Transportation* | *Neville Stanton* |

(continued)

(continued)

| | |
|---|---|
| *Advances in Artificial Intelligence, Software and Systems Engineering* | *Tareq Z. Ahram* |
| *Advances in Human Factors, Sustainable Urban Planning and Infrastructure* | *Jerzy Charytonowicz and Christianne Falcão* |
| *Advances in Physical Ergonomics & Human Factors* | *Ravindra S. Goonetilleke and Waldemar Karwowski* |
| *Advances in Interdisciplinary Practice in Industrial Design* | *WonJoon Chung and Cliff Sungsoo Shin* |
| *Advances in Safety Management and Human Factors* | *Pedro Miguel Ferreira Martins Arezes* |
| *Advances in Social and Occupational Ergonomics* | *Richard H. M. Goossens* |
| *Advances in Manufacturing, Production Management and Process Control* | *Waldemar Karwowski, Stefan Trzcielinski, Beata Mrugalska, Massimo Di Nicolantonio and Emilio Rossi* |
| *Advances in Usability, User Experience and Assistive Technology* | *Tareq Z. Ahram and Christianne Falcão* |
| *Advances in Human Factors in Wearable Technologies and Game Design* | *Tareq Z. Ahram* |
| *Advances in Human Factors in Communication of Design* | *Amic G. Ho* |

# Preface

This book is concerned with human factors and ergonomics in healthcare and medical devices. The utility of this area of research is to aid the design of systems and devices for effective and safe healthcare delivery. New approaches are demonstrated for improving healthcare devices such as portable ultrasound systems. Research findings for improved work design, effective communications, and systems support are also included. Healthcare informatics for the public and usability for patient users are considered separately but build on results from usability studies for medical personnel.

Quality and safety are emphasized, and medical error is considered for risk factors and information transfer in error reduction. Physical, cognitive, and organizational aspects are considered in a more integrated manner so as to facilitate a systems approach to implementation. New approaches to patient handling ergonomics, emergency and operating rooms, healthcare, medical device design, human factors and ergonomics measurement, and model validation are included. Recent research on special populations, collaboration and teams, as well as learning and training allow practitioners to gain a great deal of knowledge overall from this book.

Explicitly, the book is organized into four sections that contain the following subject areas:

   I. Applications in Healthcare and Medical Devices
  II. Human Factors in Healthcare
 III. Patient Safety
  IV. Human factors for Aging: Innovation for Enhanced Quality of Life

Each of the chapters of the book was either reviewed by the members of Scientific Advisory and Editorial Board or germinated by them. Our sincere thanks and appreciation go to the Board members listed below for their contribution to the high scientific standard maintained in developing this book.

Patricia Arnold, Germany
Tommaso Bellandi, Italy
Balmatee Bidassie, USA
Qammer Abbasi, UK
Fehti Calisir, Turkey
Yoel Donchin, Israel
Achim Elfering, Switzerland
Mahmut Eksioglu, Turkey
Enda Fallon, Ireland
Xin Feng, USA
Mike Fray, UK
Mazin Gadir, UAE
Anand Gramopadhye, USA
Sue Hignett, UK
Erik Hollnagel, France
Jay Kalra, Canada
Sharon Kleefield, USA
Basia Kutryba, Poland
Bruce Byung Cheol Lee, USA
Nicolas Marmaras, Greece
Jennifer L. Martin, UK
Rosângela Míriam Mendonca, Brazil
Kathy Norris, USA
Michiko Ohkura, Japan
Calvin Or, Hong Kong
Lenore Page, USA
Stavros Prineas, Australia
Paolo Trucco, Italy

This book would be of special value internationally to those researchers and practitioners involved in various aspects of healthcare delivery.

July 2018                                                                        Nancy Lightner

# Contents

## Human Factors in Healthcare

**Human Factors for Aging: Innovation for Enhanced
Quality of Life**

# Applications in Healthcare
# and Medical Devices

# Using Design to Connect Patients, Providers, and Researchers: A Cognitive Assessment and Monitoring Platform for Integrative Research (CAMPFIRE)

Paula Jacobs[✉], Dominic Anello, and Seth Elkin-Frankston

Charles River Analytics, Inc., 625 Mt. Auburn St., Cambridge, MA 02138, USA
{pjacobs, selkinfrankston}@cra.com,
dominic.anello@gmail.com

**Abstract.** There is a substantial need for an accessible suite of cognitive measures to assess and monitor signs of chemotherapy-related cognitive impairment during the treatment and survivorship phases of the cancer control continuum. To address this need we designed and demonstrated a Cognitive Assessment and Monitoring Platform for Integrative Research (CAMPFIRE), a privacy-compliant software system to support the administration of cognitive assessment measures and facilitate secure provider-patient interaction.

**Keywords:** Patient-reported outcomes
Chemotherapy-related cognitive impairment · Cognitive function
Cancer · Neuropsychology · Computerized neuropsychological assessment

## 1 Introduction

Over 14.5 million individuals in the United States today either live with or have a history of cancer [1]. Thanks to rapid advances in cancer treatments, including surgery, chemotherapy, radiation, and other targeted biological therapies, an estimated 19 million cancer survivors will live in the U.S. by the year 2024 [2]. Unfortunately, up to 70% of patients receiving chemotherapy suffer some level of cognitive decline [3–5]. While cognitive deficits can be acute, chronic impairments, including deficits in working memory, verbal memory, and psychomotor functioning, can persist for years [6–8], and may even be delayed in onset [9]. Colloquially termed "chemobrain," the neuropsychological sequelae of chemotherapy-related cognitive impairment (CRCI) include deficits in a range of cognitive domains such as learning and memory, processing speed, executive functioning and attention [10]. Despite evidence recognizing CRCI, the precise etiology, long-term impact, and specific neuropsychological deficits remain elusive. This gap in understanding may be due to the array of confounding factors contributing to CRCI, including psychological and genetic factors, oxidative stress, inflammatory responses, medication side-effects, and direct effects of chemotherapy [11, 12]. Nevertheless, the community needs a gold standard for assessing subtle cognitive changes to be able to understand, manage, and ultimately prevent chemotherapy-related cognitive impairment.

© Springer International Publishing AG, part of Springer Nature 2019
N. J. Lightner (Ed.): AHFE 2018, AISC 779, pp. 3–14, 2019.
https://doi.org/10.1007/978-3-319-94373-2_1

Given the difficulty in identifying and assessing these cognitive changes, there is a substantial need for an accessible suite of cognitive tests to assess and monitor signs of CRCI during the treatment and survivorship phases of the cancer control continuum. This assessment platform should be security-compliant (i.e., conform to HIPAA privacy and security standards), scientifically valid, and flexible enough to be administered on a variety of technology platforms, either remotely or in the clinic. To develop an electronic platform to assess cognitive changes in cancer patients via repeated administration of reliable neuropsychological measures, we must consider three primary challenges. First, the system must integrate a collection of cognitive assessment measures based on contemporary neuro- and psycho-oncology research. Detecting CRCI presents a specific challenge because of the subtle and often unique changes that can occur between individuals. Standard neuropsychological batteries can lack specificity and may not be sensitive to important covariates such as mood, stress, or anxiety. In addition, CRCI detection is reliant on assessments by trained neuropsychologists, meaning that a patient may only be assessed once or twice throughout treatment, further limiting the ability to accurately capture the scope of deficits. Therefore, an assessment suite should include a battery of well-validated measures to fully capture the gamut of cognitive impairments [13–15]. Second, the system must provide an intuitive provider/researcher portal functionality and support administration of self-guided assessment measures. Computerized assessment tools provide numerous advantages over standard pen and paper neuropsychological measures. However, wide acceptance of a new software system requires ease of accessibility, administration, interpretation, and integration. A successful approach should provide an intuitive interface to support test administration and data management for providers, researchers and patients. To address the difficulties inherent in communicating with a diverse community of health care-providers, researchers, and patients, we must also recognize that the value of computerized assessment tools may be lost if they are too difficult or confusing for the user. Third, the system must be fully security-compliant and capable of directly integrating with Electronic Medical Record systems to adequately address security issues inherent to protected health information (PHI). The use of Electronic Health Record (EHR) systems is rapidly becoming a requirement for all healthcare providers. Integrating with the EHR system affords us an opportunity to seamlessly mesh with providers' existing workflow. While integration reduces the time burden on providers and increases the efficiency of clinical research, EHR systems contain a wealth of sensitive information about patients that must be protected. Meeting these requirements will enhance the capacity for measuring cognitive changes in cancer patients, and provide a tool to address a significant gap in the understanding of chemotherapy-related cognitive impairment (Fig. 1).

To address the challenges, we designed and demonstrated a Cognitive Assessment and Monitoring Platform for Integrative Research (CAMPFIRE), a privacy-compliant software system to support the administration of cognitive assessment measures and facilitate secure provider-patient interaction. CAMPFIRE integrates well-validated cognitive assessment tools to assess and monitor subtle cognitive changes throughout the patients' cancer treatment and survivorship phases. To accomplish this goal, we relied on our expertise in healthcare information technology, neuropsychology, and clinical oncology to develop a system to support the administration, assessment, and reporting requirements of cancer treatment and research. Our technical approach is best described in terms of the following three challenges.

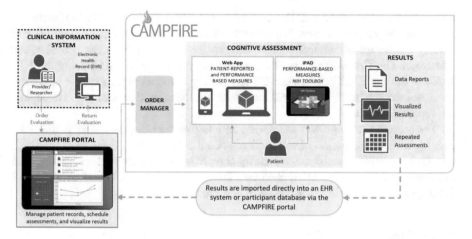

**Fig. 1.** System architecture for CAMPFIRE

Our first challenge was to identify and integrate a collection of well-validated cognitive assessment measures based on contemporary neuro- and psycho-oncology research. Despite the recognized awareness of CRCI, which spans over two decades [16–19], a unified consensus of the impact on cognition and ability to identify vulnerable individuals has remained a challenge. There are several contributing factors to this challenge, primary of which is a lack of a common core neuropsychological assessment battery. This need was first addressed by the International Cognition and Cancer Task Force (ICCTF); the ICCTF recommended a minimum core assessment battery including: (1) Hopkins Verbal Learning Test-Revised; (2) the Trail Making Test; and (3) the Controlled Oral Word Association of the Multilingual Aphasia Examination. Although this was an important first effort, several challenges remain. The core battery recommended by the ICCTF lacks specificity and may not capture all of the subtle cognitive changes associated with cancer treatment. This battery is primarily aimed at assessing objective, performance-based measures. While the predictive relationship between subjective and objective measures of cognitive performance remains a matter of debate, subjective assessments are a critical component of diagnoses, and provide important information not addressed by standard neuropsychological tests [20, 21]. Therefore, we developed a software system that integrates a suite of measures to assess and monitor cognitive function as well as other patient-reported outcome measures. We included well-validated measures to assess function in cognitive domains often affected in cancer patients, including attention, executive function, working memory, processing speed, verbal and visuospatial abilities, and motor function. Measures of subjective and objective cognitive function were selected from several instruments developed through the NIH Neurology Quality-of-Life Measurement Initiative to develop a core set of evaluation tools, including the NIH Toolbox for the Assessment of Neurological Function and Behavior [22, 23], Patient – Reporting Outcomes Measurement Information System (PROMIS) to monitor patient-perceived symptoms [24–26], and Quality of Life Outcomes in Neurological Disorders (Neuro-QoL) [27]. We also supported the three neuropsychological tests recommended by the ICCTF so that data generated by the CAMPFIRE system is comparable to previous studies. We integrated assessment measures into CAMPFIRE to develop a software system that equally supports the needs of the patient, provider, and researcher. The CAMPFIRE system monitors the full scope of CRCI using the NIH Toolbox and the ICCTF-recommended test battery to assess performance-based measures, and the PROMIS, Neuro-QOL, and NIH Toolbox Emotion item banks to capture self-reported measures.

The second challenge was to provide an intuitive provider/researcher portal functionality and administration of self-guided assessment measure and the third challenge was for CAMPFIRE to be fully security-compliant and capable of integrating with electronic health records (EHR) systems. The rest of this paper describes these two challenges and their related design tasks and products.

## 2    Designing CAMPFIRE

CAMPFIRE presented an interesting use case for balancing the needs of three user groups. Our first user group, cancer survivors, commonly report cognitive impairments following chemotherapy. They require intuitive access to their assessment tests so their providers can track these side effects. They also want to be able to access contact information for their providers. Our second group, healthcare providers, require easy access to their patient's assessment results, but are also burdened an increasing number of documentation requirements. Our final group, research investigators, require sophisticated tools to better understand the precise etiology and prevalence of cognitive changes associated with cancer and cancer treatment.

Our goal was to design a system that would make the provider's job simpler, the researchers job well informed, and the patient's job (taking the assessments) easy to navigate and intuitive, without letting the interface needs of each user type hinder the experience of the other user types. When designing each user interface (UI), we identified and explored specific use cases, developed use case diagrams showing the interaction flow for achieving tasks, prototyped and evaluated UI designs through wireframe designs, and further developed those designs that pass evaluation. We used a cognitive systems engineering (CSE) approach to ensure our UIs and designs address the needs of providers and researchers who will use the CAMPFIRE system. CSE provides a principled approach to understanding the analysts' decision-making, situational awareness, and cognitive constraints. CSE incorporates work domain analysis, cognitive task analysis, and knowledge elicitation techniques that can be used to identify needs of practitioners, as well as elements of the UI that are critical for the practitioner to achieve a high degree of success using the CAMPFIRE system. Figure 2 shows the use case diagram for the CAMPFIRE system, which allowed us to settle on the tasks each actor in the system should be able to perform (represented by each circle in the system). These informed out workflows and eventual UIs.

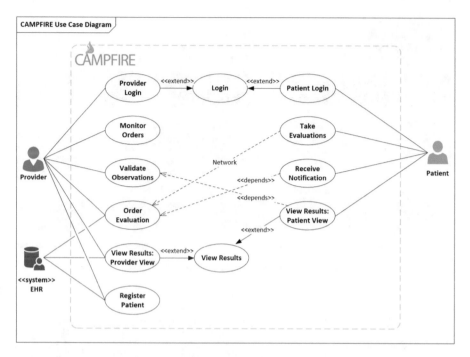

**Fig. 2.** Use case diagram for CAMPFIRE.

## 2.1  Designing for Patients

Standard paper and pencil neuropsychological tests are the cornerstone of assessing and measuring cognitive changes, many of which require the presence of an onsite neuropsychologist to both administer and provide valuable insight into an individual's cognitive abilities. While these tests are well-validated and highly reliable, the wide disparity of assessment measures administered between different studies and clinics likely contribute to inconsistencies within the literature [28]. Computerized neuropsychological assessments are being developed at a rapid pace; however, the field has been reluctant to fully embrace these technologies [29]. One of the hurdles for the successful use of software systems, especially in clinical settings, is the design of effective user interfaces (UIs) [30].

To create the UIs for the screens that would be interacting with patients (what would be the Patient Portal), we created workflows from our research efforts and use case diagram (see Figs. 2 and 3), turned those workflows into mockups, and iterated on those mockups until we had web based software prototypes ready for our initial user testing (see Fig. 4). The Patient Portal allows the user to perform two main tasks. It allows the user to contact their providers and to view and take pending evaluations. In the sample pages provided in Fig. 4, you can see the landing page (the first thing the user sees after the user logs in), a sample interaction with the provider messaging functionality (added in the workflow diagram stage), and the representative testing screen. Non-medical questions were selected for testing purposes.

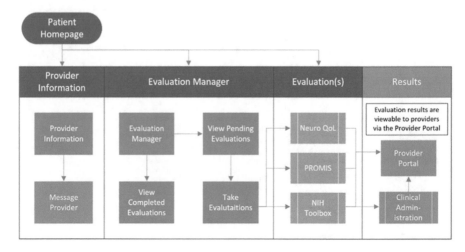

**Fig. 3.** Workflow diagram for the patient portal

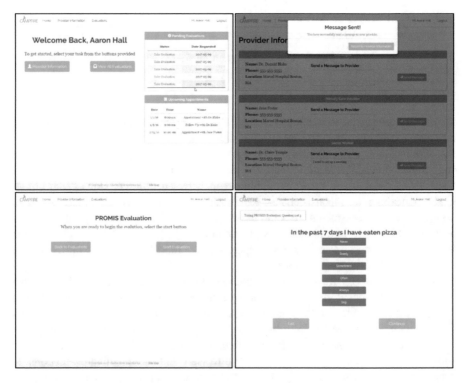

**Fig. 4.** Prototype UIs for the patient portal.

## 2.2  Designing for Providers and Researchers

A recent preliminary survey, conducted in part by the Massachusetts Neuropsychological Society, found that many of the 600 neuropsychologists interviewed spend two to three hours on average writing six-page reports. Lengthy reports serve as a critical assurance that assessments are methodical and well-reasoned; however, such extensive reports may not always be necessary. For example, due to the cost and time required for a full evaluation and report, the number of times a patient is evaluated over the course of treatment may be limited. In addition, a neuropsychological evaluation provides a snapshot of a patient's cognitive abilities at a single point in time. A more efficient way to track and monitor cognitive performance is to take many snapshots over time, allowing for a full perspective of cognitive changes throughout the course of an illness. There is a need to develop a system that enables the efficient administration of cognitive assessments in a way that reliably captures performance and likewise supplies providers and researchers valuable insight at a glance. Therefore, in Phase I, we designed the CAMPFIRE system to be compliant with multiple EHR platforms by modeling the workflow using the Integrating Healthcare in the Enterprise (IHE) Laboratory Point Of Care Testing (LPOCT) profile; that is: (1) initiating an evaluation; (2) administering the test(s) to the patient; and (3) returning the validated results to the practitioner. To maximize compatibility across multiple EHR systems, the CAMPFIRE system interface will be based on the IHE suite of integration profiles. IHE leverages existing and well supported standards for interacting with clinical information systems, notably the HL7 standard. Rather than scheduling lengthy evaluations, the LPOCT IHE profile enables ordering an evaluation to be transparently integrated into the provider's normal workflow when summarizing the encounter in their EHR.

To create the UIs for our provider facing functionality (what would become the Provider Portal), we followed the same design processed used for the Patient Portal. The Provider Portal has four main functionalities. It allows the user to manage patients, order evaluations, view/input evaluation results, and see results across patients and data sets for research purposes (Fig. 5 shows the workflow diagram for these functions). Sample screenshots from the resulting software prototype can be seen in Fig. 6. The top left shows a screen where the provider can order evaluations their patients can take. In order to accommodate test results not integrated with CAMPFIRE, we included a manual entry form, though we envision the provider using it as little as possible. On the result viewing screen (bottom left) the providers can see a table of all results and drill down to get more specific information download the results. Finally, a research view gives a provider doing research the ability to look across patients/data sets and discover trends and relationships.

## 2.3  User Testing

As the next step in our design process, we conducted a series of user tests on volunteer providers and representative patients using our software prototype. Demographics for the scenario testing are included in Table 1. Participants were instructed to complete scenarios related to tasks a patient, provider or family member would experience in the final product. Participants completed scenarios without errors and within similar time

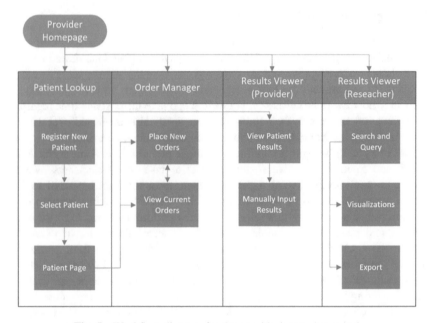

**Fig. 5.** Workflow diagram for the provider/researcher portal

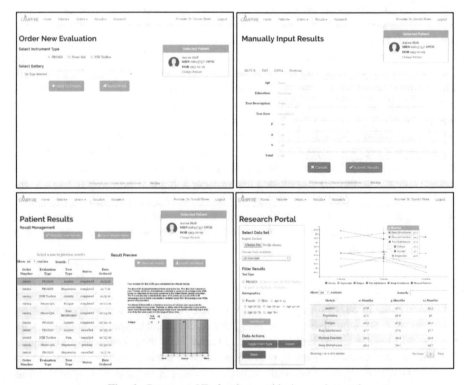

**Fig. 6.** Prototype UIs for the provider/research portal

scales. Their responses involved feedback on where to place notifications, clearer labels, and functionality. Follow-on System Usability Scale responses (Table 2) indicated positive reactions to CAMPFIRE.

**Table 1.** Participant demographics.

| Role | Sex | Age | Handedness | Backgrond |
|------|-----|-----|-----------|-----------|
| Provider | F | 38 | Left | Oncologist (MD) |
| Provider | F | 30 | Right | Oncology (RN) |
| Provider | M | 31 | Right | Oncologist (MD) |
| Patient | F | 37 | Right | Positive Family Hx (Uncle) |
| Patient | F | 33 | Right | Positive Family Hx (Uncle) |
| Patient | F | 35 | Right | Positive Family Hx (Father) |
| Patient | F | 57 | Right | Prior Diagnosis |
| Patient | M | 45 | Right | Prior Diagnosis |

**Table 2.** User testing system usability scale responses

| Question | Provider | | Patient | |
|----------|----------|-----|---------|-----|
| | Average | SD | Average | SD |
| I think that I would like to use this system frequently | 3.3 | 0.5 | 3.8 | 1.2 |
| I found the system unnecessarily complex | 1.3 | 0.5 | 1.4 | 0.5 |
| I thought the system was easy to use | 4.7 | 0.5 | 4.6 | 0.5 |
| I think that I would need the support of a technical person to be able to use this system | 1.3 | 0.5 | 1.0 | 0.0 |
| I found the various functions in this system were well integrated | 4.3 | 0.5 | 4.0 | 0.6 |
| I thought there was too much inconsistency in this system | 2.0 | 0.0 | 1.6 | 0.8 |
| I would imagine that most people would learn to use this system very quickly | 4.3 | 0.5 | 4.8 | 0.4 |
| I found the system very cumbersome to use | 1.0 | 0.0 | 1.4 | 0.5 |
| **Total** | **22.3** | **2.8** | **22.3** | **2.8** |

## 3 Discussion

The direct outcome of this program is the implementation of a web-based portal application that will enable patients, family members, and providers to better track and monitor CRCI through a collection of cognitive assessment measures that detect changes in both perceived and objective cognitive function. This technology empowers patients to monitor symptoms at home or in the clinic, and it allows providers and researchers to manage patient records, schedule assessments, and visualize results through a single system—the CAMPFIRE platform. CAMPFIRE makes patient-provider communication easier because it integrates into providers' existing workflows, and can be easily accessed and navigated by patients. Through better monitoring, the CAMPFIRE system enables better patient management by providing actionable insights though intuitive data reporting.

The CAMPFIRE platform for assessing subtle cognitive changes in a wide-range of patient populations can have a significant impact. Given the current trend for home healthcare over in-hospital care, CAMPFIRE provides an ideal approach to assess cognitive health remotely. While the focus of this effort is to detect and manage CRCI, CAMPFIRE is built on top of an extensible architecture that allows new interfaces to be brought online as needed. Along with the ability to align with standard healthcare protocols and interface with existing EHRs, CAMPFIRE provides a powerful and flexible capability for both healthcare providers and researchers. The ultimate societal and scientific benefit of CAMPFIRE will be an enhanced set of tools that help manage and monitor changes in mental status over time.

# References

1. American Cancer Society: Cancer Facts & Figures 2016. American Cancer Society, Atlanta (2016)
2. American Cancer Society: Cancer Treatment and Survivorship Facts & Figures 2014–2015. American Cancer Society, Atlanta (2014)
3. Ahles, T.A., Root, J.C., Ryan, E.L.: Cancer - and cancer treatment-associated cognitive change: an update on the state of the science. J. Clin. Oncol. **30**(30), 3675–3686 (2012). https://doi.org/10.1200/JCO.2012.43.0116
4. Ono, M., Ogilvie, J.M., Wilson, J.S., Green, H.J., Chambers, S.K., Ownsworth, T., Shum, D. H.K.: A meta-analysis of cognitive impairment and decline associated with adjuvant chemotherapy in women with breast cancer. Neuro-Oncology **5**, 59 (2015). https://doi.org/10.3389/fonc.2015.00059
5. Wefel, J.S., Schagen, S.B.: Chemotherapy-related cognitive dysfunction. Curr. Neurol. Neurosci. Rep. **12**(3), 267–275 (2012). https://doi.org/10.1007/s11910-012-0264-9
6. Ahles, T.A., Saykin, A.J., Furstenberg, C.T., Cole, B., Mott, L.A., Skalla, K., Whedon, M. B., Bivens, S., Mitchell, T., Greenberg, E.R., Silberfarb, P.M.: Neuropsychologic impact of standard-dose systemic chemotherapy in long-term survivors of breast cancer and lymphoma. J. Clin. Oncol. Official J. Am. Soc. Clin. Oncol. **20**(2), 485–493 (2002)
7. Collins, B., Mackenzie, J., Stewart, A., Bielajew, C., Verma, S.: Cognitive effects of chemotherapy in post-menopausal breast cancer patients 1 year after treatment. Psycho-Oncology **18**(2), 134–143 (2009). https://doi.org/10.1002/pon.1379
8. Yamada, T.H., Denburg, N.L., Beglinger, L.J., Schultz, S.K.: Neuropsychological outcomes of older breast cancer survivors: cognitive features ten or more years after chemotherapy. J. Neuropsychiatry Clin. Neurosci. **22**(1), 48–54 (2010). https://doi.org/10.1176/appi.neuropsych.22.1.48
9. Wefel, J.S., Saleeba, A.K., Buzdar, A.U., Meyers, C.A.: Acute and late onset cognitive dysfunction associated with chemotherapy in women with breast cancer. Cancer **116**(14), 3348–3356 (2010). https://doi.org/10.1002/cncr.25098
10. Wefel, J.S., Kesler, S.R., Noll, K.R., Schagen, S.B.: Clinical characteristics, pathophysiology, and management of noncentral nervous system cancer-related cognitive impairment in adults. CA Cancer J. Clin. **65**(2), 123–138 (2015). https://doi.org/10.3322/caac.21258

11. Janelsins, M.C., Kesler, S.R., Ahles, T.A., Morrow, G.R.: Prevalence, mechanisms, and management of cancer-related cognitive impairment. Int. Rev. Psychiatry **26**(1), 102–113 (2014). http://doi.org/10.3109/09540261.2013.864260
12. Jean-Pierre, P., Johnson-Greene, D., Burish, T.G.: Neuropsychological care and rehabilitation of cancer patients with chemobrain: strategies for evaluation and intervention development. Support. Care Cancer **22**(8), 2251–2260 (2014). https://doi.org/10.1007/s00520-014-2162-y
13. Hutchinson, A.D., Hosking, J.R., Kichenadasse, G., Mattiske, J.K., Wilson, C.: Objective and subjective cognitive impairment following chemotherapy for cancer: a systematic review. Cancer Treat. Rev. **38**(7), 926–934 (2012). https://doi.org/10.1016/j.ctrv.2012.05.002
14. Lai, J.-S., Wagner, L.I., Jacobsen, P.B., Cella, D.: Self-reported cognitive concerns and abilities: two sides of one coin? Psycho-Oncology **23**(10), 1133–1141 (2014). https://doi.org/10.1002/pon.3522
15. Wefel, J.S., Vardy, J., Ahles, T., Schagen, S.B.: International cognition and cancer task force recommendations to harmonise studies of cognitive function in patients with cancer. Lancet Oncol. **12**(7), 703–708 (2011). https://doi.org/10.1016/S1470-2045(10)70294-1
16. Jansen, C.E., Cooper, B.A., Dodd, M.J., Miaskowski, C.A.: A prospective longitudinal study of chemotherapy-induced cognitive changes in breast cancer patients. Support. Care Cancer **19**(10), 1647–1656 (2011). https://doi.org/10.1007/s00520-010-0997-4
17. Kaiser, J., Bledowski, C., Dietrich, J.: Neural correlates of chemotherapy-related cognitive impairment. Cortex **54**, 33–50 (2014). https://doi.org/10.1016/j.cortex.2014.01.010
18. van Dam, F.S., Schagen, S.B., Muller, M.J., Boogerd, W., Droogleever Fortuyn, M.E., Rodenhuis, S.: Impairment of cognitive function in women receiving adjuvant treatment for high-risk breast cancer: high-dose versus standard-dose chemotherapy. J. Natl. Cancer Inst. **90**(3), 210–218 (1998)
19. Wieneke, M.H., Dienst, E.R.: Neuropsychological assessment of cognitive functioning following chemotherapy for breast cancer. Psycho-Oncology **4**(1), 61–66 (1995). https://doi.org/10.1002/pon.2960040108
20. Schagen, S.B., Boogerd, W., Muller, M.J., Huinink, W.T.B., Moonen, L., Meinhardt, W., Van Dam, F.S.: Cognitive complaints and cognitive impairment following BEP chemotherapy in patients with testicular cancer (2008)
21. Skaali, T., Fosså, S.D., Andersson, S., Cvancarova, M., Langberg, C.W., Lehne, G., Dahl, A.A.: Self-reported cognitive problems in testicular cancer patients: relation to neuropsychological performance, fatigue, and psychological distress. J. Psychosom. Res. **70**(5), 403–410 (2011). https://doi.org/10.1016/j.jpsychores.2010.12.004
22. Weintraub, S., Dikmen, S.S., Heaton, R.K., Tulsky, D.S., Zelazo, P.D., Bauer, P.J., Carlozzi, N.E., Slotkin, J., Blitz, D., Wallner-Allen, K., Fox, N.A., Beaumont, J.L., Mungas, D., Nowinski, C.J., Richler, J., Deocampo, J.A., Anderson, J.E., Manly, J.J., Borosh, B., Havlik, R., Conway, K., Edwards, E., Freund, L., King, J.W., Moy, C., Witt, E., Gershon, R.C.: Cognition assessment using the NIH toolbox. Neurology, **80**(11 Suppl 3), S54–S64 (2013). http://doi.org/10.1212/WNL.0b013e3182872ded
23. Weintraub, S., Dikmen, S.S., Heaton, R.K., Tulsky, D.S., Zelazo, P.D., Slotkin, J.6., Carlozzi, N.E., Bauer, P.J., Wallner-Allen, K., Fox, N., Havlik, R., Beaumont, J.L., Mungas, D., Manly, J.J., Moy, C., Conway, K., Edwards, E., Nowinski, C.J., Gershon, R.: The cognition battery of the NIH toolbox for assessment of neurological and behavioral function: validation in an adult sample. J. Int. Neuropsychol. Soc. JINS **20**(6), 567–578 (2014). https://doi.org/10.1017/S1355617714000320

24. Cella, D., Riley, W., Stone, A., Rothrock, N., Reeve, B., Yount, S., Amtmann, D., Bode, R., Buysse, D., Choi, S., Cook, K., DeVellis, R., DeWalt, D., Fries, J.F., Gershon, R., Hahn, E. A., Lai, J.-S., Pilkonis, P, Revicki, D., Rose, M., Weinfurt, K., Hays, R.: Initial adult health item banks and first wave testing of the patient-reported outcomes measurement information system (PROMISTM) network: 2005–2008. J. Clin. Epidemiol. **63**(11), 1179–1194 (2010). https://doi.org/10.1016/j.jclinepi.2010.04.011

25. Cella, D., Yount, S., Rothrock, N., Gershon, R., Cook, K., Reeve, B., Ader, D., Fries, J.F., Bruce, B., Rose, M.: The patient-reported outcomes measurement information system (PROMIS). Med. Care **45**(5 Suppl 1), S3–S11 (2007). http://doi.org/10.1097/01.mlr. 0000258615.42478.55

26. Riley, W.T., Rothrock, N., Bruce, B., Christodolou, C., Cook, K., Hahn, E.A., Cella, D.: Patient-reported outcomes measurement information system (PROMIS) domain names and definitions revisions: further evaluation of content validity in IRT-derived item banks. Qual. Life Res. Int. J. Qual. Life Aspects Treat. Care Rehabil. **19**(9), 1311–1321 (2010). https:// doi.org/10.1007/s11136-010-9694-5

27. Cella, D., Lai, J.-S., Nowinski, C.J., Victorson, D., Peterman, A., Miller, D., Bethoux, F., Heinemann, A., Rubin, S., Cavazos, J.E., Reder, A.T., Sufit, R., Simuni, T., Holmes, G.L., Siderowf, A., Wojna, V., Bode, R., McKinney, N., Podrabsky, T., Wortman, K., Choi, S., Gershon, R., Rothrock, N., Moy, C.: Neuro-QOL brief measures of health-related quality of life for clinical research in neurology. Neurology **78**(23), 1860–1867 (2012). http://doi.org/ 10.1212/WNL.0b013e318258f744

28. O'Farrell, E., MacKenzie, J., Collins, B.: Clearing the Air: a review of our current understanding of "chemo fog". Current Oncol. Rep. **15**(3), 260–269 (2013). https://doi.org/ 10.1007/s11912-013-0307-7

29. Parsey, C.M., Schmitter-Edgecombe, M.: Applications of technology in neuropsychological assessment. Clin. Neuropsychol. **27**(8) (2013). http://doi.org/10.1080/13854046.2013. 834971

30. Zhang, L., Chai, X., Ling, S., Fan, J., Yang, K., Ren, Q.: Dispersion and accuracy of simulated phosphene positioning using tactile board. Artif. Organs **33**(12), 1109–1116 (2009). https://doi.org/10.1111/j.1525-1594.2009.00826.x

# Soft-Brush: A Novel Tendon Driven Tactile Stimulator for Affective Touch in Children with Autism

Zhaobo K. Zheng[1($\boxtimes$)], Dayi Bian[2], Amy Swanson[5], Amy Weitlauf[3,5], Zachary Warren[3,4,5], and Nilanjan Sarkar[1,2]

[1] Department of Mechanical Engineering, Vanderbilt University,
Nashville, TN, USA
{zhaobo.zheng,nilanjan.sarkar}@vanderbilt.edu
[2] Department of Electrical Engineering and Computer Science,
Vanderbilt University, Nashville, TN, USA
[3] Department of Pediatrics, Vanderbilt Univerisity, Nashville, TN, USA
[4] Department of Psychiatry, Vanderbilt University, Nashville, TN, USA
[5] Treatment and Research Institute of Autism Spectrum Disorders (TRIAD),
Vanderbilt University, Nashville, TN, USA

**Abstract.** Autism Spectrum Disorders (ASD) is a prevalent developmental disorder and is associated with high familial and societal cost. Early interventions during the first year can have the best developmental outcomes despite the fact that the earliest diagnosis of ASD is only possible by the age of two. Investigating brain response to basic stimuli like sight, smell and touch has proved to have the potential to find markers between individuals with ASD and their neurotypical peers during infancy. Since existing tactile stimulus delivering method tend to suffer from low accuracy, low availability and low tolerability, it is necessary to develop a precise, high-tolerable tactile stimulus delivering mechanism. The present study examined the feasibility and tolerability of Soft-Brush, a comfortable, mobile silicone tactile stimulator with tendon-driven mechanism, for delivering tactile stimulus in multisensory studies. Experiments have shown that Soft-Brush has high tolerance rate by the children during experiments resulting in reliable data collection.

**Keywords:** Autism Spectrum Disorders · Tactile stimulator
Systems engineering · Affective touch

## 1 Introduction

Autism Spectrum Disorder (ASD) has a prevalence rate of 1 in 68 among children in the United States [1] and is associated with high familial and societal cost [2]. Currently the earliest diagnosis of ASD is only possible by the age of two [3]. However, early interventions during the first year of life might have optimal developmental outcomes due to neural plasticity [4]. Although complex social and communication capabilities develop over the course of the childhood, brain response to basic stimuli like sight, smell and touch appear much earlier, even in the first few months of life [5]. In particular, affective touch,

© Springer International Publishing AG, part of Springer Nature 2019
N. J. Lightner (Ed.): AHFE 2018, AISC 779, pp. 15–22, 2019.
https://doi.org/10.1007/978-3-319-94373-2_2

which can be described as a comforting, caress-like soft touch, has been found to impact the "social brain" [6–8]. Although it is difficult to produce skin-to-skin affective touch in laboratory settings, an analogous tactile stimulation which is produced by a mechanical source (e.g., soft brushing) is comparable to affective touch that is manually produced by hand [9]. Taking advantage of this window of opportunity, researchers have recently designed a multisensory stimulus delivery (MADCAP) system to document infants' responses to stimuli [10]. Such a system can be used for exploring potential markers between individuals with ASD and their neurotypical peers during infancy.

MADCAP system has successfully presented different stimuli including tactile stimulation to the subject and collected different types of data (Fig. 1). However, only 46.15% of the infants tolerated MADCAP system mainly because the existing tactile stimulator is overwhelmingly big and rigid for infants. The existing tactile stimulator (TSD) has a box-shaped design and is 28 cm × 12 cm × 30 cm in dimensions. The box hangs on from a gravity-compensated supporting manipulator that guarantees the box could move with the infant's arm freely in 3D space. However, the inertia of the box and damping of the manipulator needs a certain force for motion and sometimes it is too much for the infants. Study with infants has shown that limitation of motion may lead infants to worse mental conditions [11] such as car seat crying. In general, the researchers need to touch the infants' arms during experimental setup with MADCAP but study has shown that almost all babies generate wariness and even fear when touched by strangers [12]. Even though there are no sharp edges in the TSD and there is cloth cover on surfaces, the contacting surfaces are still not soft and comfortable enough.

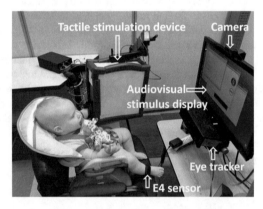

**Fig. 1.** Existing Tactile Stimulator (TSD) in MADCAP system by Bian et al.

The target population for MADCAP study is infants under the age of two. Tolerability due to comfort and safety is especially important due to the nature of the infant participants. To ensure a higher tolerance rate, a more soft and comfortable affective touch device is needed. Meanwhile, the tactile stimulator should be more compact and light-weight so that the infants do not feel constrained to move their arms.

In the present work, we have achieved the above goals by designing a novel infant-friendly silicone tactile stimulator, Soft-Brush, with a tendon-actuated mechanism that can be worn like a sleeve. This paper is organized as follows. Section 2 describes the system design of Soft-Brush. Section 3 explains the experimental setup. Section 4 presents the tolerability study results. In the final Section, we conclude the paper with a discussion and limitations of the current work.

## 2  System Design

Soft-Brush consists of three main components, which are a silicone wrap, a brushing block and an actuating part, as shown in Fig. 2. The combined weight of the silicone wrap and the brushing block is only 161 g, which is far less than the TSD. The lightweight design allows the babies to move their arms much more freely.

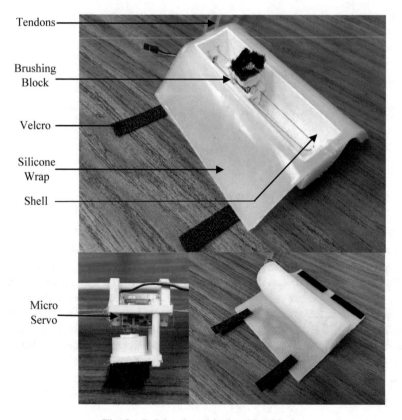

**Fig. 2.**  Soft-brush and its brushing block

The silicone wrap has a sleeve-type design and wraps around an infant's forearm. The soft plastic rubber (Ecoflex 00-30), which is skin-safe and comfortable to touch, was used to make the wrap. A mold shown in Fig. 3 was first designed and 3D printed to get the exact shape of the wrap. After curing, we sewed four strips of Velcro on both sides of the wrap to stick them together. This also allows us to use the wrap on infants with a wide range of arm sizes, from 3-months to 2-years-olds. Then we sewed a 3D-printed shell inside the chamber to keep its shape in case that the infant tries to squeeze the silicone wrap. The wrap can be soaked into warm water and it is very easy to apply Lysol and baby-wipes for disinfection.

The brushing block moves back and forth on a support axle and soft brush hair was glued on the bottom to produce affective touch [13]. The pressure and velocity are the two key factors for such affective touch. A micro servo (Hitech, HS24BB) shown in Fig. 1 with a lead screw is integrated to drive the brush up and down. By reading the encoder information of the servo, we compute the relative distance between the brush and the skin, which correlates to the brushing pressure. The brush can go 11.5 cm and 1 cm in horizontal and vertical directions, respectively. The brushing block is able to cover the 3−12 cm/s speed range that is optimal for creating affective touch [8].

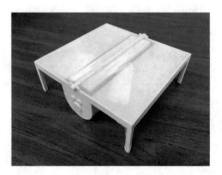

**Fig. 3.** Silicone wrap curing in 3D-printed mold

The actuating part is positioned 50 cm away from the wrap. The tendons (Brave-fisherman, 0.48 mm) stick on a disk housed on a Nema 23 stepper motor (Step-perOnline, 23HS45) and then go through plastic tubes and into the chamber, actuating the brushing block. To reduce the nonlinear friction between the tubes and the tendons, we try to keep the tubes as straight as possible during the experiments in order to achieve the smoothest brushing. Nevertheless, sufficient smooth motion can be achieved even if the tubes are bent to a circle curve. A controller (Arduino, Uno) controls both the stepper and servo motors. The Arduino connects to a workstation via serial port to deliver the tactile stimulus synchronously with audio-visual stimulus. The tendons are non-extendable so we can control the brushing velocity through the open-loop speed control of the stepper motor that is precise enough for our application (Fig. 4).

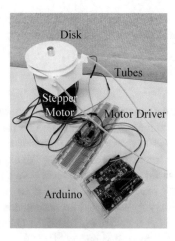

**Fig. 4.** Actuating part

# 3   Experiments

To test whether Soft-Brush can outperform TSD in terms of tolerability, we ran experiments following the same procedure as Bian et al. [10]. Before the experiment, the Soft-Brush was soaked into warm water with baby shampoo so that it is warm and fragrant. The TSD typically needs 30–45 s to put on whereas the Soft-Brush only needs 5–10 s to do so. Moreover, researchers no longer need to touch the infants' arms during the setup to avoid stranger touching effect. The experimental setup is shown in Fig. 5. The subject sits in a high chair wearing Soft-Brush on the left forearm as well as E4 sensor (Empatica, E4 wristband) on the ankle and an EEG cap (EGI, Geodesic Sensor Net) on the head. After the setup, the subject watches six sessions of videos. Tactile stimulus is applied in three of the six sessions in random orders. Throughout the experiment, EEG, physiological and eye gaze data were recorded.

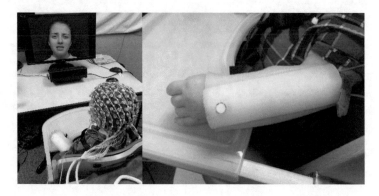

**Fig. 5.** Experimental setup and soft-brush during experiment

After the experiments, we can temporarily take the supporting axle along with the brushing block off so we can wash and disinfect the silicone wrap conveniently.

## 4   Results

We have conducted 12 experiments to date. Ten infants tolerated the entire process, which amounts to a tolerance rate of 83.33%. Note that the tolerance rate of the TSD was 46.15%. The reasons for the two infants who did not went through the whole process are as follows: One infant got upset during the experiment so we stopped the experiment; The other infant did not tolerate the EEG cap and we went through the rest of the process without EEG recording. Therefore, if we take out cases due to other causes (e.g., EEG tolerability) to compute the acceptance rate of tactile stimulators only, the acceptance rate of the Soft-Brush is 91.67% (11 out of 12). If we apply the same criteria for the TSD, the tolerance rate is 50.00%.

Moreover, the Soft-Brush created less distraction and constraint to the infants during the experiments based on our observations. They were able to move their arms freely. The shorter setup time, less stranger touching and more comfortable feeling led to a pleasant mental state in the infants. Of those infants who completed the entire procedure, 7 out of 10 infants (70%) did not display any distressed behaviors (e.g., crying) as compared to 41.67% for the TSD. The calmer and happier state of the babies during the experiments leads to a more reliable data collection.

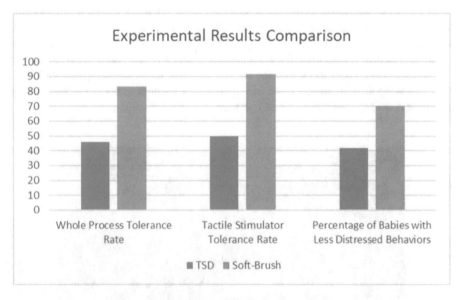

**Fig. 6.** Experimental results

The results indicate that the Soft-Brush is capable of delivering the tactile stimulus with much higher tolerance rate than the TSD. In addition, the infants wearing the Soft-Brush displayed less distress during the experiments. The observed behaviors of the infants during experiments suggest that infants feel much more comfortable wearing the Soft-Brush. In addition, feedback from the parents agrees with this observation (Fig. 6).

## 5   Conclusions and Limitations

In this paper, we have presented the design and tolerability testing of the Soft-Brush, a tendon-actuated tactile stimulator for producing affective touch, which can be worn like a sleeve. It is more comfortable for infants and more convenient for researchers to use as compared to the previous version of the affective touch device, the TSD. This current tactile stimulator (i.e., the Soft-Brush) resulted in a much higher tolerance rate and induced less distressed behaviors in the infants. Twelve infants participated the experiments using the Soft-Brush and the results indicate a significant improvement when compared to the TSD. The Soft-Brush could help collect data that are more reliable during multi-sensory stimuli presentation that could be used to find markers between children with ASD and their typically developed peers.

There are a few limitations regarding the design of the Soft-Brush and its experimental validation. First, the Soft-Brush still makes some noise when it delivers the tactile stimulus, especially when it starts. This noise sometimes attracts the attention of the subject that could confound certain experimental paradigms. Second, it will be better to add arrays of small holes for better ventilation and even lighter weight. Third, the micro-servo motor used in the system has metal parts in it and thus making the Soft-Brush not MRI-compatible and waterproof. This may limit the Soft-Brush's usage for wider experimental paradigms. In addition, more participants will be needed in the future to obtain a robust result.

**Acknowledgments.** We would like to thank all the participants and their families for their time and participation. We would also like to thank Simeng Zhao for helping hardware development for this study.

## References

1. Center for Disease Control (CDC): Community Report on Autism (2016)
2. Horlin, C., Falkmer, M., Parsons, R., Albrecht, M.A., Falkmer, T.: The cost of autism spectrum disorders. PLoS One **9**(9), e106552 (2014)
3. Zwaigenbaum, L., Bauman, M.L., Stone, W.L., Yirmiya, N., Estes, A., Hansen, R.L., McPartland, J.C., et al.: Early identification of autism spectrum disorder: recommendations for practice and research. Pediatrics **136**(Supplement 1), S10–S40 (2015)
4. Veenstra-VanderWeele, J., Warren, Z.: Intervention in the context of development: pathways toward new treatments. Neuropsychopharmacology **40**(1), 225 (2015)

5. Germani, T., Zwaigenbaum, L., Bryson, S., Brian, J., Smith, I., Roberts, W., Szatmari, P., et al.: Brief report: assessment of early sensory processing in infants at high-risk of autism spectrum disorder. J. Autism Dev. Disord. **44**(12), 3264–3270 (2014)
6. Brauer, J., Xiao, Y., Poulain, T., Friederici, A.D., Schirmer, A.: Frequency of maternal touch predicts resting activity and connectivity of the developing social brain. Cereb. Cortex **26**, 3544–3552 (2016)
7. Triscoli, C., Olausson, H., Sailer, U., Ignell, H., Croy, I.: CT-optimized skin stroking delivered by hand or robot is comparable. Front. Behav. Neurosci. **7**, 208 (2013)
8. Löken, L.S., Olausson, H.: The skin as a social organ. Exp. Brain Res. **204**, 305–314 (2010)
9. Fairhurst, M.T., Löken, L., Grossmann, T.: Physiological and behavioral responses reveal 9-month-old infants' sensitivity to pleasant touch. Psychol. Sci. **25**, 1124–1131 (2014)
10. Bian, D., Zheng, Z., Swanson, A., Weitlauf, A., Warren, Z., Sarkar, N.: Design of a multisensory stimulus delivery system for investigating response trajectories in infancy. In: International Conference on Universal Access in Human-Computer Interaction, pp. 471–480. Springer, Cham (2017)
11. Elder, D.E., Russell, L., Sheppard, D., Purdie, G.L., Campbell, A.J.: Car seat test for preterm infants: comparison with polysomnography. Arch. Dis. Child. Fetal Neonatal Ed. **92**(6), F468–F472 (2007)
12. Bretherton, I.: Making friends with one-year-olds: an experimental study of infant-stranger interaction. Merrill-Palmer Q. Behav. Dev. **24**(1), 29–51 (1978)
13. Croy, I., Geide, H., Paulus, M., Weidner, K., Olausson, H.: Affective touch awareness in mental health and disease relates to autistic traits–an explorative neurophysiological investigation. Psychiatry Res. **245**, 491–496 (2016)

# The Development of an Innovative Corneal Biopsy Tool: A Usability Comparison of Four Ergonomic Handle Prototypes

Lore Veelaert[1]([✉]), Muriel De Boeck[1]([✉]), Erik Haring[1]([✉]),
Sorcha Nì Dhubhghaill[2], Carina Koppen[2], and Guido De Bruyne[1]

[1] Department of Product Development, Faculty of Design Sciences,
University of Antwerp, Ambtmanstraat 1, 2000 Antwerp, Belgium
{Lore.Veelaert, Muriel.DeBoeck, Erik.Haring,
Guido.DeBruyne}@uantwerpen.be
[2] Department of Ophthalmology, Faculty of Medicine and Health Sciences,
Visual Optics and Visual Rehabilitation, University of Antwerp,
Universiteitsplein 1, Antwerp, Belgium
{Sorcha.NiDhubhghaill, Carina.Koppen}@uza.be

**Abstract.** Keratitis, or an inflammation of the cornea, is a common eye disease in which a biopsy of the cornea is required to determine its underlying cause. Currently, no standardized tool is available for this purpose and corneal scrapings are performed with a scalpel or wide needle, frequently with inconclusive results as too little material is removed for fear of penetration. Previous research resulted in a new cutting principle, and is used in this follow-up study. The aim of this research is to optimize the usability of the cutting principle through a user evaluation (N = 18) of four ergonomic handle prototypes. The results of this study suggest that a forceps-shaped handle provides improved usability, and propose design guidelines for further optimization.

**Keywords:** Corneal biopsy · Keratitis · Hand tool ergonomics

## 1 Introduction

Keratitis is an infection in the cornea of the eye (protecting the pupil and iris), which is caused by an agglomeration of fluids, other materials or bacteria [1–4]. Every year, between 0.046% and 1.92% of the western population is diagnosed with keratitis [5]. It can cause severe swelling and eventually blindness [1, 2]. To determine one of the various causes of the disease, it is important to verify the correct diagnosis. The current treatment procedure usually starts with the prescription of broad-spectrum antibiotics, assuming the keratitis' cause is bacterial, even though this is only the case for approximately 63% of the patients [6, 7].

When no improvement occurs, a surgeon will scrape a sample of the cornea using a standard scalpel [3, 8]. However, several difficulties may occur [9]: (i) obscured etiology of the keratitis as consequence of antibiotics [10], (ii) resistance to local therapy, and (iii) often inconclusive results as too little material is removed for fear of penetration. In the latter case, a riskier corneal biopsy using a scalpel is necessary to avoid

© Springer International Publishing AG, part of Springer Nature 2019
N. J. Lightner (Ed.): AHFE 2018, AISC 779, pp. 23–29, 2019.
https://doi.org/10.1007/978-3-319-94373-2_3

severe keratitis and penetrating keratoplasty [6, 11–13]. Unfortunately, this method is difficult and only performed by seasoned surgeons, with a relatively high risk of damaging the cornea, as no standardized tool is available.

Consequently, to ensure a better passing rate of the biopsy, it is necessary to develop a standardized tool with which the surgeon can perform the surgery on the eye. Crucial elements in this development is the guarantee of different variables, such as depth (0.1 mm), surface area (1–2 mm$^2$), and a consistency that is higher than reached with a scalpel [3].

## 1.1    Ergonomics

Surgeons frequently encounter ergonomic discomfort in areas as shoulders, wrists, thumbs, and fingertips [14]. Surgery requires a high level of intellectual preparation, an efficient and controlled workspace, fine motor skills, physical endurance, problem-solving skills and emergency response skills [15]. Due to prolonged physical endurance and motor skills, surgeons often endure pressure and fatigue in their hands [16–19] and even suffer from physical pain [15] and stiffness [14]. Previous studies have also shown that the shape of instrument handles causes discomfort. Gripping an instrument with a small contact area, for example, can put severe pressure on the fingers and palm [17–21].

Therefore, in the development of an innovative chirurgical hand tool, it is also essential to integrate ergonomic design principles for the comfort of the surgeon [18].

## 1.2    Research Objective

Previous research evaluated the effectiveness of different surgical tools for obtaining a corneal biopsy [3]. This study aims at optimizing the ergonomics of a cutting mechanism. A usability study allows evaluating four handle prototypes.

# 2    Methods and Materials

## 2.1    Construction of the Prototypes

The prototyped handles were required to enable five steps: (i) positioning the tool, (ii) vertical pressure, (iii) pinching, (iv) disconnecting the tissue, and finally (v) releasing the sample in a container. The development of the prototypes was based on the tweezers principle of the initial corneal biopsy tool, with a focus on precision of the tool. The prototypes were developed according to eight ergonomic requirements for the design of hand tools, found in ergonomic literature [18, 24]:

1. Grip opening between 65 and 90 mm;
2. Ring dimensions: length 30 mm, width 24 mm;
3. Angle between grip and cutting area between 14° and 24°;
4. Avoiding presence of a spring;
5. Opening/closing by flexors/extensors of the fingers;
6. Thumb use for rotation knob (not applicable in this study);
7. Large contact area;
8. Little opening/closing force required.

The handle prototypes were modeled with the 3D CAD software SolidWorks, after which the concepts were 3D-printed in PLA, as shown in Fig. 1. Furthermore, Table 1 shows the evaluation the prototypes according to the ergonomic requirements mentioned above.

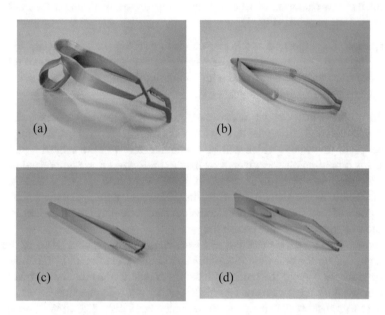

**Fig. 1.** Four handle prototypes: *(a)* hand-shaped prototype, *(b)* pipette-shaped prototype, *(c)* forceps-shaped prototype and *(d)* curved prototype.

**Table 1.** Evaluation of four prototypes according to the ergonomic handle requirements. ✓ = satisfies requirement, ✗ = does not satisfy requirement, ● = not applicable.

| Prototype model | | | | |
|---|---|---|---|---|
| 1. Grip opening | ✓ | ✓ | ● | ● |
| 2. Ring dimensions | ● | ● | ● | ● |
| 3. Angle grip-cut | ✓ | ✗ | ✗ | ✗ |
| 4. Spring | ✗ | ● | ● | ● |
| 5. Flex./ext. fingers | ✓ | ✓ | ✓ | ✓ |
| 6. Thumb use | ● | ● | ● | ● |
| 7. Large contact area | ✓ | ✓ | ✗ | ✗ |
| 8. Little force | ✓ | ✓ | ✓ | ✓ |

## 2.2  Experimental Study

**Setting and Materials.** The user tests were conducted in the usability lab on the campus of Product Development of the University of Antwerp. In order to execute the experiments, two cameras, two Petri dishes, four grains of rice and the four handle prototypes were required (Fig. 1).

**Participants.** The objective of this research is to develop a corneal biopsy tool that is suitable for both experienced and unexperienced surgeons. The evaluation of the biopsy tool was therefore conducted with 18 untrained subjects – eight women and ten men – aged between 18 and 25 years old.

**Procedure.** The study consist of two parts; a precision test and a survey. Each participant was recorded during the test by two cameras. The recordings will only be used in the scope of this study, which will be communicated with the subject at the start of the test. Each participant was given four handle prototypes in a randomized order and two Petri dishes with four grains of rice in the left Petri dish, whereby the Petri dishes were positioned 40 cm away from each other. Then, the participant was asked to pick up one grain of rice from the left Petri dish and to transport it to the right Petri dish using each of the four handle prototypes.

The different stages of the precision test were timed with a transcription of the video recordings. During the complete task, three task stages were timed: (i) the time it takes for the participant to hold the model in the correct manner, (ii) the time it takes for the participant to pick up a rice grain with the model and (iii) the time it takes for the participant to transport the rice grain to the other Petri dish. The time that each stage took for the participant with each model gives an indication of the usability and efficiency of the design.

Afterwards, each participant was given an online survey to collect qualitative data concerning the experience of the user. 6-point Likert scales were used to examine their preference regarding functionality and ergonomics of each tool. Then, a personal preference and clarification was asked based on their experiences.

**Statistics.** A one way ANOVA/Turkey HSD is used to determine if the time performance of the different models is significantly different. A non-parametric Kruskal-Wallis test is used to process the Likert-scale scores leading to the overall perception of the models regarding functionality and ergonomics.

## 3  Results and Discussion

Table 2 shows the mean time per prototype for each stage. Only the pipette-shaped model and the forceps-shaped model are significantly different ($\alpha = 0.05$) during the first stage. No significant difference is reported among the models during the other test stages. Overall, the forceps-shaped model performed best during all stages according to the average time.

**Table 2.** Mean times and standard deviations of the precision test (* = significant difference).

| Prototype model | Stage 1 (i) | SD | Stage 2 (ii) | SD | Stage 3 (iii) | SD |
|---|---|---|---|---|---|---|
| Forceps-shaped | 2.64* | 0.93 | 5.81 | 3.96 | 2.31 | 0.7 |
| Hand-shaped | 3.07 | 1.14 | 9.5 | 9.29 | 2.59 | 1.5 |
| Pipette-shaped | 4.06* | 1.81 | 7.3 | 4.23 | 2.65 | 2.0 |
| Curved-shaped | 3.44 | 1.32 | 8.79 | 6.93 | 2.32 | 0.6 |

A survey is used for obtaining information with respect to the personal preference of the models among the participants. The pipette-shaped model is preferred by most of the participants (n = 8), followed by the curved-shaped model (n = 4), forceps-shaped model (n = 3) and the hand-shaped model (n = 3). The Likert scales of functionality and grip comfort are analyzed with a Kruskal-Wallis test to check if there is a significant difference in the two comfort scores. The Kruskal-Wallis test reports only a significant difference (P 0.003) in functionality comfort; no significance is observed in grip comfort (P 0.418).

Furthermore, the precision test indicates the forceps-shaped model to be the desired design since it is overall the fastest in use. The significant difference in grasp time (stage 1) is expected to be the result of an enhanced support of this design towards precision handlings of the hand.

The different designs do not appear to be significantly different during the other two stages. However, the standard deviation in time of the hand-shaped model indicates that the design is less reliable in performance compared to the other models.

Likewise, despite the outcome of the precision test and the lack of a significantly different grip comfort, the highest preference of the participants can be found for the pipette-shaped model. Potentially, the pipette-shaped model referred to a more familiar handling for the test persons in comparison to the hand-shaped model.

In addition, an interesting discrepancy is found regarding the results of the participants' preference and the results of the Likert scales scoring functionality and grip comfort. The latter indicates that the hand-shaped model has the highest mean rank for functionality comfort instead of the overall preferred pipette-shaped model. In further research, this could be explored by means of a laddering technique during the closing survey, leading to deeper understanding of user's preference towards a certain model type. Also, several design iterations need to be created in a next step using the forceps-shaped model as a starting point as it scored best on the precision test. The benefits of the preferred (but slowest) pipette-shaped model and the functionality comfort of the hand-shaped model may be integrated within an optimized forceps-shaped designs.

## 4  Conclusion

Keratitis, or an inflammation of the cornea, is a common eye disease in which a biopsy of the cornea is required to determine its underlying cause. Currently, no standardized tool is available for this purpose and corneal scrapings are performed with a scalpel or wide needle, frequently with inconclusive results as too little material is removed for fear of penetration. Previous research resulted in a novel cutting principle of which this study aimed to optimize usability aspects through a user evaluation of four ergonomic handle prototypes: (a) a hand-shaped prototype, (b) a pipette-shaped prototype, (c) a forceps-shaped prototype and (d) a curved prototype.

The results of this study show that a forceps-shaped handle leads to the lowest average test times, that significantly differ from the pipette-shaped handle. However, the latter handle was preferred by eight participants. Finally, a significant difference among the four prototypes was found concerning the functionality comfort, whereby the hand-shaped model had the highest mean rank score, but none concerning the grip comfort. Building upon the average times in the precision test, we suggest that a forceps-shaped handle provides improved usability, for which design guidelines can be proposed for further optimization, based on the benefits of the preferred pipette-shaped handle and the most functionally comfortable hand-shaped handle.

Conclusively, an optimized corneal biopsy tool that is efficient, effective, safe and ergonomic will ensure a better passing rate of the biopsy. This will accelerate a correct diagnosis, avoiding the unsubstantiated prescription of broad-spectrum antibiotics.

**Acknowledgments.** This paper is the result of a collaborative research between the Department of Ophthalmology (UZA), Centre for Cell Therapy and Regenerative Medicine (Ophthalmology/Vaxinfectio – UA/UZA) and the Department of Product Development (UA) together with the industrial partner D.O.R.C. Additionally, we want to acknowledge all students contributing to this publication within the course of Applied Research Methods at Product Development, University of Antwerp.

# References

1. Streilein, J.W., Dana, M.R., Ksander, B.R.: Immunity causing blindness: five different paths to herpes stromal keratitis. Immunol. Today **18**(9), 443–449 (1997)
2. Yu, M.C.Z., Höfling-Lima, A.L., Furtado, G.H.C., Yu, M.C.Z., Höfling-Lima, A.L., Furtado, G.H.C.: Microbiological and epidemiological study of infectious keratitis in children and adolescents. Arq. Bras. Oftalmol. **79**(5), 289–293 (2016)
3. Veelaert, L., et al.: Usefulness of skin punch tools for corneal biopsy, vol. 590 (2018)
4. Gorski, M., Genis, A., Yushvayev, S., Awwad, A., Lazzaro, D.R.: Seasonal variation in the presentation of infectious keratitis. Eye Contact Lens Sci. Clin. Pract. **42**(5), 295–297 (2016)
5. Singh, D., Verma, A.: Fungal Keratitis: Background, Pathophysiology, Epidemiology. MedScape (2015)
6. Ibrahim, Y., Boase, D., Cree, I.: Incidence of infectious corneal ulcers, portsmouth study, UK. J. Clin. Exp. Ophthalmol. **3**(5) (2012)
7. Townsend, N., Dunbar, M.T.: The right approach. the diagnosis and the treatment rules for infectious cornea ulcers. Optom. Manag. **49**, 22, 25, 42 (2014)
8. Daschner, F.: Leitsätze der Antibiotikatherapie. In: Antibiotika am Krankenbett, pp. 15–18. Springer Heidelberg (1996)
9. Wenzel, M., Schrage, N.F.: Diagnostik bei Hornhauterkrankungen. In: Kampik, A., Grehn, F, pp. 37–50 (1996)
10. Callegan, M.C., O'Callaghan, R.J., Hill, J.M.: Pharmacokinetic considerations in the treatment of bacterial keratitis. Clin. Pharmacokinet. **27**(2), 129–149 (1994)
11. Friedlaender, M.H.: Corneal biopsy. Int. Ophthalmol. Clin. **28**(2), 101–102 (1988)

12. Newton, C., Moore, M.B., Kaufman, H.E.: Corneal biopsy in chronic keratitis. Arch. Ophthalmol. **105**(4), 577–578, April 1987. (Chicago, Ill. 1960)
13. Whitehouse, G., Reid, K., Hudson, B., Lennox, V.A., Lawless, M.A.: Corneal biopsy in microbial keratitis. Aust. N. Z. J. Ophthalmol. **19**(3), 193–196 (1991)
14. Berguer, R., Forkey, D.L., Smith, W.D.: Ergonomic problems associated with laparoscopic surgery. Surg. Endosc. **13**(5), 466–468 (1999)
15. Berguer, R.: Surgery and ergonomics. Arch. Surg. **134**(9), 1011–1016 (1999)
16. Berguer, R.: The application of ergonomics in the work environment of general surgeons. Rev. Environ. Health **12**(2), 99–106 (1997)
17. Matern, U., Eichenlaub, M., Waller, P., Rückauer, K.D.: MIS instruments: an experimental comparison of various ergonomic handles and their design. Surg. Endosc. **13**(8), 756–762 (1999)
18. Van Veelen, M.A., Meijer, D.W.: Ergonomics and design of laparoscopic instruments: results of a survey among laparoscopic surgeons. J. Laparoendosc. Adv. Surg. Tech. A **9**(6), 481–489 (1999)
19. Van Veelen, M.A., Meijer, D.W., Goossens, R.H.M., Snijders, C.J., Jakimowicz, J.J.: Improved usability of a new handle design for laparoscopic dissection forceps. Surg. Endosc. Other Interv. Tech. **16**(1), 201–207 (2002)
20. Berguer, R., Gerber, S., Kilpatrick, G., Beckley, D.: An ergonomic comparison of in-line vs pistol-grip handle configuration in a laparoscopic grasper. Surg. Endosc. **12**(6), 805–808 (1998)
21. Matern, U., Waller, P.: Instruments for minimally invasive surgery: new technology principles of ergonomic handles, pp. 174–182 (1999)
22. Daams, B.J.: Productergonomie. Ontwerpen voor nut, gebruik en beleving. Deel 2a. Uitgeverij Undesigning (2013)
23. Sancibrian, R., Gutierrez-Diez, M.C., Torre-Ferrero, C., Benito-Gonzalez, M.A., Redondo-Figuero, C., Manuel-Palazuelos, J.C.: Design and evaluation of a new ergonomic handle for instruments in minimally invasive surgery. J. Surg. Res. **188**(1), 88–99 (2014)
24. Sanders, M.S., McCormick, E.J.: Human Factors in Engineering and Design (1987)

# A Cryotherapeutic Device for Preventing Nail Toxicity During Chemotherapy: Comparison of Three Cooling Strategies

Tess Aernouts, Muriel De Boeck$^{(\boxtimes)}$, Jochen Vleugels,
Marc Peeters, and Guido De Bruyne

Department Product Development, University of Antwerp,
Ambtmanstraat 1, 2000 Antwerp, Belgium
tessaernouts@hotmail.com,
{muriel.deboeck,jochen.vleugels,marc.peeters,
guido.debruyne}@uantwerpen.be

**Abstract.** Onycholysis is a form of nail toxicity where the nail detaches from the nail bed. This medical condition is reported to appear with up to 44% of the patients undergoing a taxanes based chemotherapy. Frozen gloves can be effective in preventing nail toxicity as they enable cold-induced vasoconstriction (CIVC), or reduction of blood flow, and therefore limits the transport of chemotherapeutic agents towards the nail bed. Unfortunately, the use of frozen gloves also results in cold-induced vasodilation (CIVD), which increases blood flow and reduces the effectiveness of the preventive treatment. Moreover, the gloves induce pain and additional distress during a cancer treatment. The objective of this article is to examine the usefulness of an active local cooling device for controlling blood flow in the fingertips and reducing CIVD, while limiting pain and discomfort. Three different cooling strategies are evaluated for comparing their cooling effectiveness.

**Keywords:** Onycholysis · Chemotherapy · Cold-Induced Vasodilation
Pulsed cooling · Cryotherapy · Nail bed toxicity

## 1 Introduction

Onycholysis, a form of nail toxicity where the nail detaches from the nail bed, is observed with up to 44% of the patients undergoing a systemic cancer treatment that uses the chemotherapy chemicals anthracyclines and taxanes [1–3]. These chemicals provide a toxic effect to the bed epithelium, which will inroad the structure that holds the nail onto its nail bed. Shortage of keratin has a visible effect on Beau's lines, indicating a reduction of the strength of the nail plate [1]. Changes in the nail unit are common during the course of systemic cancer treatment and can be associated with pain and functional impairment. Chemotherapy-induced onycholysis can therefore significantly affect the daily lives of cancer patients. Hence, it is important to understand how onycholysis can be prevented during cancer treatment [4].

Cryotherapy, or cold therapy, has been found to decrease the effects of onycholysis and other chemotherapy-induced complications [5]. Localized cryotherapy invokes

© Springer International Publishing AG, part of Springer Nature 2019
N. J. Lightner (Ed.): AHFE 2018, AISC 779, pp. 30–36, 2019.
https://doi.org/10.1007/978-3-319-94373-2_4

vasoconstriction, i.e. narrowing of the blood vessels, which causes a decreased blood flow. After a certain time – generally after 5 to 10 min – the vessels start to dilate again as a protection mechanism of the body to prevent cold-induced tissue damages. This effect is called cold-induced vasodilation (CIVD) and may disrupt the effectiveness of the treatment [6]. Furthermore, during prolonged cold exposure, a so-called hunting reaction will occur which is characterized by alternating periods of vasodilation and vasoconstriction [7].

Currently, cryotherapy for the prevention of onycholysis is applied using passive cooling. Examples hereof are gel-filled frozen gloves and socks, which are usually refrigerated at −20 to −30 °C and worn for 90 min [8]. Since the cooling is applied passively, the temperature inside the gloves and socks does not remain constant and is only low during the first 15 to 20 min [9]. Hence, they are usually replaced by new ones after 45 min. These frozen gloves and socks significantly reduce nail toxicity [10, 11], with Scotté et al. reporting a drop in overall occurrence of nail toxicity from 51% to 11% [8]. Unfortunately, glove and sock temperature is not controlled during passive cooling. This may cause CIVD. Frozen gloves and socks are also painful, resulting in limited therapy adherence [4].

Tyler et al. investigated the occurrence of CIVD by comparing the thermal responses of an index finger to 0 and 8 °C water immersion [6]. They concluded that 8 °C may be more suitable when looking to optimise the CIVD fluctuations while minimising participant discomfort. Sawada et al. [12] studied the occurrence of CIVD at different ambient room temperature conditions (30, 25 and 20 °C). Their results suggest that CIVD reactivity weakens after repeated cooling of fingers in a cooler environment where the body core temperature is liable to decrease, indicating that CIVD may be the result of asymmetric cooling of the human body.

As opposed to passive cooling, an active cooling system can maintain a constant low temperature around a finger or hand over longer periods of time, with higher repeatability as cooling power and finger temperature can be balanced with the use of a cooling controller [9]. Furthermore, active cooling may allow localized finger cooling around the nail bed that may reduce pain [2, 9, 13]. Active cooling may as such allow an effective control of blood flow for reducing nail toxicity and onycholysis during cancer treatment, while inducing less pain. The underlying thermo-physiological mechanism of CIVD is nonetheless insufficiently understood for designing a cooling controller that prevents CIVD.

In this study, three localized cooling strategies are evaluated at twelve healthy persons to investigate their effect on local blood flow at the nail bed. It is hypothesized that pulsed cooling may be more effective to reduce blood flow as compared to constant cooling as it reduces asymmetric body cooling. The results of this research may help in the development of active local cooling devices to prevent onycholysis and reduce nail toxicity at cancer patients.

## 2   Methods and Materials

**Prototype.** A prototype of an active local cooling device was developed that allows cooling of the palmar side of the distal and middle phalanx of digitus IV (ring finger) and/or of the carpal area. The cooling is induced with four Peltier elements for the carpal area and two for digitus IV, whereby surface temperature is measured with NTC thermistors. The temperature of the Peltier elements is controlled by an Arduino controller. The complete test setup is shown in Fig. 1.

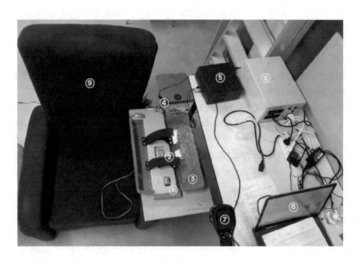

**Fig. 1.** Test setup consisting of: (1) two Peltier elements and one thermistor for digitus IV, (2) four Peltier elements and two thermistors for the carpal area, (3) cooling bath with water (18 °C), (4) Arduino, (5) power source, (6) electronic safety, (7) FLIRi7 thermal imaging camera for visual control, (8) pc with Arduino software and (9) a comfortable chair.

**Participants.** Twelve healthy test persons – six women and six men, aged between 18 and 24 years – took part in this study. In avoiding possible side effects, not everyone could participate: people who suffer from cold intolerance, perniosis, Raynaud syndrome and other cardiovascular diseases were excluded from participating. Each subject was asked not to drink any alcohol the night before the test and ensure a good and regular night's rest. Before the start of the test, each participant received a document explaining the course of the study after which they get an informed consent form to sign. By signing this form, they declared they understand the possible discomforts of participating in the study and that their participation is voluntary.

**Protocol.** The tests were conducted during three consecutive weeks. Each subject was tested three times in total, with one test per week at the same time during the day. The examination room was kept at the same temperature. The participants were asked to wear similar clothes during each test: a long pair of trousers, a T-shirt and a thin sweater. They were not allowed to eat right before or during the test. They were also not allowed to remove their finger from the test set-up. Each person retained the right to discontinue their participation in the study at any time. Before being tested, each person has to acclimatise for half an hour at a room temperature of 21 °C while being seated. Afterwards, three cooling strategies were tested.

**Cooling Strategies.** Three different cooling strategies (independent variables) were tested on the twelve subjects: (1) a cooling strategy of the finger, in which only the Peltier elements for the finger are controlled at 2 °C during a period of 60 min, (2) a pulsed cooling strategy of the finger, in which four-minute periods of cooling the finger at 2 °C alternate with two-minute periods at 20 °C and (3) a cooling strategy of the finger and carpal area, in which the Peltier elements for the finger are controlled at 2 °C and the ones for the carpal area at 10 °C. In all three strategies, the finger and carpal area are first controlled at 20 °C during five minutes prior to the test. The dependent variable is blood flow at the nail bed, quantified as the finger temperature on the dorsal side of the finger. The cooling effectiveness was quantified as the reduction in blood flow during the cooling strategy as compared to the blood flow five minutes prior to the test.

## 3 Results

First of all, a Kolmogorov-Smirnov test and Shapiro-Wilk test were performed for the assessment of normality. These normality tests indicated (Sig. > 0.05) that the data was normally distributed, which is required for further data processing.

Next, a repeated measures ANOVA was executed with the data of all entire tests (see Table 1). These results indicate that: (i) all three cooling strategies have a significant effect ($P < 0.001$) on the measured skin temperature during each 60-min trial, which implies that cooling of the palmar side of the finger and/or carpal area allowed to reduce blood flow at the nail bed. (ii) Also, a significant difference is indicated between the three cooling strategies ($F = 2.367$, $P = 0.043$). (iii) Lastly, a significant difference is shown between the data of the male and of the female subjects ($F = 3.456$, $P = 0.008$).

**Table 1.** Repeated measures ANOVA (60 min. test).

Multivariate Tests[a]

| Effect | | Value | F | Hypothesis df | Error df | Sig. |
|---|---|---|---|---|---|---|
| Time | Pillai's Trace | ,901 | 14,397[b] | 12,000 | 19,000 | ,000 |
| | Wilks' Lambda | ,099 | 14,397[b] | 12,000 | 19,000 | ,000 |
| | Hotelling's Trace | 9,093 | 14,397[b] | 12,000 | 19,000 | ,000 |
| | Roy's Largest Root | 9,093 | 14,397[b] | 12,000 | 19,000 | ,000 |
| Time * TestType | Pillai's Trace | ,897 | 1,357 | 24,000 | 40,000 | ,193 |
| | Wilks' Lambda | ,285 | 1,383[b] | 24,000 | 38,000 | ,182 |
| | Hotelling's Trace | 1,871 | 1,403 | 24,000 | 36,000 | ,175 |
| | Roy's Largest Root | 1,420 | 2,367[c] | 12,000 | 20,000 | ,043 |
| Time * Gender | Pillai's Trace | ,686 | 3,456[b] | 12,000 | 19,000 | ,008 |
| | Wilks' Lambda | ,314 | 3,456[b] | 12,000 | 19,000 | ,008 |
| | Hotelling's Trace | 2,183 | 3,456[b] | 12,000 | 19,000 | ,008 |
| | Roy's Largest Root | 2,183 | 3,456[b] | 12,000 | 19,000 | ,008 |
| Time * TestType * Gender | Pillai's Trace | ,780 | 1,065 | 24,000 | 40,000 | ,420 |
| | Wilks' Lambda | ,370 | 1,020[b] | 24,000 | 38,000 | ,468 |
| | Hotelling's Trace | 1,298 | ,974 | 24,000 | 36,000 | ,518 |
| | Roy's Largest Root | ,777 | 1,294[c] | 12,000 | 20,000 | ,295 |

Since the hunting effect occurs after 20 to 30 min, a repeated measures ANOVA between subjects was executed using only the data of the last 30 min of the test. The results indicate that the significant difference in skin temperature is still notable between the cooling strategies during the last half hour (F = 3.633, P = 0.39). Conversely, there is no significant difference between skin temperature of the male and female subjects during the last 30 min (F = 0.112, P = 0.740).

Subsequently, a post hoc test was executed in order to confirm where the differences occurred between the cooling strategies (see Table 2). These results show a significant difference between strategy 1 and 2 (P = 0.029) and between strategy 2 and 3 (P = 0.024), whereas the difference between strategy 1 and 3 was not significant (P = 0.983).

**Table 2.** Post hoc test (last 30 min. of the test).

**Multiple Comparisons**

Measure: device

LSD

| (I) TestType | (J) TestType | Mean Difference (I-J) | Std. Error | Sig. | 90% Confidence Interval | |
|---|---|---|---|---|---|---|
| | | | | | Lower Bound | Upper Bound |
| T1 | T2 | -3,0711* | 1,33873 | ,029 | -5,3433 | -,7989 |
| | T3 | ,1056 | 1,33873 | ,938 | -2,1666 | 2,3777 |
| T2 | T1 | 3,0711* | 1,33873 | ,029 | ,7989 | 5,3433 |
| | T3 | 3,1767* | 1,33873 | ,024 | ,9045 | 5,4488 |
| T3 | T1 | -,1056 | 1,33873 | ,938 | -2,3777 | 2,1666 |
| | T2 | -3,1767* | 1,33873 | ,024 | -5,4488 | -,9045 |

Based on observed means.
 The error term is Mean Square (Error) = 10,753.
 * The mean difference is significant at the, 1 level.

Finally, to determine which strategy is the most effective, the average cooling during the last 30 min of the different cooling strategies were compared (see Table 3). With an average finger temperature reduction of 8.7 °C during the last 30 min, the pulsed cooling strategy of the finger (2) is significantly more effective (P < 0.03) than the constant cooling strategy of the finger (1) which had a reduction of 5.6 °C and the constant cooling strategy of the finger and carpal area (3) which had a reduction of 5.5 °C.

**Table 3.** Means of the reduction in temperature as compared to the temperature five minutes prior to the test, i.e. cooling effectiveness (last 30 min. of the test).

**1. TestType**

Measure: device

| TestType | Mean | Std. Error | 90% Confidence Interval | |
|---|---|---|---|---|
| | | | Lower Bound | Upper Bound |
| T1 | 5,593 | ,947 | 3,986 | 7,200 |
| T2 | 8,664 | ,947 | 7,057 | 10,271 |
| T3 | 5,487 | ,947 | 3,881 | 7,094 |

# 4 Conclusion

The aim of this study was to investigate the effectiveness of local active cooling to control blood flow at the nail bed. It was hypothesized that pulsed cooling reduces cold-induced vasodilation (CIVD) and improves control of blood flow as it reduces asymmetric body cooling. Insight in CIVD may help designing a control system to prevent onycholysis at cancer patients undergoing chemotherapy treatment.

Three cooling strategies were evaluated at twelve healthy test persons: (1) a cooling strategy of the distal and middle phalanges of digitus IV, cooled at 2 °C during a period of 60 min, (2) a pulsed cooling strategy of the distal and middle phalanges of digitus IV, in which four-minute periods of cooling at 2 °C alternated with two-minute periods of 20 °C and (3) a cooling strategy of the distal and middle phalanges of digitus IV, cooled at 2 °C, in combination with a cooling of the carpal area at 10 °C. Local blood flow at the nailbed was assessed with the use of skin temperature (°C) measurements on the dorsal side of the cooled finger. The cooling effectiveness was quantified as the reduction in blood flow during the cooling strategy as compared to the blood flow five minutes prior to the test, defined as the reference period.

The results indicate that all three cooling strategies had a significant effect ($P < 0.001$) on the measured skin temperature during each 60-min trial as compared to the reference period. This showed that each cooling strategy allowed reducing blood flow at the nailbed. With an average temperature reduction of 8.7 °C during the last 30 min, the pulsed cooling strategy (2) was found to be significantly more effective ($P < 0.03$) as compared to the constant cooling strategy (1) which had a reduction of 5.6 °C and the combined cooling strategy of phalanges and carpal area.

In conclusion, this study indicates that pulsed cooling can reduce CIVD. Pulsed cooling may allow a treatment for cancer patient undergoing chemotherapy that is less painful as compared to traditional methods for preventing onycholysis as the area of cooling and duration of cooling can be reduced.

# References

1. Minisini, A.M., et al.: Taxane-induced nail changes: incidence, clinical presentation and outcome. Ann. Oncol. **14**(2), 333–337 (2003)
2. Bladt, L., et al.: Cold-induced vasoconstriction for preventing onycholysis during cancer treatment. Extrem. Physiol. Med. **4**(1), A60 (2015)
3. Hussain, S., Anderson, D.N., Salvatti, M.E., Adamson, B., McManus, M., Braverman, A.S.: Onycholysis as a complication of systemic chemotherapy: report of five cases associated with prolonged weekly paclitaxel therapy and review of the literature. Cancer **88**(10), 2367–2371 (2000)
4. Robert, C., et al.: Nail toxicities induced by systemic anticancer treatments. Lancet Oncol. **16**(4), e181–e189 (2015)
5. Kadakia, K.C., Rozell, S.A., Butala, A.A., Loprinzi, C.L.: Supportive cryotherapy: a review from head to toe. J. Pain Symptom Manage. **47**(6), 1100–1115 (2014)
6. Tyler, C.J., Reeve, T., Cheung, S.S.: Cold-induced vasodilation during single digit immersion in 0°C and 8°C water in men and women. PLoS ONE **10**(4), 1–13 (2015)

7. Daanen, H.A.M.: Finger cold-induced vasodilation: a review. Eur. J. Appl. Physiol. **89**(5), 411–426 (2003)
8. Scotté, F., et al.: Multicenter study of a frozen glove to prevent docetaxel-induced onycholysis and cutaneous toxicity of the hand. J. Clin. Oncol. **23**(19), 4424–4429 (2005)
9. Steckel, J., et al.: A research platform using active local cooling directed at minimizing the blood flow in human fingers. In: Proceedings of the ICTs Improving Patients Rehabilitation Research Techniques, pp. 81–84 (2013)
10. Scotté, F., et al.: Matched case-control phase 2 study to evaluate the use of a frozen sock to prevent docetaxel-induced onycholysis and cutaneous toxicity of the foot. Cancer **112**(7), 1625–1631 (2008)
11. Can, G., Aydiner, A., Cavdar, I.: Taxane-induced nail changes: predictors and efficacy of the use of frozen gloves and socks in the prevention of nail toxicity. Eur. J. Oncol. Nurs. **16**(3), 270–275 (2012)
12. Sawada, S., Araki, S., Yokoyama, K.: Changes in cold-induced vasodilatation, pain and cold sensation in fingers caused by repeated finger cooling in a cool environment. Ind. Health **38**, 79–86 (2000)
13. D'Haene, M., Youssef, A., De Bruyne, G., Aerts, J.-M.: Modelling and controlling blood flow by active cooling of the fingers to prevent nail toxicity, Thesis. KU Leuven, Belgium, November, p. 89 (2015)

# Design and Development of a Medical Device (Artificial Ganglio) for Aids in the Treatment of Lymphedema

Gabriela Durán Aguilar[✉], Alberto Rossa-Sierra,
and Fabiola Cortéz Chávez

Facultad de Ingeniería, Universidad Panamericana, Prolongación Calzada
Circunvalación Poniente 49, Zapopan, Jalisco 45010, Mexico
gaduran@up.edu.mx
http://www.up.edu.mx

**Abstract.** For the World Health Organization (WHO), breast cancer is the most frequent and increasing in women in both developed and developing countries. Through the studies of the American Cancer Society it can be observed that lymphedema is produced by: *Surgery, Radiation, Cancer, Infections.* If the remaining lymphatic vessels can not capture enough fluid from the area, it accumulates and causes swelling, or lymphedema. In the present document, it will be refunded in the research and development process regarding lymphedema, explaining the art prior to arriving at the final design that will derive in the medical device with aesthetic and functional characteristics.

**Keywords:** Medical devices · Artificial Ganglio · Lymphedema
Cancer · Design · Design thinking · Medical design

## 1 Introduction

According to the National Cancer Institute [1] explains that to understand the disease, it is necessary to know the functioning of the breast: "The breast is composed of glands called lobules that can produce milk and thin tubes called ducts, and carry the milk from the lobules to the nipple. The breast tissue also contains fat and connective tissue, lymph nodes and blood vessels (Fig. 1)."

"The most common type of breast cancer is ductal carcinoma, which starts in the duct cells. Breast cancer can also start in the cells of the lobules and in other tissues of the breast. Ductal carcinoma in situ is a condition in which abnormal cells are found in the lining of the ducts, but that did not spread outside the duct. Breast cancer that has spread from where it started in the ducts or lobules to the surrounding tissues is called invasive breast cancer. In the case of inflammatory breast cancer, the breast is red and swollen, and it feels hot because the cancer cells block the lymphatic vessels of the skin". The National Cancer Institute [2], determines that cancer spreads in the body in three ways: "Cancer can spread through the tissue, the lymphatic system and the blood:

© Springer International Publishing AG, part of Springer Nature 2019
N. J. Lightner (Ed.): AHFE 2018, AISC 779, pp. 37–47, 2019.
https://doi.org/10.1007/978-3-319-94373-2_5

- Tissue. Cancer spreads from where it started and extends to nearby areas.
- Lymphatic system. Cancer spreads from where it started, to enter the lymphatic system. The cancer travels through the lymphatic vessels to other parts of the body.
- Blood. Cancer spreads from where it started and enters the blood. The cancer travels through the blood vessels to other parts of the body."

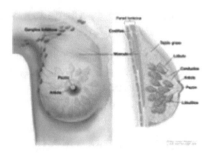

**Fig. 1.** Anatomy of the female breast (©2011, Winslow)

On the other hand, the American Cancer Society [3] mentions that "the cancer cells have spread to their lymph nodes, there is a greater probability that the cells have moved through the lymphatic system and have spread (metastasis) to other parts of the body. her body. The more lymph nodes that exist with breast cancer cells, the greater the likelihood of also finding cancer in other organs. Because of this, finding cancer in one or more lymph nodes often affects your treatment plan. Usually, surgery is performed and one or more lymph nodes are removed to see if the cancer has spread.

However, not all women with cancer cells in their lymph nodes have metastases, and some women may not have cancer cells in their lymph nodes and then metastasize."

That is to say that based on these studies, surgeries that are performed without having a more specific and/or filtered result type, run the risk of removing more lymph nodes than should be or sometimes extract more tissue of the necessary (Fig. 2).

The National Cancer Institute [4] takes into account different stages or stages to define breast cancer (Fig. 3).

## 2  Stages of Breast Cancer

1. Stage 0 (carcinoma in situ)

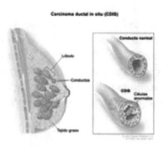

**Fig. 2.** Ductal carcinoma in situ (DCIS). Abnormal cells are found in the lining of a breast duct. (©2012, Winslow)

## 2. Stage I

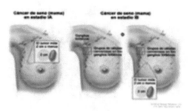

**Fig. 3.** Breast cancer (stage 1) In stage IA, the tumor measures 2 cm or less and has not spread outside the breast. In stage IB, no tumor is found in the breast or it is 2 cm or less. Small groups of cancer cells are found in the lymph nodes (greater than 0.2 mm but less than 2 mm). (©2012, Winslow)

## 3. Stage II

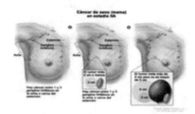

**Fig. 4.** Breast cancer (stage IIA) There are no tumors in the breast, but cancer is found between 1 to 3 lymph nodes in the armpit or in the lymph nodes near the sternum (drawing on the left); Either the tumor is 2 cm or less and cancer is found between 1 to 3 lymph nodes in the axilla or in the lymph nodes near the sternum (center drawing); Either the tumor is larger than 2 cm, but less than 5 cm, and it has not spread to the lymph nodes (drawing on the right). (©2012, Winslow)

## 4. Stage IIIA

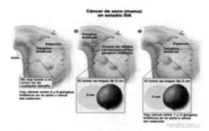

**Fig. 5.** Breast cancer (breast) in stage IIIA. No tumor is found in the breast or the tumor can be any size and cancer is found in 4 to 9 axillary lymph nodes, or in the lymph nodes near the sternum (drawing on the left); Either the tumor is larger than 5 cm and there are small groups of cancer cells (measuring more than 0.2 mm, but not more than 2 mm) in the lymph nodes (middle drawing); Either the tumor is larger than 5 cm and cancer is found in 1 to 3 lymph nodes in the axilla or in the lymph nodes near the sternum (drawing on the right)(© 2012, Winslow)

5. Stage IIIB

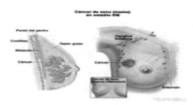

**Fig. 6.** Breast cancer (breast) in stage IIIb. The tumor can be any size and the cancer has spread to the chest wall or skin of the breast and caused swelling or an ulcer. The cancer could spread to up to nine lymph nodes in the armpit or to the lymph nodes near the sternum. The cancer that has spread to the skin of the breast can be inflammatory breast cancer. (©2012, Winslow)

6. Stage IIIC

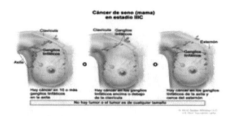

**Fig. 7.** Breast cancer (breast) in stage IIIC. No tumor is found in the breast or the tumor can be any size, and could spread to the chest wall or breast skin and cause swelling or an ulcer. In addition, the cancer spread to 10 or more axillary lymph nodes (drawing on the left); Or to the lymph nodes above or below the clavicle (middle drawing); Or to the lymph nodes in the armpit and to the lymph nodes near the sternum (drawing on the right). The cancer that has spread to the skin of the breast can be inflammatory breast cancer. (©2012, Winslow)

7. Stage IV

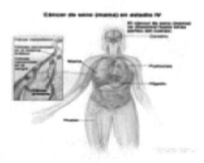

**Fig. 8.** Stage IV breast cancer The cancer has spread to other parts of the body; like the brain, the lung, the liver or the bone (©2012, Winslow)

After having analyzed the different types of stages that breast cancer has, we will explain the types of treatments that generally exist. The treatment for breast cancer depends, in part, on the stage of the disease. The National Cancer Institute [5] tells us about the different types of treatment for breast cancer patients. "Five types of standard treatment are used (Fig. 4):

- Surgery • Radiotherapy • Chemotherapy • Hormone therapy • Directed therapy
  New types of treatment are being tested in clinical trials.
- High-dose chemotherapy with stem cell transplant.

Sometimes breast cancer treatment causes side effects." Of the authors, should be checked before the paper is sent to the Volume Editors (Fig. 5).

*After breast cancer is diagnosed, according to the National Cancer Institute [6] tests are done to determine if cancer cells have spread within the breast or to other parts of the body.*

"The process used to determine if the cancer has spread inside the breast or to other parts of the body is called staging. The information obtained in the staging process determines the stage of the disease. It is important to know the stage in order to plan the treatment. The results of some of the tests used to diagnose breast cancer are also used to stage the disease. For the process of staging, you can also use tests and procedures, an example of this would be (Fig. 6):

- *Sentinel lymph node biopsy:* Extraction of the sentinel lymph node during surgery. The sentinel lymph node is the first lymph node that receives lymphatic drainage from a tumor and is the first lymph node where the cancer may spread from the tumor. A radioactive substance or blue dye is injected near the tumor. The substance or dye flows through the lymphatic channels to the lymph nodes. The first ganglion that receives the substance or dye is removed. A pathologist observes the tissue under a microscope to check for cancer cells. When cancer cells are not detected, it may not be necessary to remove more lymph nodes (Fig. 7)."

In the Science Direct database we find the following scientific article prepared by the Clinical Breast Cancer [7] on whether the sentinel lymph node biopsy should be performed or not, for its contributions.

## 3   Should We Perform an Intraoperative Biopsy of the Sentinel Lymph Node in Breast Cancer?

"The purpose of this study was to evaluate the usefulness of performing a selective intraoperative sentinel lymph node biopsy (SLNB) in patients with breast cancer. The candidate patients were women with breast cancer in our hospital in 2014. These Patients were divided into 2 groups according to clinical criteria age, tumor size and molecular subtype: (1) Group A: women with clinical criteria indicative of the need to perform an intraoperative sentinel lymph node analysis (SLN) and (2) Group B: women in whom the postoperative analysis of the SLN was performed, the anatomopathological findings obtained for the SLNs were analyzed and the sensitivity, specificity, positive predictive value and negative predictive value of the clinical criteria used were estimated. to decide between the intraoperative or postoperative analysis of SLN (Fig. 8).

A total of 170 patients were included: 106 in group A and 64 in group B. The number of positive SLNs was 29 (22 in group A and 7 in group B, P = 0.09). The sensitivity of our clinical criteria to establish the indication for performing a selective intraoperative axillary sentinel lymph node biopsy was 75.86% (95% confidence interval [CI], 56.05%–88.98%), Specificity was 40.43% (95% CI, 32.35%–49.03%), the positive predictive value was 20.75% (95% CI, 13.73%–29.95%) and the negative predictive value was 89.06% (95% CI, 78.16%–95.12%).

# 4 Conclusions

The clinical findings used to decide whether or not to perform a selective intraoperative sentinel lymph node biopsy have low sensitivity and specificity and, therefore, should not be used to decide the need for a selective intraoperative sentinel lymph node biopsy."

However, the American Cancer Society [8] reports that one of the most effective and least aggressive tests is the sentinel lymph node biopsy, avoiding minor side effects, which breast cancer itself has.

For the National Cancer Institute [9] sometimes the treatment of breast cancer causes side effects. Some breast cancer treatments cause side effects that continue or appear months or years after the end of treatment. These are called late effects.

- Inflammation of the lung after radiotherapy directed to the breast; in particular, when chemotherapy is administered at the same time.
- *Lymphedema in the arm*; in particular, when radiotherapy is administered after lymph node dissection.
- Higher cancer risk in the other breast for women younger than 45 who receive radiation therapy to the chest wall after a mastectomy.

We verified based on the research of the American Cancer Society [10] that there are side effects of aesthetic appearance, temporary physical and chronic physical.

- Falls Hair loss Leg cramps Changes in emotional and psychological state Urinary and excretion changes Fatigue/Fatigue Seizures Weakness Dehydration and lack of fluids Difficulty breathing Pain Effects on fertility and sexuality Stomas (ostomies) Fever Hiccup Swelling Infections Lymphedema Nausea and vomiting Mouth problems Skin problems Food problems Problems sleeping Low blood counts Sweating.

The design has always tried to identify and design products for the needs of the user. The current designer should be involved more intensively in the development of highly innovative products, while taking into account the aesthetic aspect and the technical function. In the field of medical design, the designer plays a very important role since it will not only contribute to the satisfaction of the user but can generate a much more emotionally significant impact, and psychologically speaking.

In the development of medical products, designers must solve: provide solutions to problems, interact with users, know their needs, manage production processes and select materials to provide the best solution within the reach of available technologies. This maybe a biomedical engineer could satisfy it. But what happens when there is a product that fulfills its function, improves the quality of life of the user, but aesthetically generates emotional, social damage to the patient? The circle of development of a product would not be generated. It is considered essential the participation of the designer in the development of medical products, which completely satisfy the user's experience without any gap.

Can we include and work in teams with all those involved and see the importance of medical design?

## 5  Statement of the Problem

After the analysis we found that for breast cancer, there are several successful treatments currently and with a view to the future. Also that most of the side effects are temporary, many of them disappear when the treatments end. However, there is a side effect little studied and treated, which decreases the quality of life of the patient, even dramatically, its name is: Lymphoedema, but to understand the problem we need to first know the functioning of the lymphatic system. The National Cancer Institute [11] tells us that "the lymphatic system is constituted by a network of lymphatic vessels, tissues and organs that transport the lymph throughout the body.

The following are the parts of the lymphatic system that play a direct role:

*Lymph:* Transparent fluid that contains lymphocytes (white blood cells) that fight infections and tumor formation. Lymph also contains plasma, the watery part of the blood that carries blood cells.

*Lymphatic vessels:* Network of thin tubes that collect lymph from different parts of the body and return it to the bloodstream.

*Lymph nodes:* Small, bean-shaped structures that filter the lymph and store white blood cells that help fight infection and disease. The lymph nodes are located throughout the network of lymphatic vessels throughout the body. Clusters of lymph nodes are found in the axilla, pelvis, neck, abdomen and groin. The spleen, thymus, tonsils and bone marrow are also part of the lymphatic system.

### 5.1  "Lymphedema Occurs When the Lymph Cannot Circulate Through the Body as It Should."

For the American Cancer Institute [12] "One possible long-term side effect of a lymph node surgery is swelling in the arm or chest, called lymphedema. Because any excess fluid in the arms normally returns to the bloodstream through the lymphatic system, the removal of the lymph nodes sometimes blocks the drainage of the arm, which causes the accumulation of this fluid. This is less common after a sentinel lymph node biopsy than an axillary lymph node dissection. Up to 30% of women who undergo an axillary lymph node dissection have lymphedema. In addition, it also occurs in up to 3% of women who undergo a sentinel lymph node biopsy. It may be more common if radiation is given after surgery. Sometimes a swelling occurs that lasts only a few weeks and then goes away. But in some women, the swelling can last for a long time.

## 5.2  Limited Arm and Shoulder Movement

You may also have limitations in the movement of the arm and shoulder after surgery. This is more common after an axillary lymph node dissection than after a sentinel lymph node biopsy. The doctor may advise exercises to help prevent permanent problems (a "frozen" shoulder). Some women notice a rope-like structure that begins under the arm and can extend up to the elbow, sometimes called scar adhesion or lymphatic cords. This is more common after an axillary lymph node dissection than a sentinel lymph node biopsy. Symptoms may not appear for weeks or even months after surgery. It can cause pain and limit movement of the arm and shoulder. Often, this problem goes away without the need for treatment, although some women may benefit from physical therapy.

## 5.3  Numbness

Numbness of the skin in the upper inner portion of the arm is a common side effect, since the nerves that control this sensation in this place travel through the area of the lymph nodes. "In the Science Direct database, we found the following scientific article: "Reliable prediction of postmastectomy lymphedema: The Risk Assessment Tool Assessing Lymphoedema" [13].

## 5.4  Background

Lymphedema related to breast cancer remains a major complication after mastectomy. Identifying patients at higher risk may be better to inform the allocation of health resources and improve results. This study aims to identify the predictors of lymphedema after mastectomy to develop a simple and accurate risk assessment tool.

## 5.5  Methods

An institutional retrospective review identified all women with breast cancer who underwent a mastectomy between January 2000 and July 2013 with postmastectomy lymphedema as the primary outcome. Multivariate Cox regression by stages identified independent predictors of lymphedema. A simplified risk assessment tool was derived and the composite risk was estimated for each patient.

# 6  Results

Of the 3,136 patients included, 325 (10.4%) developed lymphedema after a follow-up of 4.2 years. Significant predictors included the diagnosis of invasive cancer (HR = 2.25), postmastectomy radiation (HR = 2.05), age over 65 years (HR = 1.90) and axillary dissection (HR = 1.79). The risk of lymphedema stratified by group was defined as follows: low 6.2%, moderate 10.0%, high 16.4% and extreme 36.4%. The model demonstrated excellent risk discrimination (C = 0.78). Conclusions: The incidence of postmastectomy lymphedema was 10.4%. Invasive cancer diagnosis, chemoradiation and axillary dissection gave a significant risk. The risk assessment tool that assesses lymphedema offers accurate risk discrimination ranging from 6.2% to 36.4%. Selective treatment approaches can improve outcomes and provide cost-effective healthcare. "For researchers Wernicke, Goltser, Shamis and Swistel, from Weill Cornell Medical College, Department of Radiation Oncology, in the USA, in their article published by INTECH Open Science [14]" In general, lymphedema is a serious condition that requires timely intervention and proper treatment. The multidisciplinary approach is important for a patient with lymphedema risk It is important that early education about lymphedema is a standard of management and care for all patients. Prevention, detection and measurement are all important for the early detection of lymphedema related to breast cancer. The surgical conservator minimizes the long-term risk of lymphedema in patients with cancer as well as hormone therapy. Chemotherapy, on the other hand, may have risks developing lymphedema after breast cancer. "The quality of life of patients with lymphedema is compromised depending on how much the disease affects them. Dr. Blanca Alicia Meza León [15], founding president of the "Asociación Mexicana de Linfología y Linfedema AC" (Amlylac) mentions in an interview for the newspaper Milenio that "out of every eight women undergoing breast cancer treatment, four can develop it (lymphedema) immediately; and in a term of five years until 70, 80% will have it very evident. The majority of people who remove their lymph nodes is a fact that they will enter the subclinical stage of lymphedema at any time ".

## 6.1   Investigation Questions

Can lymphedema be avoided? Is it possible once you have the disease to improve the quality of life of the patient? Can this side effect of the treatment be permanently reduced? Is there any type of permanent treatment/surgery for its cure and without having to go through the patient several times due to processes that are already invasive? Could a lymph node transplant be done? Could surgery in the same surgery remove as many lymph nodes as needed, and be replaced by a mechanism/function identical to that performed by the ganglion per se? Is there a bio-compatible material that does not reject the patient's organism and that can be produced with everything and the system in the approximate size of a real ganglion (4 mm)? Is it possible that this mechanism is on the outside of the patient's body? How should hygiene be in people suffering from this disease? If there are treatments such as sentinel lymph node biopsy, massages, short and medium stretch bandages of various sizes, bandages, tubular bandages, foam foams of different densities, sleeves or circular or flat weave stockings, and sometimes even treatment sessions that include pneumatic compression pumps, ultrasonotherapy and other special techniques applied by Physiotherapists, which are so affordable for all patients in economic question, geographical area?

# 7 Hypothesis

With the advance of the technology applied to the design and development of medical devices, the design and development of an artificial ganglion for help in the treatment of lymphedema is feasible.

Develop a solution to improve the quality of life in patients suffering from lymphedema through a medical device

To investigate the functioning as a lymph node mechanism and its development.

Investigate the current temporary and permanent treatment worldwide, its operation and implementation. Analysis of testimonies of patients with lymphedema.

Investigate the procedures in treatments and surgeries against breast cancer in its different stages. Comparison of alternatives of medical devices and devices for the supply of medicines and replacement of physiological processes. Analysis of existing biocompatible materials for possible use in the device. Comparison of costs for treatments Research and analysis of procedures in surgeries to remove lymph nodes in public and private institutions Development of the artificial ganglion with its mechanism of operation at the smallest possible scale.

## 7.1 Scopes of the Project

- Analysis and Research with special emphasis in Mexico in order to make a better one available to everyone who suffers from this disease and who do not have the financial means to face it.
- Development of the prototype with its operating mechanism at the smallest possible scale.
- Medical device for anyone who undergoes a procedure such as breast cancer.

# References

1. National Cancer Institute: Tipos de cancer, Octubre 2017. de National Cancer Institute Sitio web (2017). https://www.cancer.gov/espanol/tipos/seno
2. National Cancer Institute: El cáncer se disemina en el cuerpo de tres maneras. E.U.A (2017). National Cancer Institute, Estadios del cáncer de mama. E.U.A (2017g). https://www.cancer. gov/espanol/tipos/seno/paciente/tratamiento-seno-pdq#section/_24. Recuperado el 17 de junio del, Recuperado el 10 de Julio del 2017
3. American Cancer Society: ¿Cómo se propaga el cáncer de seno? E.U.A (2016). https://www. cancer.org/es/cancer/cancer-de-seno/acerca/que-es-el-cancer-de-seno.html. Recuperado el 23 de Julio de 2017
4. National Cancer Institute: Estadios del cáncer de mama. Julio 2017, de National Cancer Institute Sitio web (2017). https://www.cancer.gov/espanol/tipos/seno/paciente/tratamiento-seno-pdq#section/_24
5. National Cancer Institute: Aspectos generales de las opciones de tratamiento. E.U.A (2017). https://www.cancer.gov/espanol/tipos/seno/paciente/tratamiento-seno-pdq#section/_52. Recuperado el 10 de Junio del 2017

6. National Cancer Institute: Después de que se diagnostica el cáncer de mama, se realizan pruebas para determinar si las células cancerosas se diseminaron dentro de la mama o hasta otras partes del cuerpo., E.U.A (2017). https://www.cancer.gov/espanol/tipos/seno/paciente/tratamiento-seno-pdq#section/_24. Recuperado el 10 de julio del 2017

7. Ceberio, N., Cuadra, M., Mendizabal, J.L., Gorostiaga, J., Lete, I.: Clinical Breast Cancer "Should We Perform the Intraoperative Sentinel Lymph Node Biopsy in Breast Cancer?", Volumen 16, Problema 6, Diciembre 2016, Páginas e175-e180 (2016). http://www.sciencedirect.com/science/article/pii/S1526820916301410. Recuperado el 01 de septiembre de 2017

8. American Cancer Society: Cirugía de ganglios linfáticos para el cáncer de seno. Julio 2017, de American Cancer Society Sitio web (2017). https://www.cancer.org/es/cancer/cancer-de-seno/tratamiento/cirugia-del-cancer-de-seno/cirugia-de-ganglios-linfaticos-para-el-cancer-de-seno.html

9. National Cancer Institute: Efectos Secundarios., E.U.A (2017). https://www.cancer.gov/espanol/tipos/seno/paciente/tratamiento-seno-pdq#section/_52. Recuperado el 15 de julio del 2017

10. American Cancer Society: Efectos Secundarios. E.U.A (2016). https://www.cancer.org/es/tratamiento/tratamientos-y-efectos-secundarios/efectos-secundarios-fisicos.html. Recuperado el 18 de julio del 2017

11. National Cancer Institute: Sistema Linfático, E.U.A. (2017). https://www.cancer.gov/espanol/cancer/tratamiento/efectos-secundarios/linfedema/linfedema-pdq. Recuperado el 15 de junio del 2017

12. American Cancer Institute: Cirugía de ganglios linfáticos para el cáncer de seno., E.U.A (2016). https://www.cancer.org/es/cancer/cancer-de-seno/tratamiento/cirugia-del-cancer-de-seno/cirugia-de-ganglios-linfaticos-para-el-cancer-de-seno.html. Recuperado el 16 de junio del 2017

13. Basta, M.N., Wu, L.C., Kanchwala, S.K., Serletti, J.M., Tchou, J.C., Kovach, S.J., Fosnot, J., Fischer, J.P.: Science Direct "Reliable prediction of postmastectomy lymphedema: The Risk Assessment Tool Evaluating Lymphedema" presentado ante American Society of Plastic Surgeon's Annual Meeting, en Octubre de 2015, en Boston, Massachusetts. (2015). http://www.sciencedirect.com/science/article/pii/S0002961016305153. Recuperado el 31 de Julio del 2017

14. Wernicke, A.G., Goltser, Y.: Arm Lymphedema as a Consequence of Breast Cancer Therapy, Novel Strategies in Lymphedema. In: Vannelli, A. (ed.) InTech (2012). https://doi.org/10.5772/33014. https://www.intechopen.com/books/novel-strategies-in-lymphedema/arm-lymphedema-as-a-consequence-of-breast-cancer-therapy. Recuperado el 07 de junio del 2017

15. León, B.A.M.: Tras cancer de mama, 50% de mujeres sufren linfedema, Presidenta fundadora de la Asociación Mexicana de Linfología y Linfedema A.C (Amlylac) (2016). http://www.milenio.com/region/linfedema-cancer_mama_Mexico-prendas_comprension_0_716328408.html. https://www.amlylac.org/. Recuperado el 25 de Agosto del 2017

# Squatting Support Device for Labor

Ghi-Hwei Kao[1,2(✉)], T. K. Philip Hwang[1,3], Yi Lin[4],
and Yu-Ching Lin[5]

[1] National Taipei University of Technology, Taipei, Taiwan
aghi.box@gmail.com
[2] Oriental Institute of Technology, New Taipei, Taiwan
[3] Da-Yeh University Dacun Township, Changhua County, Taiwan
bphwang@mail.dyu.edu.Tw
[4] Takming University of Science and Technology, Taipei, Taiwan
celaine5201@gmail.com
[5] MacKay Memorial Hospital, Taipei, Taiwan
dm037@mmh.org.tw

**Abstract.** Women have a high mortality rate and pain in childbirth before modern medicine. Current natural childbirth might take 12–16 h on labor, the body weight on the spine and pelvic make pregnant women fatigue, it might cause to use medical drugs to relieve pain, or cesarean delivery way. If women use birth squatting allows the pelvis to expand exports about 25% reduction in the second stage of labor, there is less pain, reduce the use of analgesics, increase comfort, increased fetal blood oxygen and carbon dioxide to reduce the value of fetal blood, significantly reduce perineal laceration, and there is less use of episiotomy surgery and auxiliary equipment. Squatting is not easy to maintain even in minutes, therefore, this study used "squatting support device" to provide women with a ramp birth squatting 20–30°, so that the body forward, the body's center of gravity and support points remained at the same paw on the vertical axis, so that women can effectively contraction of the abdominal muscles to help viviparous through the birth canal. As comparing the time from starting pushing to crowning, ergonomics ankle support squatting is 25.52 min (F = 6.02, p < .05) shorter than semi-recumbent group in average. The time from starting pushing to fetal childbirth is 25.21 min shortened (F = 6.14, p < .05). Score of ergonomics ankle support squatting group is 5.05 to 3.22 (rating from 0 to 10) lower than semi-recumbent group in average as showing in visual analogue scale (VAS). The overall score of ergonomics ankle support squatting group is lower than semi-recumbent group and squatting group (F = 18.12, p < .001) as measured with short form McGill pain questionnaire (MPQ-SF). Ergonomics ankle support squatting group expressed better labor pushing experiences than other groups.

**Keywords:** Squatting · Labor · Universal design

## 1 Introduction

### 1.1 R&D Background

Until the mid-18th century, women were encouraged to give birth in any positions they preferred. During the period from 377 BC to 460 AD, birth chairs were used for helping

© Springer International Publishing AG, part of Springer Nature 2019
N. J. Lightner (Ed.): AHFE 2018, AISC 779, pp. 48–55, 2019.
https://doi.org/10.1007/978-3-319-94373-2_6

women to deliver in upright position. Francois Mauricean (1637–1709), a French obstetrician, pointed out that using reclining position was the most comfortable position for both women about to give birth and their helpers, but he did not endorse it as a common practice. The reason he gave was that multiple activities and the weight from the baby moving downward were instrumental in making the cervix open widely [1]. Experiments confirmed that giving birth lying down was the worse position as it prevented the head of the baby from falling down to the pelvic cavity due to the weight of the mother being put on the sacral bone and the tail bone [2]. Besides, the stirrup position taken by laboring women when exerting may result in pressure on bones, damage to nerve, and thrombus formation in four limbs [3]. A better position for the laboring mother in the second stage of labor was squatting [3] as it could help widen pelvic opening by 25% [4], and help reduce the length of the second stage of labor {1}, [5]. In addition, squatting could also help ease labor pains, reduce the use of analgesics and instruments such as forceps and vacuum extractors, provide comfort, increase blood oxygen for the baby and lower the degree of its blood carbon dioxide, and decrease tearing wounds to perineum [6, 7].

## 1.2  Motive for R&D

In July, 2014, Lin Yu-chin, a head nurse in a delivery room at Mackay Hospital, found that primiparas suffered from a prolonged period of labor when using positions, in the second stage of labor, such as supine, prone, semi-prone, or squatting-in-bed ones. She also discovered that a prolonged squatting position would not only cause limp and numb of lower limbs as well as loss of balance but also lessen the effects of exerting in the second stage of labor and even lead to a final decision for cesarean section. As of now, nurses would encourage primiparas to take the squatting position in bed when exerting. But the position would cause soreness in lower limbs, resulting in being unable to maintain balance. And sometimes because of the mattress being too soft or it being pressed too close to the mattress, it was difficult for professional midwives to precisely observe the progress of delivery.

When learning of the delivery procedures currently used in various hospitals in Taiwan, this author suggested that, by adopting the design concept in successfully developing patented ankle supports for squatting pan, a similar assistive device tallying with human body mechanics be designed for the benefits of squatting for birth, a gadget that was able to relieve muscle burden, maintain balance, allow primiparas to exert easily, shorten the period of exerting in the second stage of labor, lessen soreness and backache, and help gain a pleasant experience in delivery.

## 1.3  Conclusion

In coordination with the general delivery methods and the specifications of hospital beds, this ankle support device is intended for use when the laboring mother entering the second stage of labor and the exposure of the head of the baby reaching a +1 level, or the exerting becoming involuntary. It is hoped that this supporter will help shorten the length of the second-stage labor, promote the call for a smooth delivery in baby friendly hospitals, and avoid unexpected incidents during delivery or cesarean section because of unbearable pains.

## 2   Research on Human Squatting

When making a comparison between the center of gravity in the human body and the center of pressure as to which can better reflect the balance function of the body, Odenrick [8] found in his research that the position of the center of gravity shows less change than that of the center of the body and that the act of keeping the center within the range of support will cause the position of the center of pressure to bring about a bigger change.

Zhuo Min-xian explained that the center of pressure refers to the delivery of the body weight to the center of pressure on the ground when standing on two feet and that, when squatting, if the center of gravity and the center of pressure are on the vertical axis, the balance function of the body can be greatly improved. In daily life, people usually adopt a squatting position when picking up things or using squatting pans. In order to maintain squatting for a longer time, they will make it feasible by either reaching out two arms or levering up back heels (Fig. 1).

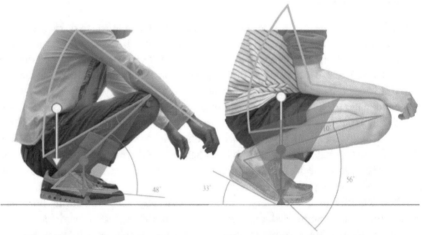

The distance between the axis of gravity and the center shaft is greater.

The gravity center of bodyweight shift to the foot support center shaft into same line.

**Fig. 1.** The equilibrium principle of ankle and squatting

### 2.1   Angle of Ankle Support

When squatting, people tend to level up their back heels to maintain balance. When not doing so, they have to reach out two arms to allow the center of the body and the support of the tiptoes to form a vertical line for balance. For this reason, the author of this report worked in 2010 with two students to divide evenly the 45° angle into four levels – 11.25°, 22.5°, 33.75° and 45°. Fifty people taking part in the test were asked to squat on the assistive device for support at the four angles. Most participants said they felt that the most suitable angle for levering up the human body was situated between 22.5° and 33.75° and that the best inclination of the ankle support was 22.5°, which allows the center of gravity and the force bearing point to form a vertical line, making the point of application move from the heel to the tiptoe and therefore reducing the pressure of the calf and ankle and lowering the level of being uncomfortable (Fig. 2).

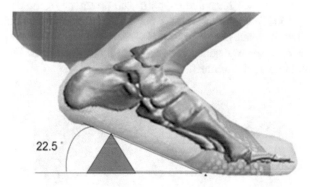

**Fig. 2.** A 22.5° foot

# 3  Human Body Test

This project, conducted between February and July of 2015, was approved by the Ethics Committee on Human Body Research through the assistance of Dr. Ong Shuanlong and Lin Yu-chin, a head nurse, at the Hsinchu Branch of Mackay Hospital.

Project name: Effects of Assistive Device for Squatting in Body Mechanics on Exerting in the Second Stage of Labor

Test content: Compared the ways of exerting in semi-recumbent and squatting positions or the squatting position by use of assistive device for ankle support, and how the three different methods affected primiparas in their delivery of new-born babies and their experience in exerting. When the laboring mother entered the second stage of labor, the exposure of the head of the baby reached a 1+level, or the exerting became involuntary, all participants in the three different groups began to exert.

## 3.1  Test Target and Venue

Venue: A delivery room at a regional teaching hospital in northern Taiwan, with samples collected randomly.

Requirements for samples: Primiparas, bearing their first babies, planned to make vaginal spontaneous delivery. Accompanied by their family members, these mothers were able to listen, speak, read, and write Chinese or to chat in Taiwanese and to fill out questionnaires as well. And they all agreed to participate in this research project (Fig. 3).

Those excluded: Included those who were unable to squat because they decided to have a cesarean or an epidural, or suffered from fetal distress, bleeding, or needed an urgent cesarean.

### 3.2    Research Tools and Reliability

Ergonomic assistive device for ankle support: The prototype of the device was made from synthetic wood boards that were 1 cm thick or over. Its chassis was 60 cm x 60 cm, with two inclined planes of roughly 22.5° attached with slip proof mats. In addition, a mantle mirror was added between the planes to be placed on the mattress, with the hospital bed as the armrest.

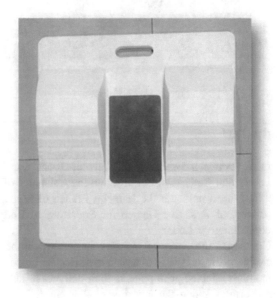

**Fig. 3.**   Test tool: ergonomic assistive device for squatting

### 3.3    Data Collection: Method and Procedure

1. This project was approved by the IRB of Mackay Hospital (Serial No: 14MMHIS173), with data being collected between January 29 and June 25, 2015.
2. Explained to all obstetricians and nurses at delivery rooms about the objective of this research and the way data were collected.
3. Timing of intervention: When cervix opened to the fullest and the mother had a strong desire for exerting, fetal parts reached the stage of station: +1, or uterine contraction maintained at least at 50 mmHg.

4. Mothers in the two groups (test group and control group) were sent to the delivery room when crowning of the baby head reached 2–3 cm. They were requested to give birth in a semi-recumbent position of $> 45°$.
5. Closing procedure: Mothers and their spouses were accompanied by researchers to ensure safety. The procedure may be terminated at the request of the participating mothers.

### 3.4  Attributes of Cases

A comparison showed there were no distinct differences among the three groups in nationality, education, religion, profession, history of disease, age, height, pregnancy (planned or not planned), fever conditions during delivery, gaining of weight during pregnancy, and average sleeping time before checking in at the hospital. This result indicated homogeneity, so as to reduce the effects of discrepancy in sampling.

### 3.5  Variables Before and After Delivery

- No distinct differences showed among the three groups in whether the mother was told about the delivery process or the way of exerting before delivery, experience in accompanying during the bearing course, whether painkiller was applied when waiting for delivery, weeks of pregnancy, and the duration of the first-stage labor.
- No distinct differences showed in EP wound, bleeding after delivery, and weight of newborn babies.

### 3.6  Differences in Effects of Exerting in Second Stage of Labor

- Time used for exerting from the beginning to the expulsion of the baby: Time used by the mothers in the test group was shorter by 25.21 min on average in comparison with that used by those who adopted the semi-recumbent position.
- Exerting time until the crowning of head was shorter by 25.52 min on average in comparison with that used by those adopting the semi-recumbent position.

## 4  Conclusion and Discussion

In terms of time used from the beginning of exerting to the crowning of head by both the squatting group using assistive device for ankle support and the group adopting the semi-recumbent position, the former spent 25.52 min less ($F = 6.02$, $p < .05$) on average compared with the latter, and time spent from the beginning of exerting to the delivery was 25.21 min less ($F = 6.14$, $p < .05$). In terms of the pain level felt, the difference was between 5.05 and 3.22, with the lower score registered for the group using the assistive device. As for the total scores recorded on the scale, the group using the assistive device had a lower score than both the semi-recumbent group and the regular squatting group ($F = 18.12$, $p < .001$). The experience in exerting gained by the group using the assistive device was generally more positive than that shared by the other two groups.

It was found in this research that adopting the ergonomic assistive device for ankle support enabled women to shorten their time used for exerting, reduce pains suffering during the delivery, and arouse more positive feeling toward exerting in delivery.

## 4.1    Shorter Time for the Process of Delivery

For the test group, the exerting time used from the beginning of exerting to the crowning of head was 25.52 min less compared with that used by the semi-recumbent group, and the exerting time used until the delivery was 25.21 min less in the same comparison between the two groups. A comparison with the previous shows:

- Time used in exerting when taking the squatting position was less than that when adopting the supine position [9].
- The second stage of labor was shorter by 23 min when adopting the squatting position, compared with the semi-recumbent position [10].
- A 90-degree upright position above waist with open glottis pushing was able to save exerting time by 54 min, compared with the semi-recumbent position with breathing suspended.

## 4.2    Less Pain Felt

Less pain was felt among those in the group using the assistive device in comparison with that felt by those groups without the device and adopting the semi-recumbent position – 3.57 points less than the semi-recumbent group and 3.27 points less than the group without the device.

- Research findings were the same as those gained by Waldenstrom and Gottvall [11]: 6.9 and 7.6 points. By allowing thigh to support abdomen, abdomen was able to be effectively raised up, so that the angle between the body of the baby and the entrance of pelvic could be readjusted, resulting in the pressure from the head of the baby directly exerted on the pelvic, increasing the pelvic contraction, accelerating the delivery process, and reducing the pain in sacrum.
- Research findings were different from those gained by Chang [12]: As the attention to the pain was transferred and the sense in self-control and confidence was increased because of involvement in the first stage of labor, the effects were not significant in the second stage of labor.

## 4.3    Clinical Application and Suggestion

We suggest that the ergonomic assistive device for ankle support be used in clinical nursing in order to lessen leg pain, redress imbalance in the squatting position, and to increase the effectiveness in exerting, so that the exerting time can be shortened during the second stage of labor. Also, exerting with the help of the said assistive device leads to a positive feeling toward the experience in exerting. The findings are identical to those compiled by Chang and others [12], leading to the gaining of confidence and being able to adjust strategies on one's own during the process of birth.

The exerting position by the help of the assistive device relieves discomfort of waist when waiting for delivery in the supine position. Like the feeling toward waist pain tested using the pain scale, the feeling level felt by the test group is lower than that by the regular squatting group, but is still ranked fifth, a phenomenon that is caused by the pressure put on waist and back during pelvic contraction.

The findings are different from those announced by Crowley and others [13], owing to the fact that delivery measures adopted in delivery rooms are told during attending outpatient treatment by the mothers. The discrepancies occur between the random distribution and expectation. In other words, caution must be exercised when explaining the delivery procure in detail and the timing for random distribution.

# References

1. Shermer, R.H., Raines, D.A.: Positioning during the second stage of labor: Moving back to basics. J. Obstet. Gynecol. Neonatal. Nurs. **26**(6), 727–734 (1997)
2. Holland, R.L., Smith, D.A.: Management of the second stage of labor: a review (Part II). Maternal positioning as it relates to the management of the second stage of labor is reviewed. South Dakota. J. Med. **42**(6), 5–8 (1989)
3. Mayberry, L.J., Wood, S.H., Strange, L.B., Lee, L., Heisler, D.R., Neilson-Smith, K.: Managing second-stage labor. Obstet. Neonatal Nurs. **3**(6), 28–34 (1999)
4. Smith, M.A., Ruffin, M.T.T., Green, L.A.: The rational management of labor. Am. Family Phys. **47**(6), 1471–1481 (1993)
5. Romney, M.: Midwifery: chair versus bed. Nurs. Mirror **160**(3), 35–36 (1985)
6. Gould, D.: Normal labour: a concept analysis. J. Adv. Nurs. **31**(2), 418–427 (2000)
7. Roberts, J.E.: The "push" for evidence: management of the second stage. J. Midwifery Womens Health **47**(1), 2–15 (2002)
8. Odenrick, P., Tropp, H., Ortengren, R.: A method for measurement of postural control in upright stance. Biomechanics **10-A**, 437–443 (1987)
9. Allahbadia, G.N., Vaidya, P.R.: Squatting position for delivery. J. Indian Med. Assoc. **91**(1), 13–16 (1993)
10. Golay, J., Vedam, S., Sorger, L.: The squatting position for the second stage of labor: effects on labor and on maternal and fetal well-being. Birth **20**(2), 73–78 (1993)
11. Waldenstrom, U., Gottvall, K.: A randomized trial of birthing stool or conventional semirecumbent position for second-stage labor. Birth **18**(1), 5–10 (1991)
12. Chang, S.C., Chou, M.M., Lin, K.C., Lin, L.C., Lin, Y.L., Kuo, S.C.: Effects of a pushing intervention on pain, fatigue and birthing experiences among Taiwanese women during the second stage of labour. Midwifery **27**(6), 825–831 (2011). https://doi.org/10.1016/j.midw.2010.08.009
13. Crowley, P., Elbourne, D., Ashurst, H., Garcia, J., Murphy, D., Duignan, N.: Delivery in an obstetric birth chair: a randomized controlled trial. Br. J. Obstetr. Gynaecol. **98**(7), 667–674 (1991)

# Glaucoma and Short-Wavelength Light Sensitivity (Blue Light)

Sandra Preto[1(✉)] and Cristina Caramelo Gomes[2]

[1] Faculdade de Arquitectura da Universidade Técnica de Lisboa,
Lisbon, Portugal
sandrapreto@hotmail.com
[2] Faculdade de Arquitectura e Artes,
Universidade Lusíada de Lisboa, Lisbon, Portugal
cris_caramelo@netcabo.pt

**Abstract.** Glaucoma is caused by a group of different eye diseases and is in the group of neurodegenerative diseases and is a major cause of blindness. Glaucoma occurs mainly by an increased pressure within the eye, due to excessive fluid (aqueous humor), which over time induce damage in the optic nerve. Recent studies suggest that ipRGC (intrinsically photosensitive retinal ganglion cells), one of the types of retinal ganglion cells (RGC), are damaged in glaucoma. Besides, ipRGCs contain melanopsin and have a peak sensitivity within the short-wavelength light (blue light), at 480 nm (nanometers) in humans and are involved in non-visual responses to light. The aim of the present paper is to contribute to a better knowledge about the impact of short-wavelength light on visual and non-visual systems in glaucoma. In order to accomplish such goals, the research will be conducted throughout literature review.

**Keywords:** Daylight · Artificial light · Visual and Non-visual system
Blue light · Glaucoma · Workplace · ipRGCs

## 1 Introduction

The present paper seeks a better understanding between the relation of short-wavelength light sensitivity and glaucoma. We will start with the definition of glaucoma, and, since there is some connection between glaucoma and retinal ganglion cells damage, we will describe what we know so far. It seems that short-wavelength light has an important role and for that same reason, we will explore the impacts of it in our visual and non-visual systems. Then, we will remark the artificial light sources that we are exposed all the time in our residences, workplace and so forth. Lastly, we will evidence the major signs that are linked to glaucoma and have a relation with blue light, such as, the impact in pupil size and sleep quality, since they are non-visual facts that can jeopardizes the quality of life of those who suffer from glaucoma.

© Springer International Publishing AG, part of Springer Nature 2019
N. J. Lightner (Ed.): AHFE 2018, AISC 779, pp. 56–67, 2019.
https://doi.org/10.1007/978-3-319-94373-2_7

# 2   Literature Review

## 2.1   Glaucoma

First of all, we must clarify what Glaucoma is and how it appears. It all start with alterations on the aqueous humor, the fluid that nourishes the tissues of the eye, in a continuous circulation through the anterior chamber, and maintain the eyeball from collapsing. Aqueous humor is produced by the ciliary body, which is located behind the iris. It flows between the iris and the lens and nourishes the cornea and lens and then flows out through the trabecular meshwork situated where the iris and cornea meet. (Fig. 1) [1] Glaucoma is, in fact, a result of increased intraocular pressure (IOP), that can damage the optic nerve cupping and then the damage spreads from one nerve cells to another creating "blind spots" that start to appear in the visual field. Primarily it affects the peripheral field of vision and afterwards the central visual, leading to a worse quality of life (Fig. 2). [2–4] Fortunately, not all people that have high IOP level develop glaucoma. Recent studies suggest that ipRGCs are damaged in glaucoma [4, 5].

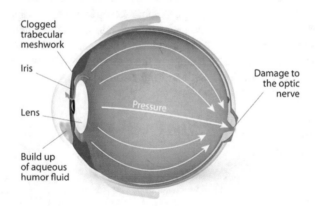

**Fig. 1.**   Glaucoma [6].

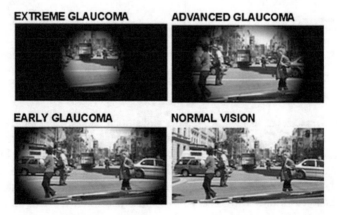

**Fig. 2.**   Normal Vision, Early, Advanced and Extreme Glaucoma [7].

## 2.2    Types of Glaucoma

There are several types of Glaucoma: Primary Open-Angle Glaucoma (POAG), Angle-closure (closed angle) glaucoma, Low-tension glaucoma (normal-tension glaucoma), Congenital glaucoma, Secondary glaucoma, Pigmentary Glaucoma, Exfoliation Syndrome and Trauma-Related Glaucoma. POAG occurs when the optic nerve fibers die one by one, and normally the person does not realize because the vision is lost over the time, gradually and it could happen unnoticed and it is the most common (Fig. 3). The Angle-closure occur when a sudden protrusion of the iris blocks all drainage channels and it is most common in Asia than in the West (Fig. 4). These sudden attacks happen, frequently, in darkened places, like at cinema, and happens because the pupil dilate (when the contact between the iris and lens is minimal) which narrows the angle that could trigger an attack. It happens mostly to Asian people descent and who are far-sighted (near-sighted, e.g. myopia). When the optic nerve is damaged despite the tension, low or high, pressure in the eye it gives rise to the low-tension glaucoma. Congenial glaucoma is when the subject is born with a narrow drainage angle. Secondary glaucoma, like the denomination induces, is a consequence of other disease like diabetes. Pigmentary glaucoma is a type of inherited open-angle that appears mostly in men in the early twenties and thirties. Exfoliation Syndrome in more common in people of Europe, over fifty years old. Trauma-related glaucoma which is caused due to a mechanical disruption or physical change in the eye, such as a blow to the eye, which, can cause a chemical burn that may lead to glaucoma [1, 3, 4].

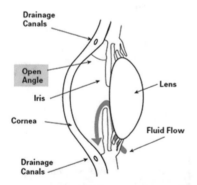

**Fig. 3.**  Open-Angle Glaucoma [8].

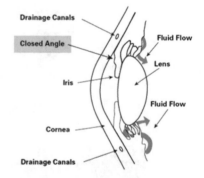

**Fig. 4.**  Angle-Closure Glaucoma [8].

## 2.3    Retinal Ganglion Cells (RGCs)

Retinal Ganglion Cells have several subtypes and among them we can find Parvocellular (P), Magnocellular (M) and recent anatomic evidence suggest that there is, also, Koniocellular (K) (Fig. 5). Whereas parvocellular pathways are activated by low temporal and high spatial frequencies, and have smaller receptive fields, represents 80–90%, magnocellular are triggered by high temporal and low spatial frequencies, and have large receptive fields, constitute 10%, and koniocellular pathway seems to be involved in processing information from the short-wavelength cones (S-cones) and represent 8-10% of RGCs. Early glaucoma affects M-pathway but recent studies suggest that it may not be so. Many of glaucoma patients have a decrease in short-wavelength sensitivity, which suggests that there are degeneration of type-I and type-II P cells and K cells. Therefore, we have to comprehend why the short-wavelength is so important in humans [2].

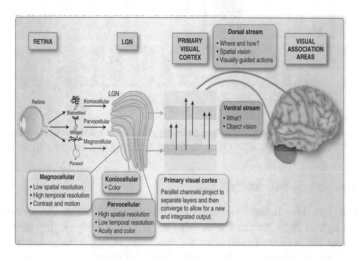

**Fig. 5.** Primary Visual Pathway [9].

## 2.4   Blue Light and Melanopsin

The visible spectrum goes from 360 to 720 nm, situated between the ultraviolet (UV) and infrared (IR) radiation. Visible spectrum comprises the short- (blue), medium- (green) and long- wavelength (red) radiation. Blue light comprehends the radiation between 380 and 500 nm, and it is present in natural light and artificial lighting sources [10]. Blue light have a greater impact in our visual and non-visual systems. Circadian rhythms in humans are most sensitive to short-wavelength light, and these responses are driven by ipRGCs which contains the photopigment melanopsin. The greatest damage of blue light occurs between 415 and 455 nm (Fig. 6). Blue light, also, stimulates connections between areas of the brain that process emotion and language which may help people to better react to emotional challenges and regulate mood [11]. During the exposure to blue light there is a significant reduction in both breath rate and the diastolic blood pressure, thus blue light reduces physiological arousal, supporting the claim that blue light can be used to induce physiological rest [12]. Emotional tasks were shown to be stronger with blue light exposure (473 nm or 480 nm), to which melanopsin ipRGCs and the non-image-forming system is maximally sensitive [11].

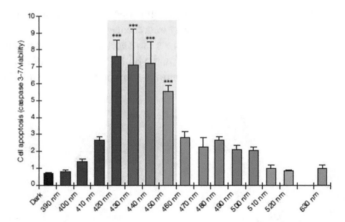

**Fig. 6.** Phototoxic action (apoptosis) spectrum on A2E-loaded RPE cells and morphological changes of the REP cells. ***p < 0.001 as compared to control cells maintained in the dark [10].

## 2.5    Visual and Non-visual Systems

The human eye has natural defenses against the UV radiation, whereas short-wavelength light is right next to UV-A (also known as near blue light), all together are blue light, and IR. As for the visual mechanisms of defense o the retina, there are the cornea block to ultraviolet radiation (UVR) below 300 nm, which is absorbed by the iris, while the crystalline lens block UVR between 300 and 400 nm [12, 13]. Despite the eye's age, (Figs. 7 and 8) the light absorption and transmission changes, first the crystalline lens becomes gradually more yellow, which in turns make the elderly eyes more sensitive to blue light since the mechanisms of repair become less effective. Secondly, the pupil decreases in size, and the result is the elderly become more sensitive to disorders of circadian entrainment. Retinal pigmental epithelial (RPE) absorbs blue light and supply to the rods and cones (photoreceptors) nutrients [10]. On the other hand, we have lipofuscin, which accumulates in the eye and contributes to permanent cellular damage [12–14]. Besides, reactive oxygen species (ROS) just like lipofuscin, also builds up all over the years, and it can induce photochemical damage, which leads to death by apoptosis of the RPE and then of the cones and rods [10]. Furthermore, light is also essential for non-visual systems, comprehending the synchronization of circadian cycles, which reflects on thermoregulation, endocrine and cardiovascular functions, sleep/awake cycle and quality (through melatonin production), immune system, cognitive performance, memory, fight-and-flight response (cortisol, epinephrine and norepinephrine production), pupil constriction, and in mood (serotonin production) [15–17].

The visual system is mainly driven by the cones (peak sensitivity at 505 nm) and rods (peak sensitivity at 555 nm) whereas the non-visual systems is mediated by the intrinsically photopigment retinal ganglion cell (ipRGCs), which contain melanopsin (peak sensitivity at 420–480 nm). ipRGCs are more sluggish than cones and rods [18], and as the exposure to light increases in time the contribution (with cones) decreases. The longer the exposure of ipRGCs to short-wavelength light more effective is the alertness and performance levels. The ipRGCs are more responsive to short-wavelength light and this reflects in the production of cortisol (stress hormone), by the adrenal gland (as response to bright light) increases, and no production of melatonin (its antagonistic hormone, the dark hormone, often associated with sleep) occurs. Along with cortisol production, serotonin (mood hormone) is activated by light and have a positive effect on human, although over the time its production decreases somewhat like 10% less per decade. IpRGCs have a spectral sensitivity very similar to rods but need much brighter light for its activation [19–21].

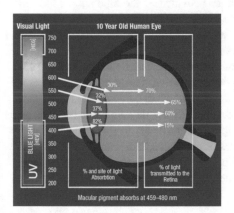

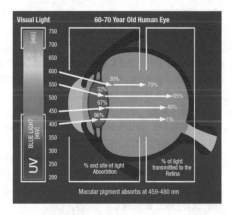

**Fig. 7.** Excessive blue light exposure can permanently damage your eyes and retina: 10-year-old Human Eye [11].

**Fig. 8.** Excessive blue light exposure can permanently damage your eyes and retina: 60–70-year-old Human Eye [11].

## 2.6    Ageing, Pupil Constriction and Sleep Quality

Biological ageing is associated with the structural changes of the lens which becomes yellowing by 0.6–0.7 percentage point per year of life [22] On the other hand, when blue light transmission to the retina is reduced due the yellowing of the lens, which provoke that people could have an increased risk of sleep disturbances. Furthermore, under blue light, or bright light, the pupil decreases in size, which protects our eye since it allows less light penetration. However, Pupil size decreases over the time [20] and in reaction to short-wavelength light the reduction in pupillary response do not means that we are prone to glaucoma, but rather that there is a reduction in ipRGC activation [4]. Glaucoma is associated with a worse sleep quality, a daytime sleepiness and a circadian dysfunction [5]. All these aspects could result disruption in the photoentrainment of circadian rhythm. So, it worth to comprehend how much blue light is essential to promote the photoentrainment of circadian rhythm [22]. When we have to consider artificial lighting systems we have to have in mind other kind of facts, which are stated below.

## 2.7    Artificial Light

Nowadays, we are more exposed to artificial than to natural light, since we spend most of our lifetime indoors. While the Kyoto Protocol induce the abandoning of incandescent light sources and gradually, also, the fluorescent light sources, the LEDs (Light Emitting Diodes) will be the light of the next future. But, for now, the lighting systems existing in our residences and workplaces is mainly based on fluorescent system's type, which have a spectrum in the green (550 nm). Our circadian rhythms respond better to the blue light spectrum. At this point, the LEDs seems to be the best answer, especially, for our productivity and performance, which are activated by the blue range (460 nm), since they promote our alertness, cognitive performance, improves our mood and contribute to our non-visual responses. Besides, LEDs are less expensive than fluorescent lighting systems. So, LEDs try to stimulate our non-visual needs, while the fluorescent light are more concerned with our visual ones. The downside is that LEDs [21], at the present moment, have many characteristics that should be revised, like, for example, the flickering that our nervous system acknowledge even though our visual systems seems to ignore it. LEDs also contribute to the development of ROS and damage RPE, and since, it is mostly blue light, it contributes to the damage of outer nuclear layer (ONL) which destroys 4/5 layers of photoreceptors (cones and rods) from the 12/13 layers over the time (39 weeks) (Fig. 9) [14]. This destruction of the rods and cones leads to a loss of vision and night blindness. In order to overcome this loss, the IOLs (intraocular lens), sunglasses or some kind of filters for the glasses could be a response but not at all times.

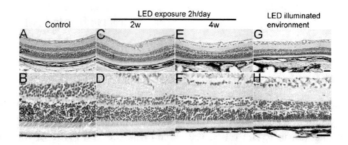

**Fig. 9.**  Representative images of hematoxylin staining for retina section in control and [24]

LED-exposure mice. Light micrographs were taken from the mouse retinas. Sections of control and light-exposed retinas stained with hematoxylin. In control retinas (A and B), the ONL shows the photoreceptor nuclei normally (B). The arrangement of photoreceptor cells in the outer nuclear layer was slightly distorted and the thickness of the outer nuclear layer was decreased after 2 weeks (C and D) and 4 weeks (E and F) exposure. At 39 weeks after light exposure (G and H), with a significant reduction in the thickness of the outer nuclear layer (G), and the photoreceptor cell loss is evident (H). After light exposure, noted that the outer nuclear layer becomes thinner over time. ONL, outer nuclear layer. Scale bars = 50 um [24].

However, if we avoid blue light we will not have the advantages of it, such as cognitive performance or a better mood and even a greater visual acuity (Fig. 10). So, we cannot ignore these facts but we should balance the exposure to blue light, from natural and artificial light, the best option that we have is manage the lighting systems and try to, just like the daylight, vary during the day [23]. Another effect of blue light is the increase of cortisol and serotonin production, which is a good thing, but only in the right amounts. If we are under blue light too much time, the cortisol production, which make us more energetic, will turn out in more nervous and stressful, and when this levels are higher they promote the norepinephrine and epinephrine levels, which lead us to the negative part of the stimulation curve.

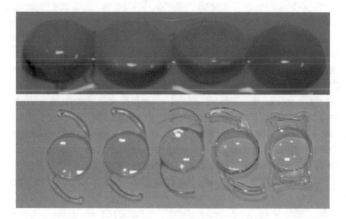

**Fig. 10.** Colour photographs of four of the donor lenses [aged 18, 35, 63 and 76 years (from left to right)] and the five intraocular implant lens (IOLs) IOLS [SA60AT, SN6/WF, Hoya-PS AF-a (UY), EYECRYL. HFY 600, CT Asphina 404V (from left to right)] [23].

## 2.8   Workplace

Contemporaneous working places differs from the traditional ones because of the new methods of work enhanced by technology. Interacting with technology improve human productivity and encouraged new activities and functions; however, these new tools demand different spatial layout configurations from which the development of a task in a vertical and auto-illuminated plan emerge as one of the major changes and challenges. Despite the awareness of this reality, working places are still following traditional design principles. There is a significant progress with the ergonomic questions, related to desks and chairs, the opposition of the computer, monitor and mouse; questions related to the inclusion of individuals with limitations are being answered. Yet, when considering the lighting design, it seems that the aesthetical demands come together with the accomplishment of parameters of a data sheet, neglecting its effect on human being particularly on the non-visual effects, which have a strong impact on comfort and health of the user.

Recurrently, the support for this reality is a push game between professionals from different background, but the result is a deficient lighting solution for spaces oriented to work.

Moreover, is important to highlight that a lighting design which neglects its impact on user health and comfort, answering to numeric requirements that spot a quantity of lux and lumens to an activity, and disregard the colour spectrum of the light contribute to the increase of glaucoma incidents.

Furthermore, the ageing population is a reality that draft new challenges to build environment and working places are not an exception, mostly when the retirement age is changing for higher values. There is a natural relation between the emergence of glaucoma and age that requires an answer from lighting designers.

It is a document fact that we spend 70% to 90% of our lifetime indoors [22, 25, 26] in indoor spaces, like homes, and workplaces, where daylight only penetrates the building for less than 4 h, especially in winter which have a negative impact on individual mood (SAD, Seasonal Affective Disorder) and on neurocognitive processes.

Unfortunately, the lighting recommendations for indoors are based on visual criteria [23, 27, 28]. SAD, for instance, improves under bright-light exposure. Exposure to blue light/bright light in the morning and evening also improve alertness and productivity; the lack of daylight exposure to whom spend many hours indoors, especially in winter, may compromise health and wellbeing [28]. We must not forget that we are outdoor animals, so it is in outdoors places that we feel balanced biological and psychologically. There is a great difference between outdoor (2.000 and 100.000 lx) and indoor illuminance, where norms suggests 200 and 500 lx. Moreover, in the last two decades, we move from paper source (horizontal plane) to computer tasks (vertical plane) [29]. Nevertheless, as already stated, older eyes need more time to adapt to brightness differences due to the reduced elasticity of the iris. At workplaces, for instance, dynamic artificial lighting, like the natural light, could help to prevent diseases, disorders and promote employees' productivity and performance, and mood, which also protects our eyes from the blue light, since the extent of our exposure to it is lesser [30].

## 3  Conclusions

It seems that short-wavelength light sensitivity has in fact relation with glaucoma, however there are not certainties about how it occurs and what is the relation. Although, K cells are involved with short-wavelength, rods have similar peak with ipRGCs. There are more questions that emerge than answers. If ipRGCs are fewer it makes sense that the melatonin levels are higher and this results in more melatonin production, which makes us drowsier and sleepy. But, if pupil size decreases the light that passes through the lens and reach the retina is also less, so it may not be the ipRGCs that are less effective but the pupil size that allows less blue light to reach the retina. Besides, the yellowing of the crystalline, also, avoids that blue light damage the retina. Even though, the glaucoma initially affects the peripheral visual field (M cells), but recent evidence suggest that may be not be so.

It appears that the only certainty is that we must keep the aqueous humor circulating within the eye, since it maintains the trabecular meshwork healthy. Another fact is that RPE can help to control the lipofuscin and ROS formation, and in that way, we can keep the eye well. There is, also, the need to continue to study the RGCs (Retinal Ganglion Cells) role in the short-wavelength sensitivity since there is some evidences that suggests that there is a cause-effect relation. Block the short-wavelength light must not be the answer since we need it in order to maintain our circadian rhythms synchronizes and all that concerns.

Considering the knowledge about the impact of short-wavelengths on human beings a new consciousness must support indoors lighting design particularly workspaces. Working tasks require different types of light which usually are selected regarding their intensity and energy consumption neglecting their impact on human performance and well-being. Beside the segregation of the user requirements for the selection of lighting sources it is also mistreated the shift from traditional forms of work to the intensive use of digital equipment where monitors emerge as a new working surface. Moreover, it is important to accept that population is ageing and retirement age is increasing bringing along new challenges towards the lighting design.

## 4 Discussion

This paper aims to high spot the need to control one of the major causes of human blind: glaucoma. The available information allows to relate this disorder with its cause: and light contributes significantly to its emergence and development. However, although the available information lighting design performs aesthetically remarkable solutions, answering to established parameters that determine the amount of light quantity required by different tasks, however, lighting design solutions overlook user requirements, namely the ones related with user non- visual system, which, by the way affect considerably human health and the sensation of comfort.

Thus, emerge the need to bring this subject to light towards a broader discussion and to challenge professionals from different background towards innovative solutions. Research is needed to confirm (or not) the available information once, as many other aspects in science, there are different approaches, some antagonistic.

Experiences to orient an innovative path to the right lighting design, answering to function as user requirements are needed. From these will be easier to achieve information to support new data sheets to be accomplish in every lighting design project.

Professionals from architecture and design areas ought to be moved to new approaches beyond the aesthetical or performative (traditional) ones.

## References

1. Lighthouse International: What is Glaucoma? http://li129-107.members.linode.com/about-low-vision-blindness/vision-disorders/glaucoma/
2. Karwatsky, P., Overbury, O., Faubert, J.: Red-Green chromatic mechanisms in normal aging and glaucomatous observers. Invest. Ophthalmol. Visual Sci. **45**(8), 2861–2866 (2004)

3. The Glaucoma Foundation: Patient Guide. https://www.glaucomafoundation.org/docs/PatientGuide.pdf
4. Rukmini, A.V., et al.: Pupillary responses to high-irradiance blue light correlate with glaucoma severity. Ophthalmology **122**, 1777–1785 (2015)
5. Gracitelli, C.P.B., et al.: Relationship between daytime sleepiness and intrinsically photosensitive retinal ganglion cells in glaucomatous disease. J. Ophthalmol. **2016**, 1–9 (2016)
6. SightMD: Glaucoma. https://www.google.pt/search?client=firefox-b-ab&dcr=0&biw=1366&bih=635&tbm=isch&sa=1&q=Glaucoma%2Cjpeg&oq=Glaucoma%2Cjpeg&gs_l=psy-ab.3...14096.15009.0.15394.5.5.0.0.0.0.144.617.0j5.5.0....0...1.1.64.psy-ab..0.2.265...0j0i19k1j0i8i30i19k1j0i30i19k1.m_KTmjm__zE#imgrc=8Sr2UMoXh3VLGM
7. Natures Gist: Causes, Symptoms and How to Naturally Treat Glaucoma. https://naturesgist.com/2017/02/11/causes-symptoms-naturally-treat-glaucoma/
8. Glaucoma.org: types of Glaucoma. http://www.glaucoma.org/glaucoma/types-of-glaucoma.php
9. Essilor: blue light hazard: new knowledge, new approaches to maintaining ocular health. http://www.crizalusa.com/SiteCollectionDocuments/Crizal-Literature/Blue%20|Light%20Roundtable_White%20Paper.pdf
10. Garbus, C.: Functional visual field assessement and management. http://slideplayer.com/slide/5279716/
11. Health-e.com: symptons of digital eye strain include. http://health-e.com/pages/theproblem
12. Chang, A.-M.M., et al.: Human responses to bright light of different durations. J. Physiol. **590**(13), 3103–3112 (2012)
13. Cuthbertson, F.M., et al.: Blue light-filtering intraocular lenses: review of potential benefits and side effects-. J. Cataract Refract. Surg. **2009**(35), 1281–1297 (2009)
14. Essilor Inc.: protecting the eye against sunlight - more than just blocking UV? http://www.xperiouvusa.com/SiteCollectionImages/Protectyoureyesunderthesun/d7102537_lumiere_bleu_16x21_gb_MD.pdf
15. Vandewalle, G., Djik, D.-J.: Neuroimaging the effects of light on non-visual brain functions. http://orbi.ulg.ac.be/bitstream/2268/149605/1/Vandewalle%20%26%20Schmidt%202013.pdf
16. Philips: physiological effects of light – how light regulates sleep, mood and energy. http://www.newscenter.philips.com/pwc_nc/main/standard/resources/corporate/press/2009/winter_blues/Blue_light_white_paper_Europe_Final.pdf
17. Gronfier, C.: The good blue and chronobiology – light and non-visual functions. http://www.crizalusa.com/content/dam/crizal/us/en/pdf/blue-light/The_Good_Blue_andChronobiology.pdf
18. Bizjak, G.: Nonvisual effects of light. http://ip2013.eap.gr/pdf/SI_Bizjak_Nonvisual_efects_of_light_1.pdf
19. Burnett, D.: Circadian adaptive lighting. http://www.photonstartechnology.com/Main_Upload/2012_Circadian_Adaptive_Lighting_Burnett.pdf
20. Bmcophthalmol.bioledcenntral.com: intrinsically photosensitive retinal ganglion cell function in relation to age: a pupillometric study in humans with special reference to the age-related optic properties of the lens. http://bmcophthalmol.biomedcentral.com/articles/10.1186/1471-2415-12-4
21. Chamorro, E.: Photoprotective Effects of Blue Light Absorbing Filter against LED Light. Exposure on Human Retinal Pigment Epithelial Cells In Vitro. J Carcinog Mutagen S6: 008. https://doi.org/10.4172/2157-2518. S6-008 (2013)
22. Mahnke, F.: Color, Environment & Human Response. Wiley, New York (1996)

23. Brøndsted, A.E., Lundeman, J.H., Kessel, L.: Short wavelength light filtering by the natural human lens and IOLs – implications for entrainment of circadian rhythm (2013)
24. Peng, M., et al.: The influence of low-powered family LED lighting on eyes in mice experimental model. http://www.lifesciencesite.com/lsj/life0901/072_8366life0901_477_482.pdf
25. Hobday, R.: Healing Sun: Sunshine and Health in the 21st Century. Findhorn Press Ltd. (1999)
26. Kuller, R.: Physiological and psychological effects of illumination and colour in the interior environment. https://www.jstage.jst.go.jp/article/jlve/10/2/10_2_2_1/_article
27. Ámundadottir, M.L., Hilaire, M.A., Lockley, S.W., Andersen, M.: Modelling non-visual responses to light: unifying spectral and temporal characteristics in a single model structure. http://infoscience.epfl.ch/record/186074/files/Amundadottir_OP16_CIE2013_EPFL.pdf
28. Mills, P.R., Tomkins, S.C., Schlangen, L.J.M.: The effect of high correlated colour temperature office lighting on employee wellbeing and work performance http://www.biomedcentral.com/1740-3391/5/2/
29. Gooley, J.J., et al.: Melanopsin and rod-cone photoreceptors play different roles in mediating pupillary light responses during exposure to continuous light in humans. J. Neurosci. 32(41), 4242–14253 (2012)
30. Braun, H.: Photobiology - the biological impact of sunlight on health & infection control (2008). https://phoenixprojectfoundation.us/uploads/BioLight-Sunlight___Infection_Control.pdf

# Evaluation of the Hemodynamic Effects of AC Magnetic Field Exposure by Measurement of an FMD and a Microscope

Tsukasa Kondo[1], Hideyuki Okano[2(✉)], Hiromi Ishiwatari[3], and Keiichi Watanuki[1,2,4]

[1] Graduate School of Science and Engineering,
Saitama University, Saitama, Japan
[2] Advanced Institute of Innovative Technology,
Saitama University, Saitama, Japan
hideyukiokano@aol.com
[3] Soken Medical Co., Ltd., Tokyo, Japan
[4] Brain and Body System Science Institute, Saitama University, Saitama, Japan

**Abstract.** This study focuses on the acute influence of an AC electromagnetic field (ELF-EMF) exposure (50 Hz, $B_{max}$ 180 mT) on flow-mediated dilation (FMD) and peripheral capillary flow velocity in healthy human subjects. In a randomized, double blind and crossover design, the sham control (CTL) and the EMF exposures were carried out. For FMD study, exposure of the left upper arm to EMF was performed for 30 min in a supine position. In the case of the measurement of microcirculation, exposure of the left forearm to EMF was conducted for 15 min in a sitting position. The FMD values were significantly increased from the baseline value in the presence of EMF exposure. The values of the microcirculation were significantly increased by the EMF exposure. These results imply that the EMF-enhanced vasodilation and microcirculation might help eliminate the metabolic waste products and endogenous pain producing substances inducing muscle stiffness and pain.

**Keywords:** Electromagnetic field · Flow-Mediated Dilatation (FMD)
Microcirculation

## 1 Introduction

Many researches for exploring biological and health hazardous effects on extremely low frequency electromagnetic fields (ELF-EMF) ranging 1–300 Hz have been done [1–10]. However, there are only a few reports evaluating the exposure mechanisms for medical therapeutic applications [9, 10]. When focusing on Japan alone, non-thermal noninvasive alternating current (AC) EMF therapy with a sinusoidal frequency of 50/60 Hz has been used to relieve chronic pain, muscle stiffness, muscle fatigue and so on, for more than 30 years, since approved by Japanese Ministry of Health, Labour and Welfare for improvement of muscle stiffness and blood circulation in the EMF-exposed area, in which the peak magnetic flux density $B_{max}$ of the surface area on the approved EMF therapeutic device should be ranging between 35 and 180 mT.

© Springer International Publishing AG, part of Springer Nature 2019
N. J. Lightner (Ed.): AHFE 2018, AISC 779, pp. 68–79, 2019.
https://doi.org/10.1007/978-3-319-94373-2_8

Despite the inadequate scientific evidence, ELF-EMF therapy including pulsed EMF with low frequency has been proposed by practitioners of alternative medicine for a variety of purposes, including cell growth promotion, pain reduction, improved blood circulation, bone repair, increased wound healing, sedative effects, enhanced sleep, and arthritic relief [11]. Because clinical evidence and the physiological mechanisms are not clear enough to support the effectiveness of the therapeutic approach, especially due to AC EMF-enhanced blood circulation and recovery of muscle fatigue and pain, we have been investigated the hemodynamic effects of non-thermal AC EMF exposure (50 Hz, peak magnetic flux density $B_{max}$ 180 mT, up to 30-min duration of exposure). It has recently been found that the values of forearm blood flow velocity in an ulnar artery were significantly increased by forearm exposure to an AC EMF (50 Hz, $B_{max}$ 180 mT, for 15 min) [12]. However, the effects of the EMF on flow-mediated dilation (FMD) in the brachial artery and microcirculation in capillaries have not been examined. Therefore, this study focuses on the acute influence of the EMF on FMD and peripheral capillary flow velocity in healthy human subjects.

## 2 Methods

### 2.1 Subjects

Healthy volunteer subjects (10 males, age range 21–24 years, heights 155–175 cm, weights 48–72 kg) participated after signing an informed consent form approved by the university's institutional review board. During the study period, subjects were not used any form of physical therapy and were not taking any vasoactive medication. Subjects' body temperature, and systolic and diastolic blood pressures were within normal ranges.

### 2.2 Study Protocol

In a randomized, double blind and crossover design, the sham control (CTL) and the EMF exposures were carried out under the conditions of switching off and on, respectively. The measurements of the FMD and the blood flow velocity were conducted in different protocols and therefore were not done simultaneously. The both measurements were performed on different days. The values of both measurements were compared with two different exposures.

### 2.3 Measurement of FMD

The FMD measurement has been reported elsewhere [13–15]. Briefly, an FMD monitoring device (UNEXEF18G, UNEX, Nagoya, Aichi, Japan) has a high-resolution linear artery transducer coupled to computer assisted analysis software that used an automated edge detection system for measurement of the brachial artery diameter (Fig. 1a). A blood pressure cuff was placed around the forearm (Fig. 1b).

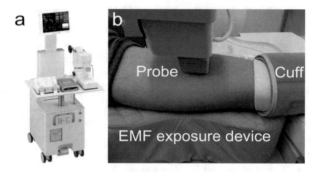

**Fig. 1.** An FMD monitoring device (a) and FMD measurement/EMF exposure device (b).

The brachial artery was scanned longitudinally 5–8 cm above the elbow. When the clearest B-mode image of the anterior and posterior intimal interfaces between the lumen and vessel wall was obtained, the transducer was held at the same point throughout the scan by a special probe holder (UNEX) to ensure consistency of the imaging. Depth and gain setting were set to optimize the images of the arterial lumen wall interface. When the tracking gate was placed on the intima, the artery diameter was automatically tracked, and the waveform of diameter changes over the cardiac cycle was displayed in real time using the FMD mode of the tracking system. This allowed the ultrasound images to be optimized at the start of the scan and the transducer position to be adjusted immediately for optimal tracking performance throughout the scan. Pulsed Doppler flow was assessed at baseline and during peak hyperemic flow, which was confirmed to occur within 15 s after cuff deflation. Blood flow velocity was calculated from the Doppler data and displayed as a waveform in real time. The baseline longitudinal image of the artery was acquired for 30 s, and then the blood pressure cuff was inflated to 50 mmHg above systolic pressure for 5 min. The longitudinal image of the artery was recorded continuously until 2 min after cuff deflation. Pulsed Doppler velocity signals were obtained for 20 s at baseline and for 10 s immediately after cuff deflation. Changes in brachial artery diameter were immediately expressed as a percentage change relative to the vessel diameter before cuff inflation. FMD was automatically calculated as the percentage change in peak vessel diameter from the baseline value using the following equation.

$$\text{FMD } [\%] = \frac{\text{peak diameter} - \text{baseline diameter}}{\text{baseline diameter}} \times 100 \tag{1}$$

For FMD measurement, exposure of the dorsal side of the left upper arm to EMF was carried out for 30 min in a supine position (Fig. 1b). The brachial artery FMD values in the left upper arm were monitored at the baseline (pre-exposure) and post-exposure.

The protocol of FMD measurement is shown in Fig. 2. After putting on the dorsal side of the left upper arm on an AC EMF exposure device and attaching the cuff around the left forearm about at least 5-min resting period, the FMD values were measured for about 7 min at pre-exposure and post-exposure periods (time points I–II). The EMF or CTL exposure was performed continuously for 30 min.

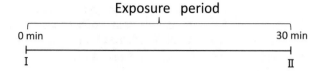

**Fig. 2.** Protocol of FMD measurement.

## 2.4 Measurement of Capillary Flow Velocity

The measurement of blood flow velocity in nailfold capillaries has been reported elsewhere [16–19]. Briefly, the ring finger of the left hand were examined using a nailfold video capillaroscopy (Bscan Z, Toku, Tokyo, Japan) with a 350 × optic magnification (Fig. 3). Exposure of the ventral side of the left forearm to EMF was performed for 15 min in a sitting position (Fig. 3).

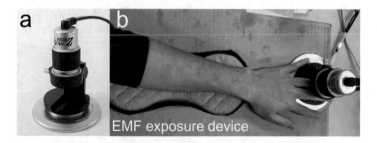

**Fig. 3.** A capillaroscopy (a) and measurement of blood flow velocity/EMF exposure device (b).

The protocol of measurement of capillary flow velocity is shown in Fig. 4. After putting on the ventral side of the left forearm on an AC EMF exposure device and setting the ring finger of the left hand on the capillaroscopy for about at least 5-min resting period, the microcirculation of nailfold capillaries in the ring finger was observed and the image of the microcirculation was recorded at pre-exposure, during and post-exposure periods at 5-min intervals (time points I–VI) for 25 min. The EMF or CTL exposure was conducted continuously for 15 min (time points I–IV).

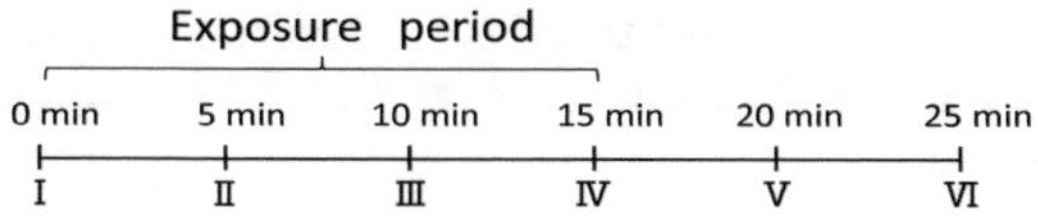

**Fig. 4.** Protocol of measurement of capillary flow velocity.

The values of velocity of leukocytes or white blood cells (WBCs) were analyzed as an indicator of blood flow velocity using image acquisition and analysis software (Capiscope II, KK Technology, Colyton, Devon, UK), because the legible trajectories of WBSs were easier to trace than those of erythrocytes or red blood cells. Thereafter, the centerline velocity of WBCs ($\mu$m s-1) was determined on acquired images in black and white using the additional calibrated ruler function of image analyzing software (Beta 4.0.3 of Scion Image; Scion, MD, USA). At 25 frames s-1, the distance of WBCs moved over time, was measured within a relatively straight vessel. The velocity was measured over 3–4 frames for capillaries. Ten centerline velocity measurements were made and the three fastest values were used to calculate mean values.

## 2.5    AC EMF Exposure Device

An AC EMF exposure device (Soken MS), which was manufactured by Soken (Toride, Ibaraki, Japan), was utilized for research purpose. Two separate electromagnetic coils are set horizontally inside the EMF exposure device and the value of the $B_{max}$ is 180 mT on the surface of the EMF exposure device above the center of the coils. The spatial distribution of the $B_{max}$ from the surface of the EMF exposure device is shown in Fig. 5. The magnetic flux density values of AC EMF decrease exponentially with distance. The estimated $B_{max}$ value in ulnar artery and brachial artery is approximately 13 mT and 8 mT, in which the distance from the surface $B_{max}$ 180 mT of the EMF exposure device is approximately 3 cm and 4 cm, as shown in Fig. 5.

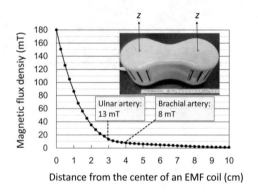

**Fig. 5.** Spatial distribution of the peak magnetic flux density $B_{max}$ values along $z$-axis.

The measurement of root mean square (rms) values ($a$) was made by means of a Hall probe magnetometer in AC mode (AC/DC Magnetometer, AlphaLab, Salt Lake City, UT, USA). Here, the $B_{max}$ values ($b$) of AC EMF were calculated using the following the equation:

$$b = \sqrt{2}a \qquad (2)$$

The room temperature and the temperature in the surface of the EMF exposure device during the EMF exposure period was maintained at 25 ± 0.5 °C. The relative humidity was controlled at 50 ± 10%.

## 2.6  Statistical Analysis

Statistical analysis of differences in mean values of the sham control and EMF exposure groups was made by using the Wilcoxon rank-sum test (between groups) and Wilcoxon paired signed rank test (within group) for non-parametric data. In addition, post-hoc differences were analyzed by two-way ANOVA for repeated measures (experimental groups and time points). For all comparisons, a P value less than 0.05 was considered significant.

# 3  Results and Discussion

## 3.1  Measurement of FMD

Nine individuals have been assessed in duplicate measurements on different days for the EMF exposure and the CTL exposure, and average values were calculated for each individual. The changing rate (%) from the baseline value of FMD was analyzed because the variability of the baseline values were very large between individuals, which can be associated with fluctuations in blood pressure over time. These results were shown in Fig. 6.

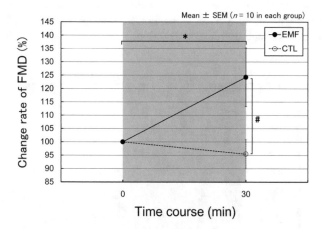

**Fig. 6.** The time course of the change rate of FMD in EMF exposure group and sham control (CTL) exposure group. The measurements of each individual were repeated in duplicate on different days, and the average values were calculated for each individual. Solid black circles represent the EMF exposure group; and open black circles represent the CTL exposure group. The gray color zone indicates the 30-min duration of EMF or CTL exposure. Values are expressed as mean ± SEM ($n = 10$ in each group). The FMD values were significantly increased by the EMF exposure compared with the CTL exposure. *$P < 0.05$ (within group) and #$P < 0.05$ (between groups) were considered statistically significant.

The FMD values were significantly increased from the baseline value in the presence of EMF exposure. There were significant differences between EMF and CTL exposures. FMD is an indicator of endothelial function and shear stress-induced nitric oxide (NO) production [14, 15]. Therefore, EMF-induced increase of FMD values indicates enhancement of NO production. In contrast, in CTL exposure, there was no significant change in the FMD values during experimental period. For this reason, for example, it has been reported that both values of forearm blood flow velocity and vascular resistance were not changed for at least 5 h in the supine position without any intervention [20].

## 3.2    Measurement of Capillary Flow Velocity

Eight individuals have been assessed in duplicate measurements on different days for the EMF exposure and the CTL exposure, and average values were calculated for each individual. As is the same case with FMD measurement, the changing rate (%) from the baseline value of blood flow velocity was analyzed due to the large variability of the baseline values between individuals. These results were shown in Fig. 7. The values of the blood flow velocity were significantly increased by the EMF exposure compared with CTL exposure. There were significant differences between EMF and CTL exposures at 15-min exposure and 5-min and 10-min post-exposure periods. In contrast, in CTL exposure, there was no significant change in the values of blood flow velocity during experimental period. Therefore, the results suggest that EMF induced increase in peripheral capillary microcirculation.

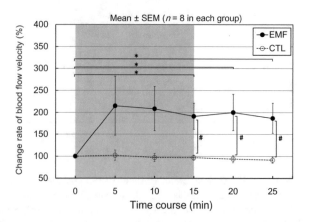

**Fig. 7.** The time course of the change rate of blood flow velocity in EMF exposure group and sham control (CTL) exposure group. The measurements of each individual were repeated in duplicate on different days, and the average values were calculated for each individual. Solid black circles represent the EMF exposure group; and open black circles represent the CTL exposure group. The gray color zone indicates the 15-min duration of EMF or CTL exposure. Values are expressed as mean ± SEM ($n$ = 8 in each group). The FMD values were significantly increased by the EMF exposure compared with the CTL exposure. *$P < 0.05$ (within group) and #$P < 0.05$ (between groups) were considered statistically significant.

### 3.3    Plausible Biophysical Mechanisms of AC EMF on Hemodynamics

The nerve stimulation and increased blood flow by eddy current has been evaluated using transcranial magnetic stimulation (TMS) [21–25]. In contrast, however, the decreases in regional blood flow induced by TMS have been reported [21, 25–28]. Thus, the effects of TMS on blood flow are variable and fluctuating depending on the stimulus conditions, e.g., stimulus frequency, intensity, duration, and, to date, the optimal stimulus conditions have not been established. The eddy current density ($J$) is based on the Lenz's law, and in this study the estimated values of eddy current for an AC EMF of $B_{max}$ 180 mT were calculated using the following equation [29, 30]:

$$J = \pi f \, \sigma \, Br \tag{3}$$

where $f$ is the frequency (Hz), $\sigma$ is the conductivity of living tissue (S/m), the $B$ is the magnetic flux density (T), and $r$ is the electromagnetic coil radius (m).

Measurement results of each parameter were that $f = 50$ Hz, $\sigma = 0.7$ S/m in blood [30], $B = 0.008$ T (4 cm depth from the surface of the EMF exposure device) to 0.18 T (on the surface), and $r = 5 \times 10^{-2}$ m.

The current density in blood has not been estimated and discussed in the context of TMS and EMF. The calculated values of $J$ were ranged from 44.0 to 989.6 mA/m$^2$ in blood. Here the maximum value of 989.6 mA/m$^2$ was 1/3 or less of the maximum current density of the standard TMS method used for brain stimulation to gray and white matters, i.e., the peak values for coil positions are 2.82 A/m$^2$ in the dorsal lateral prefrontal cortex and 3.57 A/m$^2$ in the motor strip [31]. As dominant biophysical mechanisms of EMF, the EMF-induced eddy current of EMF exposure may be enough to induce changes in blood flow, probably via nerve stimulation, although the values of current density were under those of the standard TMS method.

### 3.4    Plausible Biochemical Mechanisms of AC EMF on Hemodynamics

Acetylcholine can effect vasodilation by several mechanisms, including activation of endothelial nitric oxide synthase (NOS) and prostaglandin (PG) production [32]. The plausible biochemical mechanisms of AC EMF for the promotion of hemodynamic responses have been reported in experimental studies [33]. Most importantly, the inhibitory effect of AC EMF on acetylcholinesterase (the lytic enzyme of acetylcholine) was observed in the magnetic flux density of 0.74 mT or more [34]. For other pathways, the exposure of HaCaT cells to AC EMF (50 Hz, $B_{rms}$ 1 mT, for 3 h) increased inducible nitric oxide synthase (iNOS) and endothelial nitric oxide synthase (eNOS) expression levels [35]. These AC EMF-dependent increased expression levels were paralleled by increased NOS activities and increased NO production.

### 3.5    Plausible Integrated Mechanisms of AC EMF on Hemodynamics

Considering both plausible biophysical and biochemical mechanisms of AC EMF on hemodynamics, we speculate the following integrated mechanisms as shown in Fig. 8.

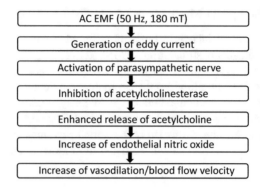

**Fig. 8.** Plausible integrated mechanisms of AC EMF on hemodynamics.

Here, the eddy current induced by AC EMF could play a crucial role in the initiation of a series of the physiological response processes involved in hemodynamic responses. Further studies should be needed to investigate the EMF-based therapeutic applications and elucidate the underlying mechanisms of EMF effects on blood flow and blood vessels.

## 4   Conclusions

The values of the FMD as well as peripheral capillary microcirculation were significantly increased by the EMF exposure after exposure period compared with the CTL exposure. When considering the physiological significance of the non-thermal EMF effects, these results imply that the EMF-enhanced vasodilation and microcirculation might help eliminate the metabolic waste products and endogenous pain producing substances inducing muscle stiffness and pain.

## References

1. McKay, J.C., Prato, F.S., Thomas, A.W.: A literature review: the effects of magnetic field exposure on blood flow and blood vessels in the microvasculature. Bioelectromagnetics **28**, 81–98 (2007)
2. Ohkubo, C., Okano, H., Masuda, H., Ushiyama, A.: EMF effects on microcirculatory system. Environmentalist **27**, 395–402 (2007)
3. McNamee, D.A., Corbacio, M., Weller, J.K., Brown, S., Prato, F.S., Thomas, A.W., Legros, A.G.: The cardiovascular response to an acute 1800-μT, 60-Hz magnetic field exposure in humans. Int. Arch. Occup. Environ. Health **83**, 441–454 (2010)
4. McNamee, D.A., Corbacio, M., Weller, J.K., Brown, S., Stodilka, R.Z., Prato, F.S., Bureau, Y., Thomas, A.W., Legros, A.G.: The response of the human circulatory system to an acute 200-μT, 60-Hz magnetic field exposure. Int. Arch. Occup. Environ. Health **84**, 267–277 (2011)

5. Ueno, S., Okano, H.: Static, low frequency and pulsed magnetic fields in biological systems. In: Lin, J.C. (ed.) Electromagnetic Fields in Biological Systems, pp. 115–196. CRC Press, Boca Raton (2011)

6. Mattsson, M.O., Simko, M.: Grouping of experimental conditions as an approach to evaluate effects of extremely low-frequency magnetic fields on oxidative response in In Vitro studies. Front. Public Health. 2, Article 132 (2014)

7. Ohkubo, C., Okano, H.: Magnetic field influences on the microcirculation. In: Markov, M.S. (ed.) Electromagnetic Fields in Biology and Medicine, pp. 103–128. CRC Press, Boca Raton (2015)

8. Pilla, A.A., Muehsam, D.J., Markov, M.S., Sisken, B.F.: EMF signals and ion/ligand binding kinetics: prediction of bioeffective waveform parameters. Bioelectrochem. Bioenerg. 48, 27–34 (1999)

9. Pilla, A.A.: Weak time-varying and static magnetic fields: from mechanisms to therapeutic applications. In: Stavroulakis, P. (ed.) Biological Effects of Electromagnetic Fields, pp. 34–75. Springer, New York (2003)

10. Pilla, A.A.: Mechanisms and therapeutic applications of time-varying and static magnetic fields. In: Barnes, F., Greenebaum, B. (eds.) Handbook of Biological Effects of Electromagnetic Fields, 3rd edn, pp. 351–411. CRC Press, Boca Raton (2007)

11. Begue-Simon, A.M., Drolet, R.A.: Clinical assessment of the RHUMART system based on the use of pulsed electromagnetic fields with low frequency. Int. J. Rehabil. Res. 16, 323–337 (1993)

12. Okano, H., Fujimura, A., Ishiwatari, H., Watanuki, K.: The physiological influence of alternating current electromagnetic field exposure on human subjects. In: IEEE International Conference on Systems, Man, and Cybernetics (SMC), pp. 2442–2447 (2017). ISBN 9781538616451

13. Kajikawa, M., Maruhashi, T., Iwamoto, Y., Iwamoto, A., Matsumoto, T., Hidaka, T., Kihara, Y., Chayama, K., Nakashima, A., Goto, C., Noma, K., Higashi, Y.: Borderline Ankle-Brachial Index value of 0.91–0.99 is associated with endothelial dysfunction. Circ. J. 78, 1740–1745 (2014)

14. Stoner, L., Sabatier, M.J.: Use of ultrasound for non-invasive assessment of flow-mediated dilation. J. Atheroscler. Thromb. 19, 407–421 (2012)

15. Bleeker, M.W., De Groot, P.C., Poelkens, F., Rongen, G.A., Smits, P., Hopman, M.T.: Vascular adaptation to 4 wk of deconditioning by unilateral lower limb suspension. Am. J. Physiol. Heart Circ. Physiol. 288, H1747–H1755 (2005)

16. Brookes, Z.L., Kaufman, S.: Effects of atrial natriuretic peptide on the extrasplenic microvasculature and lymphatics in the rat in vivo. J. Physiol. 565, 269–277 (2005)

17. Brookes, Z.L., Stedman, E.N., Guerrini, R., Lawton, B.K., Calo, G., Lambert, D.G.: Proinflammatory and vasodilator effects of nociceptin/orphanin FQ in the rat mesenteric microcirculation are mediated by histamine. Am. J. Physiol. Heart Circ. Physiol. 293, H2977–H2985 (2007)

18. Nakagami, G., Sanada, H., Matsui, N., Kitagawa, A., Yokogawa, H., Sekiya, N., Ichioka, S., Sugama, J., Shibata, M.: Effect of vibration on skin blood flow in an in vivo microcirculatory model. Biosci. Trends. 1, 161–166 (2007)

19. Mihara, K., Shindo, H., Ohtani, M., Nagasaki, K., Nakashima, R., Katoh, N., Kishimoto, S.: Early depth assessment of local burns by videomicroscopy: 24 h after injury is a critical time point. Burns. 37, 986–993 (2011)

20. Fox, J.S., Whitehead, E.M., Shanks, R.G.: Cardiovascular effects of cromakalim (BRL 34915) in healthy volunteers. Br. J. Clin. Pharmacol. **32**, 45–49 (1991)
21. Loo, C.K., Sachdev, P.S., Haindl, W., Wen, W., Mitchell, P.B., Croker, V.M., Malhi, G.S.: High (15 Hz) and Low (1 Hz) frequency transcranial magnetic stimulation have different acute effects on regional cerebral blood flow in depressed patients. Psychol. Med. **33**, 997–1006 (2003)
22. Speer, A.M., Willis, M.W., Herscovitch, P., Daube-Witherspoon, M., Shelton, J.R., Benson, B.E., Post, R.M., Wassermann, E.M.: Intensity-dependent regional cerebral blood flow during 1-Hz Repetitive Transcranial Magnetic Stimulation (rTMS) in healthy volunteers studied with $H_2^{15}O$ positron emission tomography: II. Effects of prefrontal cortex rTMS. Biol. Psychiatry **54**, 826–832 (2003)
23. Mesquita, R.C., Faseyitan, O.K., Turkeltaub, P.E., Buckley, E.M., Thomas, A., Kim, M.N., Durduran, T., Greenberg, J.H., Detre, J.A., Yodh, A.G., Hamilton, R.H.: Blood flow and oxygenation changes due to low-frequency repetitive transcranial magnetic stimulation of the cerebral cortex. J. Biomed. Opt. **18**, 067006 (2013)
24. Thomson, R.H., Cleve, T.J., Bailey, N.W., Rogasch, N.C., Maller, J.J., Daskalakis, Z.J., Fitzgerald, P.B.: Blood oxygenation changes modulated by coil orientation during prefrontal transcranial magnetic stimulation. Brain Stimul. **6**, 576–581 (2013)
25. Cao, T.T., Thomson, R.H., Bailey, N.W., Rogasch, N.C., Segrave, R.A., Maller, J.J., Daskalakis, Z.J., Fitzgerald, P.B.: A near infra-red study of blood oxygenation changes resulting from high and low frequency repetitive transcranial magnetic stimulation. Brain Stimul. **6**, 922–924 (2013)
26. Rollnik, J.D., Düsterhöft, A., Däuper, J., Kossev, A., Weissenborn, K., Dengler, R.: Decrease of middle cerebral artery blood flow velocity after low-frequency repetitive transcranial magnetic stimulation of the dorsolateral prefrontal cortex. Clin. Neurophysiol. **113**, 951–955 (2002)
27. Aoyama, Y., Hanaoka, N., Kameyama, M., Suda, M., Sato, T., Song, M., Fukuda, M., Mikuni, M.: Stimulus intensity dependence of cerebral blood volume changes in left frontal lobe by low-frequency rTMS to right frontal lobe: a near-infrared spectroscopy study. Neurosci. Res. **63**, 47–51 (2009)
28. Vernieri, F., Altamura, C., Palazzo, P., Altavilla, R., Fabrizio, E., Fini, R., Melgari, J.M., Paolucci, M., Pasqualetti, P., Maggio, P.: 1-Hz repetitive transcranial magnetic stimulation increases cerebral vasomotor reactivity: a possible autonomic nervous system modulation. Brain Stimul. **7**, 281–286 (2014)
29. Gustrau, F., Bahr, A., Rittwenger, M., Goltz, S., Eggert, S.: Simulation of induced current densities in the human body at industrial induction heating frequencies. IEEE Trans. Electromagn. Compat. **41**, 480–486 (1999)
30. Li, Y., Hand, J.W., Wills, T., Hajnal, J.V.: Numerically-simulated induced electric field and current density within a human model located close to a Z-gradient coil. J. Magn. Reson. Imaging **26**, 1286–1295 (2007)
31. Wagner, T., Eden, U., Fregni, F., Valero-Cabre, A., Ramos-Estebanez, C., Pronio-Stelluto, V., Grodzinsky, A., Zahn, M., Pascual-Leone, A.: Transcranial magnetic stimulation and brain atrophy: a computer-based human brain model study. Exp. Brain Res. **186**, 539–550 (2008)
32. Kellogg Jr., D.L., Zhao, J.L., Coey, U., Green, J.V.: Acetylcholine-induced vasodilation is mediated by nitric oxide and prostaglandins in human skin. J. Appl. Physiol. **1985**(98), 629–632 (2005)

33. Robertson, J.A., Thomas, A.W., Bureau, Y., Prato, F.S.: The influence of extremely low frequency magnetic fields on cytoprotection and repair. Bioelectromagnetics **28**, 16–30 (2007)

34. Ravera, S., Bianco, B., Cugnoli, C., Panfoli, I., Calzia, D., Morelli, A., Pepe, I.M.: Sinusoidal ELF magnetic fields affect acetylcholinesterase activity in cerebellum synapto-somal membranes. Bioelectromagnetics **31**, 270–276 (2010)

35. Patruno, A., Amerio, P., Pesce, M., Vianale, G., Di Luzio, S., Tulli, A., Franceschelli, S., Grilli, A., Muraro, R., Reale, M.: Extremely low frequency electromagnetic fields modulate expression of inducible nitric oxide synthase, endothelial nitric oxide synthase and cyclooxygenase-2 in the human keratinocyte cell line HaCat: potential therapeutic effects in wound healing. Br. J. Dermatol. **162**, 258–266 (2010)

# A Comparative Usability Study of a Commercially Acquired and a Locally Developed Prototype of a Newborn Hearing Screening Device

Joanna Nicole Yu[(⊠)], James II Curtney Li, Eireen Ng, and Benette Custodio

Department of Industrial Engineering and Operations Research, University of the Philippines Diliman, 1101 Quezon City, Philippines
dugeporkie@gmail.com, jamesli_24@yahoo.com, ngeireen@gmail.com, bpcustodio@up.edu.ph

**Abstract.** With present laws requiring all newborns in the Philippines to be screened for hearing loss, an affordable biomedical device is being developed locally to increase the rates of newborn hearing screening that will lead to possible early treatment. The main objective of this study was to determine whether the hearing screening device prototype was usable for a Filipino screener. The study was executed through user testing of the prototype and a commercially acquired hearing screening device, followed by post-test interviews of the participants. The effectiveness and satisfaction of the users between the two devices were compared. Findings of the study suggested that several modifications must be made on the current design of the prototype to improve its the usability.

**Keywords:** Comparative usability study · Newborn hearing screening
Device design

## 1 Introduction

### 1.1 Background of the Study

In the Philippines, 1.38 per 1000 neonates are suffering from congenital hearing loss, which may affect the child's linguistic, emotional, and intellectual development [1]. In 2009, Republic Act 9709, also known as the "Universal Newborn Hearing Screening and Intervention Act", required all newborns in the Philippines to be screened for hearing loss. However, the lack of availability for newborn hearing screening devices limits the number of infants who are able to undergo these tests. As such, an affordable biomedical device is being developed in order to increase the rates of newborn hearing screening by utilizing the automated auditory brainstem response (AABR) screening procedure.

A number of research reports, medical error reports, and other official documents exhibit an evident connection between usability problems and user error [2]. With the nature of the development of the device, a thorough usability study of the product must be achieved in order to identify and mitigate use and use-error related hazards [3] as the

© Springer International Publishing AG, part of Springer Nature 2019
N. J. Lightner (Ed.): AHFE 2018, AISC 779, pp. 80–87, 2019.
https://doi.org/10.1007/978-3-319-94373-2_9

primary concern for usability engineering is for the device to be safe and effective for its intended users, uses, and use environment [4].

## 1.2 Rationale of the Study

Device usability studies form an important part of the device production process. There is a link between poor device design, which fails to account for the needs of users, and what is traditionally classified as user error [5]. With this, usability studies are needed in order to assess device design or instruction deficiencies for the reduction of user errors and potential harm; and to save time, money, and resources in the long run [4].

Currently, a newborn hearing screening device is being developed. A usability analysis is critical to identify possible problems for the users of these devices, as well as for the subjects and their families. If the hearing screening device is not properly attached to the subject, a number of effects may happen such as weaker device signal and higher electrode impedance; which may lead to a greater chance for a false-positive result and an incorrect diagnosis for the newborn.

## 1.3 Problem

There is a need to conduct a comparative usability study on a locally developed prototype and a commercially acquired newborn hearing screening device in order to identify possible user errors, to ensure that the device is user-centered, and to make appropriate adjustments on the design if necessary.

## 1.4 Scope and Limitations

The study only focused on the usability and the design of the hearing screening devices since a working prototype of the device was not available during the project timeframe. With this, the accuracy of test results between devices, along with their testing time, could not be compared. Lastly, mannequins were used to represent the different head sizes of infants, which were based on previous studies regarding anthropometric measurements for newborns.

# 2 Methodology

Sixteen (16) participants, with varying occupational backgrounds, were asked to participate in the study [6]. Participants were 18 years old and above, and have at least graduated from high school since these were the minimum requirements for the intended users of the prototype.

## 2.1 Phase 1 of the Study

The first phase of the study focused on analyzing the design of the parts of both hearing screening devices and identifying the problematic parts while the device was fitted on a mannequin having a head circumference of 32 cm, which was within range of the measurement of infants at zero months of age [7]. Half of the participants were asked to use the benchmark device while the other half used the prototype. Critical activity in using the devices was fitting the electrodes.

Each of the participants was requested to accomplish two tasks: (1) fit the ear electrodes, and (2) fit the head electrodes. For each of the tasks, all possible errors that may be committed were listed, and the researchers took note of the number of errors committed by the subject while performing the tasks. Moreover, participants either received no training (Type 1) or full training (Type 2) on how to use the device assigned to them. Thus, the parameters used for comparison were the number of errors committed by the participants while accomplishing the tasks.

## 2.2 Phase 2 of the Study

The second phase of the study was concerned with the ease of use for both devices. The participant was trained by showing a video demonstrating the functions of the device parts and the proper way of attaching the device. The task was to fit the device on all of the mannequins with varying head sizes. The head circumference of the mannequins were 31 cm, 32 cm, and 35 cm for the small, medium and large mannequins, respectively; and all sizes were within the range of measurements of actual infants at zero months of age [7].

Quantitative and qualitative data were also gathered. These included the number of errors committed when the device was attached on the mannequin's head; and the overall satisfaction rating (ranging from 0 to 3 with 3 being the highest) which was obtained from the questionnaire given to the subject after the test. The latter was collected by open-ended questions that asked for the participant's suggestions on how the device can be improved.

## 2.3 Possible Errors Per Device Type

The tables below classified the possible errors to be observed per device part on each of the devices (Tables 1 and 2).

**Table 1.** Errors for benchmark device

| Benchmark device | | | |
|---|---|---|---|
| Device part | Errors | | |
| Forehead electrode | Not in contact with head | Forced rotation | Wrong placement |
| Cushion | Having a significant gap | | |
| Ear electrode | Not in contact with head | Wrong placement | |
| User error | Inverted device | | |

**Table 2.** Errors for prototype device

| Prototype device | | |
|---|---|---|
| Device part | Errors | |
| Forehead electrode | Not in contact with head | Wrong placement |
| Cushion | Having a significant gap | |
| Ear electrode | Not in contact with head | Wrong placement |
| User error | Electrode is placed inside the ear | Inverted earpieces |

## 3   Results and Discussion

### 3.1   Errors Due to Training Type for Phase 1

As mentioned, participants for both devices may either receive no training (Type 1) or full training (Type 2). Afterwards, they proceeded with performing the tasks. The errors that were committed and the parts of the device associated with these errors were noted.

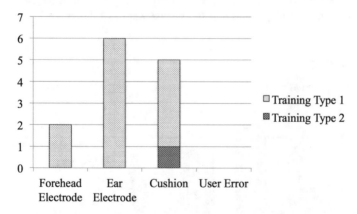

**Fig. 1.** Comparison of total errors between training types for commercially acquired device

Figure 1 showed that most of the participants who used the commercially acquired device committed errors when they received no training. However, if training was received, the likelihood of committing errors decreased significantly.

Figure 2, on the other hand, presents the errors committed while using the prototype. The graph showed that even if full training was already received, the participants still committed errors while attaching the device to the mannequin contributing to 46% of the total errors.

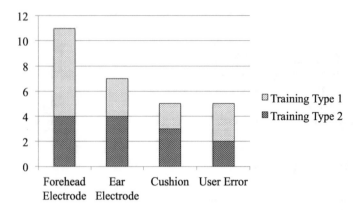

**Fig. 2.** Comparison of total errors between training types for prototype device

## 3.2 Errors Due to the Device Used for Phase 1

Other than training type, the device parts corresponding to each of the errors observed for both devices were also noted and the results were as follows:

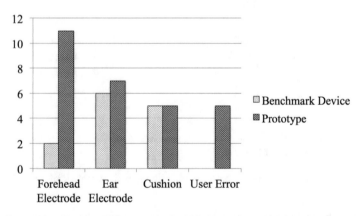

**Fig. 3.** Comparison of total error between devices

Figure 3 showed that more errors were committed when using the prototype accounting for more than 68% of the total errors for Phase 1. Moreover, the most frequent error observed in the parts of the prototype device were as follows: for the ear and forehead electrodes, the misplacement of these electrodes; for the cushion, having a significant gap between the device and the mannequin; and the most common user error observed was inverting the device.

### 3.3    Errors Due to Varying Head Sizes for Phase 2

For Phase 2, all of the participants were given the second type of training and the task was to fit the device on mannequins of varying head sizes. The researchers took note of the device parts that caused the errors and the results for both devices were as follows:

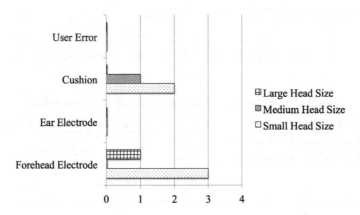

**Fig. 4.** Comparison of total errors between head sizes for the commercially device

Figure 4 showed that for the commercially acquired device, most of the user errors were committed when positioning the forehead electrode and the cushion. It was observed that participants had difficulties in properly attaching the forehead electrodes for the small and large mannequins, and the cushion was problematic for the small and medium mannequins.

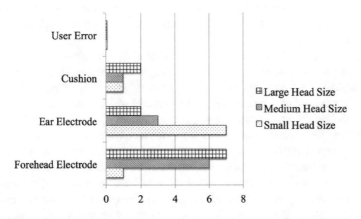

**Fig. 5.** Comparison of total errors between head sizes for the locally developed prototype

Figure 5, on the other hand, showed that for locally developed prototype, most of the participants encountered difficulties while attaching the forehead and ear electrodes. For the forehead electrode, it was most difficult to attach the part on the medium and large mannequins. Moreover, for the ear electrode, the participants had a hard time fitting them on the small mannequin.

### 3.4    Feedback for the Devices Used (Phase 2)

After the participants accomplished the tasks for Phase 2, to assess user satisfaction, a device feedback form was given and questions with rating scales were included.

**Table 3.** Comparison of mean feedback scores between devices

| Factor | N | Mean score (Out of 18) | Standard deviation |
|---|---|---|---|
| Commercially acquired device | 8 | 14.625 | 1.408 |
| Locally developed prototype | 8 | 8.125 | 2.949 |

Table 3 showed that the benchmark device received a much higher feedback score of 14.625 out of 18 as compared to the prototype, which only received a score of 8.125. This would indicate that users were more satisfied with using the benchmark device and the prototype still needs a lot of improvement to increase user satisfaction.

## 4    Conclusion

The study was conducted to make a comparative usability study of a commercially acquired and locally developed prototype of a newborn hearing screening device. Effectiveness was quantified by noting the mistakes committed by the users while accomplishing the critical tasks, and satisfaction of the users was quantified using a questionnaire [8–11].

The results showed that in using the commercially acquired device, the type of training received influenced the number of errors; it was observed that participants who received no training committed most of the errors. However, for the locally developed prototype, regardless of whether the participant had training or not, most of the participants still had difficulties while using the device.

The results also showed that most participant who used the commercially acquired device mostly committed the error of wrongly placing the ear electrodes on the infant's head. This error was also prevalent for the users of the locally developed prototype, along with the additional mistake of misplacing the head electrodes on the mannequin.

Participants were given the task of fitting the device on mannequins of varying head sizes; and the results showed that for the commercially acquired device, the forehead electrode and cushion were the problematic areas when attaching the device to the small mannequin. For the prototype, the forehead electrodes were difficult to fit on both the medium and large mannequins, while the ear electrodes were difficult to attach on the small mannequin.

Lastly, based on the user satisfaction form that was given to the participants after the completion of the two phases, results showed that the commercially acquired device received a much higher mean feedback score compared to the prototype.

Therefore, the findings suggest several modifications must be made with regards to the current design of the locally developed prototype.

# References

1. Chiong, C., Ostrea Jr., E., Reyes, A., Gonzalo, E., Uy, M.E., Chan, A.: Correlation of hearing screening with developmental outcomes in infants over a 2-year period. Acta Otolaryngologica **127**(19), 384–388 (2007)
2. Zhang, J., Johnson, T., Patel, V., Paige, D., Kubose, T.: Using usability heuristics to evaluate patient safety of medical devices. J. Biomed. Inform. **36**, 24 (2003)
3. Wiklund, M., Kendler, J., Strochlic, A.: Usability Testing of Medical Devices. CRC Press, Florida (2011)
4. Food, U.S., Administration, Drug: Applying Human Factors and Usability Engineering to Medical Devices. CDRH, Maryland (2011)
5. Ward, J.R., Clarkson, P.J.: An analysis of medical device-related errors: prevalence and possible solutions. J. Med. Eng. Technol. **28**, 2–21 (2004)
6. Faulkner, L.: Beyond the five-user assumption: benefits of increased sample sizes in usability testing. Behav. Res. Methods Instrum. Comput. **35**(3), 379–383 (2003)
7. De Onis, M., Onyango, A., Borghi, E., Siyam, A., Pinol, A.: World Health Organization Child and Growth Standards. WHO Press, France (2006)
8. Georgsson, M., Staggers, N.: Quantifying usability: an evaluation of a diabetes mhealth system on effectiveness, efficiency, and satisfaction metrics with associated user characteristics. J. Am. Med. Inform. Assoc. **23**(1), 5–11 (2016)
9. Schnittker, R., Schemettow, M., Verhoeven, F., Schraagen, J.M.C.: Combining situated cognitive engineering with a novel testing method in a case study comparing two infusion interfaces. Appl. Ergonomics **55**, 16–26 (2016)
10. Garmer, K., Liljegren, E., Osvalder, A., Dahlman, S.: Application of usability testing to the development of medical equipment: usability testing of a frequently used infusion pump and a new user interface for an infusion pump developed with a human factors approach. Int. J. Ind. Ergon. **29**, 145–159 (2002)
11. Walji, M., Kalenderian, E., Piotrowski, M., et al.: Are three methods better than one? A comparative assessment of usability evaluation methods in an EHR. Int. J. Med. Inform. **83**, 361–367 (2014)

# The Feasibility of Ontological Description of Medical Device Connectivity for Laparoscopic Surgery

Kazuhiko Shinohara[✉]

School of Health Sciences, Tokyo University of Technology,
Tokyo 1448535, Japan
kazushin@stf.teu.ac.jp

**Abstract.** This study develops an ontological description of medical electronic (ME) device connectivity for endoscopic surgery, and discusses some problems and the feasibility of the approach. The connection status and human–machine interface of ME devices for endoscopic surgery, considered in the operating room, are investigated and classified, from the upper level down to sub-class concepts. These aspects are then ontologically described within a resource-description framework. The connection status of ME devices was successfully described within ontological concepts, and these ontological descriptions were possible to derive via either device-centered or Human (patient or surgeon)-centered descriptions. Endoscopic surgery requires a wider variety of medical devices than conventional open surgery does, and so the ME device connectivity during endoscopic surgery can impose a heavy burden on surgeons and nurses. Thus, an ontological description of the ME devices and their network could find application in many areas, including education and training, navigation systems for the operating room, and medical safety. As well, such descriptions could aid artificial-intelligence research about surgery itself.

**Keywords:** Medical device · Connectivity · Endoscopic surgery
Ontology

## 1 Introduction

For artificial intelligence (AI) to be applied to human activities, ontological analysis is necessary. Ontological investigation has been applied to the health care field in several areas, including disease terminology, nursing services, and clinical guidelines. However, few reports have adopted an ontological approach to clinical surgery that strongly depends on advanced medical electrical devices. This study attempts an ontological description of the connection of ME devices during endoscopic surgery.

## 2 Materials and Methods

The connectivity and network between ME devices (electric surgical unit, harmonic scalpel, endoscope unit, insufflation unit, aspiration machine, anesthesia machine) are investigated with the aim of constructing an ontological description of the network of

© Springer International Publishing AG, part of Springer Nature 2019
N. J. Lightner (Ed.): AHFE 2018, AISC 779, pp. 88–95, 2019.
https://doi.org/10.1007/978-3-319-94373-2_10

ME devices, the patient, and energy-supply outlets during endoscopic surgery, using the concept of a resource description framework for this.

## 3  Results

An ontological description of the connection status of ME devices was constructed. The system (connection and network of ME devices, patient, and energy-supply-outlets) for endoscopic surgery was ontologically described as follows. The connection of ME devices for cutting and hemostasis are shown in Fig. 1.

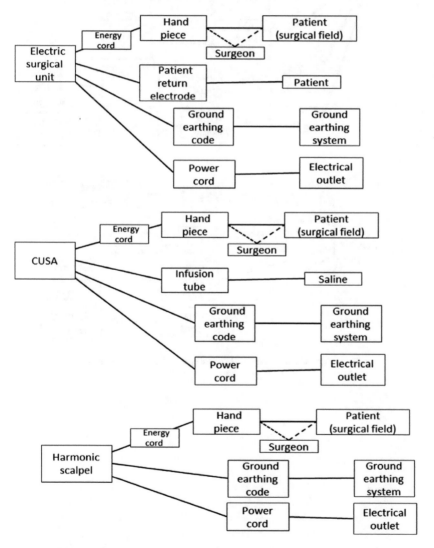

**Fig. 1.** The connectivity of ME devices for cutting and hemostasis

The connection of the endoscope unit and insufflation unit, which are specific to endoscopic surgery, are shown in Fig. 2.

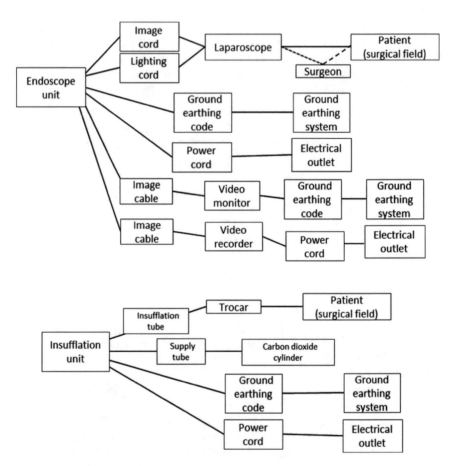

**Fig. 2.** The connectivity of Endoscope unit and insufflation unit

The connections of the anesthesia machine and the aspiration machine are shown in Fig. 3. The electric power supply and ground-earthing system are important for all these ME devices. From another viewpoint, the patient-centered description of the network of ME devices is shown in Fig. 4.

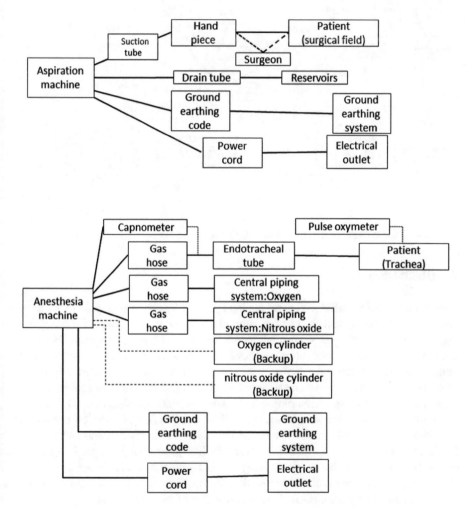

**Fig. 3.** The connectivity of Anesthesia machine and Aspiration machine

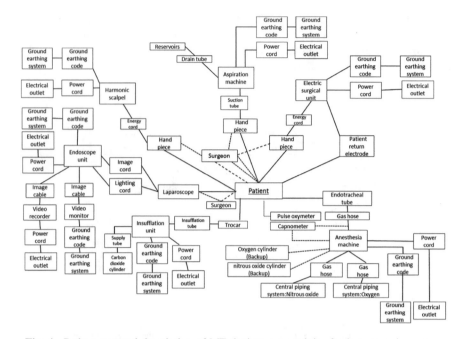

**Fig. 4.** Patient-centered description of ME devices connectivity for laparoscopic surgery

# 4 Discussion

Application of AI to ME devices and medical practice has been attempted many times, starting in the 1960s. Several fields of internal medicine and diagnostic radiology now rely on automated diagnosis from laboratory results and medical imaging. However, there have been few successful applications of AI to surgery. In recent years, AI has attracted renewed interest for use in various industries, and ontological investigation of medical domains has been proposed. Some medical domains have been analyzed in this way, including disease terminology, automated diagnosis, education, and clinical guidelines. Several ontologies, including OGEM and POID, that focus on ontological definitions of diseases have been proposed for use in medical information systems [1–3]. In the field of clinical guidelines, research has produced computer-interpretable ontological guidelines based on existing clinical guidelines. Nishimura et al. have already reported ontological activity models for nursing guidelines; these are suitable for integrated use by the CHARM model created by OntoGear [4, 5].

Despite these advances, ontological analysis has not previously been applied to the activities of surgical field except for ontological analysis of surgical endoscopy [6, 7]. Human-machine interactions in the operation room are rapidly increasing in this era of endoscopic surgery compared with in the era of conventional open surgery. Since modern endoscopic surgery began in the 1990s, indications for its use have greatly increased. The main merit of endoscopic surgery for the patient is minimal invasiveness, but it brings the disadvantage that surgeons have to operate on the internal organs via small-caliber channels with restricted tactile sense and visual information. To compensate for this, many types of ME devices have been developed (Figs. 5 and 6). So monitoring ME device connectivity during endoscopic surgery can impose a heavy burden on surgeons and nurses. In this study, the connection status of ME devices was successfully described via ontological concepts, and these ontological descriptions were possible to derive with descriptions centering on either the device or a human. Despite the preliminary nature of this study, the feasibility of taking an ontological approach to endoscopic surgery is demonstrated by these results.

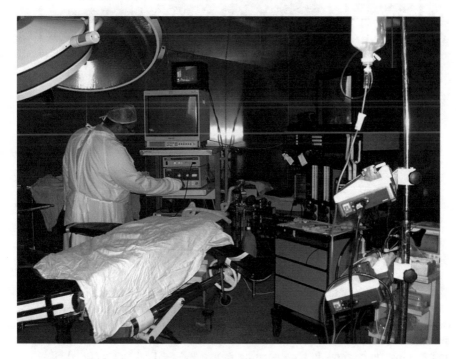

**Fig. 5.** A scene of preparation for laparoscopic surgery

The concepts of ontology are ultimately logical and essential for application of AI. An ontological description of the ME devices and their network could thus find application in many areas, including education and training, navigation and automation systems for the operating room, and medical safety. As well, such descriptions could aid AI research about surgery itself. Despite these benefits, the process of ontological analysis of clinical maneuvers has proved troublesome, and particularly so for intuitive human activities such as surgery. Difficulties therefore remain in mapping human–machine interactions. These difficulties show the need for simple and practical methods of finding a clinical ontology for the further analysis of the workflow of medical devices and the surgical staff involved.

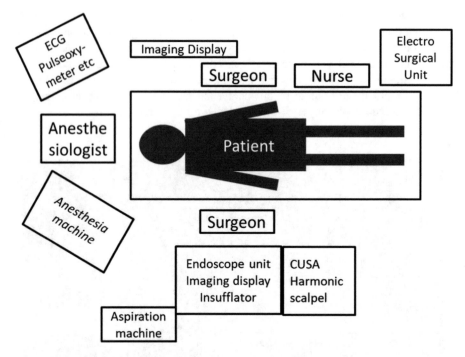

**Fig. 6.** Layout of ME devices for Laparoscopic surgery (example)

## 5   Conclusion

This study applies ontological analysis to the network of ME devices for endoscopic surgery. The ontological descriptions of the network are possible as either ME-device-centered description or human-centered description. Ontological description of the ME devices network can be applied in many areas, including medical training, navigation and automation systems in the operating room, and medical safety, in addition to AI research itself. The need for simple and practical methods of clinical ontology was also revealed in this study.

## References

1. Kozaki, K., et al.: Browsing causal chains in a disease ontology. In: 11th International Semantic Web Conference on Poster and Demo Notes, Boston, USA, 11–15 November 2012
2. Scheuermann, R., et al.: Toward on ontological treatment of disease and diagnosis. In: Proceedings of the 2009 AMIA Summit on Translational Bioinformatics, San Francisco, pp. 116–120 (2009)
3. Osborne, J., et al.: Annotating the human genome with disease ontology. BMC Genomics **10**(1), S6 (2009)
4. Kumar, A., et al.: An Ontological Framework for the Implementation of Clinical Guidelines in Healthcare Organization: Ontologies in Medicine. IOS Press, Amsterdam (2004)

5. Nishimura, N., et al.: CHARM as activity model to share knowledge and transmit procedural knowledge and its application to nursing guidelines integration. J. Adv. Comput. Intell. Intell. Inf. **17**(2), 208–220 (2013)
6. Shinohara, K.: Ergonomic considerations on the implementation of small-caliber trans-nasal gastroduodenoscopy. In: Advances in Human Factors and Ergonomics in Healthcare, pp. 730–735, CRC Press (2011)
7. Shinohara, K.: Preliminary study of ontological process analysis of surgical endoscopy. In: Advances in Human Factors and Ergonomics in Healthcare and Medical Devices, pp. 455–461. Springer (2017)

# Human Factors in Healthcare

# User-Centered Design of a National Medical Registry for Tick-Borne Diseases

Berglind Fjola Smaradottir[1]([✉]), Randi Eikeland[2], Harald Reiso[2], and Rune Werner Fensli[1]

[1] Department of Information and Communication Technology, University of Agder, Jon Lilletuns vei 9, 4879 Grimstad, Norway
{Berglind.Smaradottir,Rune.Fensli}@Uia.no
[2] The Norwegian National Advisory Unit on Tick-Borne Diseases, Sørlandet Hospital, Post Box 783 Stoa, 4809 Arendal, Norway
{Randi.Eikeland,Harald.Reiso}@Sshf.no

**Abstract.** Tick-borne diseases are increasing in a global perspective, with Lyme disease and tick-borne encephalitis as the most frequent. The Norwegian National Advisory Unit on Tick-borne Diseases is preparing the development of a national medical registry for clinical follow-up of patients with tick-borne diseases based on the best practice guidelines and for research purposes. This paper presents the methodological approach of a user-centered design process applied in the initial phase of the registry development. A user workshop identified user needs, requirements and proposed a service workflow for the registry operation. As the next step, a simulation of the proposed service workflow was performed in a clinical laboratory together with end-user groups. The main contribution of this paper lies on the methodological descriptions of the user-centered design process, and how to facilitate the active contribution of end-users in a technical development process within a health care context.

**Keywords:** User-centered design · Medical registry · Simulation Tick-borne diseases

## 1 Introduction

Ticks are arachnid organisms that can act as vectors for a broad range of human pathogens, see Fig. 1 [1, 2]. Tick-borne diseases (TBD) are an increasing health burden in a global perspective [3, 4] impacted by climate- and environmental changes and leisure habits, that expose more people to tick-bites [2, 5, 6]. The most prevalent tick-borne disease in the northern hemisphere is Lyme disease, caused by the Borrelia burgdorferi bacterium [4]. Lyme disease is a multistage and multisystem disorder, with a variety of clinical symptoms that predominantly affect the skin (erythema migrans), but can also manifest in joints, the heart and the nervous system (neuroborreliosis). 7000 persons are treated for erythema migrans and 400 for more disseminated disease, whereof about 300 neuroborreliosis, per year in Norway [7]. Globally, neuroborreliosis is reported in 3–12% of the borrelia patients [4, 8]. The Lyme disease diagnosis is guided by clinical examination and analysis of antibodies in blood and cerebrospinal fluid. Antibiotics are the main treatment.

© Springer International Publishing AG, part of Springer Nature 2019
N. J. Lightner (Ed.): AHFE 2018, AISC 779, pp. 99–108, 2019.
https://doi.org/10.1007/978-3-319-94373-2_11

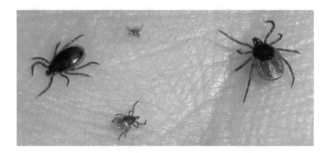

**Fig. 1.** The castor bean tick, Ixodes ricinus, at different stages of the development (photo: Per Eikeseth Knudsen).

In Norway, disseminated disease has been a nationally notifiable disease since 1995 [9]. The tick-borne infection of the brain, the Tick-borne Encephalitis (TBE) is also increasing. It is caused by a flavivirus that is transmitted by ticks in a geographic area from western Europe to the eastern Japan. TBE can cause acute meningoencephalitis and long-lasting sequelae occur among a third of the patients, with substantial impairment in quality of life and cognitive function. The diagnosis is based on antibodies in blood. There is no existing specific treatment. Vaccination is the main preventive measure for TBE [6, 10].

Previous studies have reported that there are constraints related to the diagnosis and clinical management of tick-borne diseases [2, 4] and that there is a lack of reliable data on the economic global impact [1, 11]. This brings to light challenges with decision support following evidence-based clinical guidelines, particularly for diagnosed patients with remaining symptoms [12].

In this context, The Norwegian National Advisory Unit on Tick-borne Diseases [13] took the initiative to develop a National Medical Registry for Tick-borne Diseases, together with the Centre for eHealth at the University of Agder, the Norwegian Lyme Borreliosis Organization and the industry partner Egde Consulting. The National Medical Registry for Tick-borne Diseases has the aim to provide support in the follow up of patients with a verified tick-borne disease, based on an algorithm developed from international clinical guidelines. In addition, the registry will provide data for research on the prevalence of tick-borne diseases and the management in a long-term perspective.

In the initial project phase, a User-centered Design process was made that consisted of two steps: (1) user workshop with end-users and stakeholders, and (2) simulation of the registry service workflow in a clinical laboratory. This paper presents the methodology of the User-centered Design process in the initial project phase. The research questions (RQs) stated for this study were:

RQ1: *Which methodological procedures facilitate active end-user involvement in technical development projects within a health care context?*

RQ2: *What are the lessons learned that are transferable to other technical development projects within a health care context?*

Following this introduction, the methodology with a research background is presented. In the third and fourth section, the procedures from the User-centered Design process are described, also focusing on the infrastructure for laboratory simulation. The discussion and conclusion reflect on lessons learned and study contributions.

## 2 Methodology

The communication and information flow in health care services and between organizations are complex by nature, and Health Information Technology (HIT) plays an important role for coordination, information processing and decision support [14, 15]. Development of efficient and user-friendly HIT, such as a National Medical Registry, requires a detailed analysis of the needs and preferences of the end-user groups and stakeholders.

In the system development cycle, the approach of User-centered Design has the aim to actively involve end-users in every step and allowing them to provide suggestions and evaluations regarding design and functionality [16–18]. For the National Medical Registry for Tick-borne Diseases development, a User-centered Design approach was chosen to develop technology well-adapted to the clinical work processes of tick-borne disease management, and considered easy to use.

### 2.1 The Data Collection

Qualitative research methods [19] were used for data collection and analysis of the User-centered Design process that was applied in the National Medical Registry for Tick-borne Diseases development. The data collection was executed from August until November 2017 and included the methods observation and focus group interview in the initial development phase. The User-centered Design process was divided into two parts: (1) the user workshop and (2) the simulation in laboratory, both were audio-visually recorded with a total amount of 6 h recorded data. In the data analysis, the recordings were viewed and analyzed qualitatively [20]. In addition, the research team made annotations during the different parts of the study, which is also included in the data collection.

### 2.2 Ethical Considerations

Carrying out evaluations in real clinical environments is not recommended for legal, ethical and privacy reasons [21]. Instead, user-based simulation with evaluation and test of an application can be made in a clinical laboratory, which has the strength of providing a controlled environment for the variables studied [22]. In a simulation, the end-users are asked to perform a role-play and do pre-defined tasks using a system, while being observed and recorded. The goal is to test conceptual ideas and analyze how new technology influences the existing clinical workflow. Measurements can be made on time for task solving and number of errors. The aim is to provide a better understanding of the user interactions and the technology involved in clinical work process [23, 24]. Actors are often used, such as in the patient role, to increase the realism [25].

The Norwegian Centre for Research Data approved the study, with project number 55163 [26]. The participation in the study was voluntary and the informants received written information about the project and signed an individual consent form. The authors declare that there are no conflicting interests with any of the participants, organizations or industry.

# 3   User Workshop

A user workshop with participants from end-user groups and stakeholders was hosted by The Norwegian National Advisory Unit on Tick-borne Diseases and lead by two researchers from the University of Agder, see Table 1 for overview of participants.

**Table 1.** The workshop participants

| Profession | N = 12 |
|---|---|
| Neurologist hospital | 2 |
| Nurse hospital | 1 |
| Microbiologist hospital | 1 |
| IT department hospital | 1 |
| Innovation unit hospital | 1... |
| Research unit hospital | 1... |
| Industry partner | 1 |
| Patient representative | 2 |
| Researcher University | 2 |

The aim was to understand the context of use of the National Medical Registry for Tick-borne Diseases, and to work out the user requirements and make a conceptual plan for the service workflow of the registry. In addition, the workshop was a source of information and familiarization for people involved in the project.

The workshop lasted 4 h, including a break, and was divided into two parts. In the first part of the workshop, participants were introduced to the project National Medical Registry for Tick-borne Diseases with a presentation of the most common diseases and how the registry could support the clinical treatment. The conceptual idea for the National Medical Registry was that it should work as a two-way communication platform, connecting the patient with the clinician and provide decision support based on clinical guidelines.

The workshop participants were asked to describe and write down user needs and how they expected the registry to function on colorful post-it notes for 10 min. Afterwards, each participant presented their suggestions to the group. The patient representatives described their preferred way of interacting with the registry application in a home setting. A digital versus paper-based consent form was discussed, and the clinicians suggested digital consent to avoid double registrations and increase of the daily workload.

In the second part of the workshop, a white board was used to identify the different user roles involved. A sketch was made to describe the service procedure and the operation of the National Medical Registry, where the case was a patient with a tick-borne disease making registrations for a period of 12 months. The topics discussed were the administration of the consent form, what kind of information a patient would be expected to register, and what kind of feedback should be provided from the health care services or automatically from the system to the patient at home.

## 4 Laboratory Simulation

The service operation of the National Medical Registry for Tick-borne Diseases was carried out as a realistic clinical situation simulated in a laboratory environment together with end-user groups and stakeholders, see Table 2 for distribution of participants. The scenarios were constructed based on information gathered from the previous workshop, and led by two researchers experienced in simulation of health care services and usability evaluation.

**Table 2.** The simulation participants

| Profession | N = 11 |
|---|---|
| Neurologist hospital | 1 |
| GP/TBDs specialist | 1 |
| Nurse hospital | 1 |
| Adviser TBDs hospital | 1 |
| Industry partner | 3 |
| Patient representative | 2 |
| Researcher University | 2 |

The simulations were executed in the clinical laboratory of the Centre for eHealth at the University of Agder, Norway. The laboratory consisted of two rooms; the control- and observation room and the test room that simulated an office at the neurological outpatient ward at hospital. The rooms were connected through a one-way mirror with visualization towards the test room, see Fig. 2. In the control- and observation room one researcher was in charge of the recordings and the remote control for the fixed camera. The simulation was followed simultaneously on four 55" large monitors and through the one-way mirror.

Recordings in the test room were made by the fixed camera and a document camera placed on a stand for the mobile phone. The recordings from the camera sources were merged into one single video file using the software Tricaster, to ease the analysis.

In the test room, the patients' own Samsung smartphone device were used to access the National Medical Registry prototype application, which was developed with the software program proto.io. The smartphone application had a suite of modules that were separated by color coding and designed to support self-management activity, see Fig. 3.

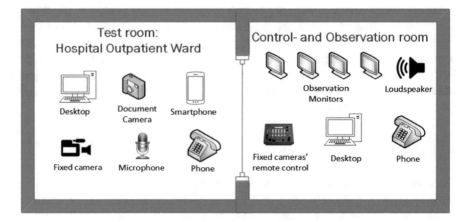

**Fig. 2.** The physical and technical infrastructure used in the laboratory simulations.

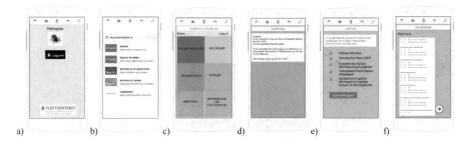

**Fig. 3.** (a) Start screen, (b) Secure log in, (c) The modules, (d) Patient's diagnose and last appointment, (e) Patient's administration of the clinicians' access, (f) Patient's health information input.

Considering the user group, accessibility precautions were important as neuroborreliosis patients can have decreased strength and sensation in fingers, and the design goal was a meaningful presentation with a smooth navigation flow. For the clinician in the test room, a web-based clinical portal was used to access the Medical Registry prototype, see Fig. 4.

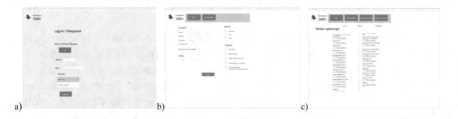

**Fig. 4.** (a) Start screen with log in procedure, (b) Registration of a new patient into the registry, (c) Registration of clinical symptoms.

Two sessions with simulations were run during one day. In each simulation, there were three different role-based scenarios, each with a description of a situation and tasks to perform. The roles were: (a) patient at a first-time consultation the neurological outpatient ward, (b) doctor at the neurological outpatient ward, (c) nurse at the neurological outpatient ward, (d) observer in the observation room following the role-play and technology interactions. The first three roles were assigned to one person at each time. The doctors played the doctor's role, the nurse had the nurse's role and the patient representatives acted the patient's role. The observers were a group of 5–6 persons having the role at the same time. In the test room, a moderator from the research team guided through the scenarios and asked the participants to speak aloud, as a think aloud protocol was used [27, 28]. In the control- and observation room, one member from the research team instructed the observers.

In each simulation session the scenario was: (1) a patient with tick-borne disease symptoms having a first-time consultation at the neurological outpatient ward with a doctor, (2) consultation with a nurse for guidance with installing the National Medical Registry application on patient's own smartphone and (3) a second consultation with the doctor for medical results, instructions for treatment and use of the application. The information flow and the interactions with technology across the roles were especially observed and the time for each scenario and potential errors were annotated. A debrief session was organized after each simulation together with the participants. The aim was to use the group dynamics for discussing how the scenarios worked out, how the actions related to existing workflow and improvements were suggested.

## 5   Discussion

This paper has presented how to involve end-users in technical development, based on the experiences from the National Medical Registry for Tick-borne Disease project. The lessons learned by the research team showed that the User-centered Design process was an efficient way of involving end-users and stakeholders in the initial phase of the development. The research questions (RQs) formulated are answered below based on the results from the study.

About the RQ1, which methodological procedures that facilitate active end-user involvement in technical development projects. The workshop which was organized in an early project phase together with end-user groups and stakeholders, efficiently outlined user needs and the context of use. It was the key to elicit users' requirements of the application and taking on board different user roles and patient groups. In the second part of the workshop, a process model of the workflow was presented as a swimming lane diagram. That provided a good foundation for discussion, showing the participants the details in the service workflow, the user roles and what actions that were suggested. Such visual representations are meaningful in workflow discussions, to show who is supposed to do what and at what time. The outcome of the workshop provided the scenarios for the simulations performed later, where the service workflow and operation of the proposed technology was tested.

The RQ2, lessons learned that are transferable and applicable in similar contexts. It was experienced in the User-centered Design process that the user workshop and simulations were of high importance for the project, providing a deeper understanding on the National Medical Registry's mission and aims. The organization with active end-user involvement in the workshop and laboratory simulation was considered as well structured and can be recommended to other development projects. In the simulation, the role-play and use of real patients as actors to create a realistic scenario was positively evaluated and can be recommended. Regarding the distribution of roles, the role as observer in the control- and observation room was important and allowed the participants to actively follow the information flow and the interactions with technology in the test room. The observers made notes and contributed at a detailed level to the group debrief after the simulations.

This study had some limitations such as a reduced number of simulations (n = 2) to test the service operation of the National Medical Registry prototype. However, a significant number of participants, with a total of 17 people belonging to different user groups and stakeholders, meaningfully represented the end-user groups of the application.

## 6 Conclusion

This paper was made within the project National Medical Registry for Tick-borne Diseases, in order to share experiences on how end-users can be involved in technical development and how clinical scenarios can be simulated in a laboratory environment. The main contribution lies on the descriptions of how a User-centered Design approach can facilitate the active contribution of the end-user groups in a development process. In addition, the methodological procedures for simulation and the technical descriptions are applicable and transferable to other projects within a health care context. The results presented are congruent with other studies of User-centered Design [16, 29], highlighting the importance of involving the end-user groups early in the development. They also showed that simulation with low fidelity software prototypes allows a low-cost test of proposed service workflow and operation [22]. The role-play with real patients as actors in the simulations was useful and informative, and provided realism to the scenarios [24]. The clinical laboratory provided a controlled environment, with audio-video recordings to retrospectively analyze the collected data. In terms of future work, a full development of the National Medical Registry for Tick-borne Diseases is proposed, with an active end-user involvement in all phases.

**Acknowledgments.** The authors thank the participants of the study for their disinterested contribution. Special thanks to Åsmund Rodvig Somdal for technical support and assistance in the laboratory simulations. Financial support was provided by the Regional Research Fund of Agder [30] in Norway with Grant number 272978.

# References

1. Jongejan, F., Uilenberg, G.: The global importance of ticks. Parasitology **129**(S1), S3–S14 (2004)
2. Dantas-Torres, F., Chomel, B.B., Otranto, D.: Ticks and tick-borne diseases: a one health perspective. Trends Parasitol. **28**(10), 437–446 (2012)
3. Gray, J.S., Dautel, H., Estrada-Peña, A., Kahl, O., Lindgren, E.: Effects of climate change on ticks and tick-borne diseases in Europe. Interdiscip. Perspect. Infect. Dis. (2009)
4. Koedel, U., Fingerle, V., Pfister, H.W.: Lyme neuroborreliosis—epidemiology, diagnosis and management. Nat. Rev. Neurol. **11**(8), 446 (2015)
5. Danielová, V., Schwarzová, L., Materna, J., Daniel, M., Metelka, L., Holubová, J., Kříž, B.: Tick-borne encephalitis virus expansion to higher altitudes correlated with climate warming. Int. J. Med. Microbiol. **298**, 68–72 (2008)
6. Lindquist, L., Vapalahti, O.: Tick-borne encephalitis. Lancet **371**(9627), 1861–1871 (2008)
7. Eliassen, K.E., Berild, D., Reiso, H., Grude, N., Christophersen, K.S., Finckenhagen, C., Lindbæk, M.: Incidence and antibiotic treatment of erythema migrans in Norway 2005–2009. Ticks Tick Borne Dis. **8**(1), 1–8 (2017)
8. Wilking, H., Stark, K.: Trends in surveillance data of human lyme borreliosis from six federal states in Eastern Germany, 2009–2012. Ticks Tick Borne Dis. **5**(3), 219–224 (2014)
9. Norwegian Institute of Public Health: Report on Ticks and Tick-borne Diseases (2015). https://www.fhi.no/globalassets/dokumenterfiler/moba/pdf/flatt-og-flattbarne-sykdommer-pdf2.pdf
10. Lindquist, L.: Tick-borne encephalitis. In: Handbook of Clinical Neurology, vol. 123, pp. 531–559. Elsevier (2014)
11. Müller, I., Freitag, M.H., Poggensee, G., Scharnetzky, E., Straube, E., Schoerner, C., Norris, D.E.: Evaluating frequency, diagnostic quality, and cost of lyme borreliosis testing in Germany: a retrospective model analysis. Clin. Dev. Immunol. (2012)
12. Lorentzen, Å.R., Forselv, K.J., Helgeland, G., Salvesen, R.E., Sand, G., Flemmen, H.Ø., Bø, M.H., Nordaa, L., Roos, A.K., Jim, M.W., Owe, J.F., Nyquist, K.B., Schüler, S., Eikeland, R., Mygland, Å., Ljøstad, U.: Lyme neuroborreliosis: do we treat according to guidelines? J. Neurol. **264**(7), 1506–1510 (2017)
13. The Norwegian National Advisory Unit on Tick-borne Diseases. https://xn--flttsenteret-ucb.no/in-english/
14. Goldzweig, C.L., Towfigh, A., Maglione, M., Shekelle, P.G.: Costs and benefits of health information technology: new trends from the literature. Health Aff. **28**(2), w282–w293 (2009)
15. U.S. Department of Health and Human Services: Office of the National Coordinator for Health Information Technology. https://www.healthit.gov/patients-families/basics-health-it
16. Vredenburg, K., Mao, J., Smith, P.W., Carey, T.: A survey of user-centered design practice. In: Conference on Human Factors in Computing Systems (SIGCHI 2002), pp. 471–478 (2002)
17. Lazar, J.: Web Usability- a User-Centered Design Approach. Pearson Education, Boston (2006)
18. Nielsen, J.: Usability Engineering. Elsevier, Amsterdam (1993)
19. Denzin, N.K., Lincoln, Y.S.: Handbook of Qualitative Research. SAGE Publications, Inc., Thousand Oaks (1994)
20. Kushniruk, A.W., Borycki, E.M.: Development of a video coding scheme for analyzing the usability and usefulness of health information systems. In: CSHI, pp. 68–73 (2015)

21. Svanæs, D., Alsos, O.A., Dahl, Y.: Usability testing of mobile ICT for clinical settings: methodological and practical challenges. Int. J. Med. Inf. **79**(4), e24–e34 (2010)
22. Smaradottir, B., Fensli, R.W., Boysen, E.S., Martinez, S.: Infrastructure for health care simulation: recommendations from the model for telecare alarm services project. In: The International Conference on Health Informatics and Medical systems (HIMS 2017), pp. 64–69, CSREA Press, Las Vegas (2017)
23. Li, A.C., Kannry, J.L., Kushniruk, A., Chrimes, D., McGinn, T.G., Edonyabo, D., Mann, D.M.: Integrating usability testing and think-aloud protocol analysis with "near-live" clinical simulations in evaluating clinical decision support. Int. J. Med. Inf. **81**(11), 761–772 (2012)
24. Borycki, E., Kushniruk, A.: Identifying and preventing technology-induced error using simulations: application of usability engineering techniques. Healthc. Q. **8**(Sp) (2005)
25. Smaradottir, B.F.: The steps of user-centered design in health information technology development: recommendations from a PhD research study. In: International Conference on Computational Science and Computational Intelligence (CSCI), pp. 116–121. IEEE (2016)
26. The Norwegian Centre for Research Data. http://www.nsd.uib.no/personvern/en/index.html
27. Kushniruk, A.W., Patel, V.L.: Cognitive and usability engineering methods for the evaluation of clinical information systems. J. Biomed. Inf. **37**(1), 56–76 (2004)
28. Jaspers, M.A.: Comparison of usability methods for testing interactive health technologies: methodological aspects and empirical evidence. Int. J. Med. Inf. **78**(5), 340–353 (2009)
29. Ritter, F.E., Baxter, G.D., Churchill, E.F.: Foundations for Designing User-Centered Systems. Springer, London (2014)
30. Regional Research Fund Agder. http://www.regionaleforskningsfond.no/prognett-rff-hovedside/RFF_in_English/1253976860326

# Towards Playful Monitoring of Executive Functions: Deficits in Inhibition Control as Indicator for Cognitive Impairment in First Stages of Alzheimer

Lucas Paletta[1(✉)], Martin Pszeida[1], and Mariella Panagl[2]

[1] Institute for Information and Communication Technologies,
JOANNEUM RESEARCH Forschungsgesellschaft mbH DIGITAL,
Steyrergasse 17, 8010 Graz, Austria
{lucas.paletta,martin.pszeida}@joanneum.at
[2] Sozialverein Deutschlandsberg, Unterer Platz 7b,
8530 Deutschlandsberg, Austria
m.panagl@sozialverein-deutschlandsberg.at

**Abstract.** Meaningful treatment of dementia today consists of multi-component interventions, such as, cognitive and also physical, sensomotoric stimulation. A serious game was developed for multimodal training performed by clients and caregivers using easily configurable services on a Tablet PC. A key problem in developing substantial knowledge about dementia and impacting factors is lack of data about mental processes evolving over time. For this purpose, eye tracking data were captured from non-obtrusive sensing during games to enable daily monitoring of dementia profiles. An anti-saccade measuring paradigm was used to detect attention inhibition problems that typically occur in executive function related neurodegenerative diseases, such as, in Alzheimer. In a 6 month study with 12 users a classifier was developed that enables to discriminate dementia stages from extracted eye movement features received from training at home. The playful training and its diagnostic toolbox offer affordances for entertaining users, measuring and analyzing mental process parameters, and enabling people with dementia to stay longer at home to slow down the progress of disease.

**Keywords:** Alzheimer intervention system · Eye movement features
Playful diagnostics · Executive functions

## 1 Introduction

Dementia is a broad category of neurocognitive disorders that cause a long term and often gradual decrease in the ability to think and remember that is great enough to affect a person's daily functioning. Adequate, sufficient and economically feasible care is currently one of the greatest technological and social challenges [1]. A key problem in developing knowledge about dementia and its impacting factors is the lack of data about the mental processes and the psychophysiological dependencies as they evolve

© Springer International Publishing AG, part of Springer Nature 2019
N. J. Lightner (Ed.): AHFE 2018, AISC 779, pp. 109–118, 2019.
https://doi.org/10.1007/978-3-319-94373-2_12

over time. The individual trajectories of dementia are often suspected to be rather specific, however, longitudinal quantitative studies about dementia are rare.

There is no cure for dementia [2], however, cognitive and behavioral interventions may be appropriate, educating and providing emotional support to the caregiver is important. Physical exercise programs are beneficial by activities of daily living and potentially improve outcomes [3].

Cognitive and also physical, sensomotoric stimulation is decisive for a meaningful treatment of dementia, however, lack of exercise is one of the major risk factors for the dementia development [4]. Therefore, multi-component interventions are important, even being accompanied by community settings [5, 6].

A key problem in developing knowledge about dementia and impacting factors is lack of data about mental processes evolving over time. Cognitive and behavioral interventions, emotional support by caregivers and physical exercise programs are beneficial to activities of daily living [3]. However, lack of exercise is a major risk factor in dementia development [4] (Fig. 1).

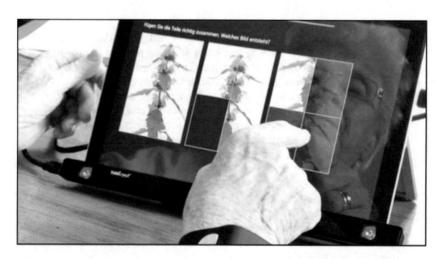

**Fig. 1.** Playful multimodal training using a tablet PC with eye tracking device for executive functions diagnostics.

The presented playful training presents an integrated theratainment solution for the growing market of care, rehab and diagnostics. In a serious game performed by persons with dementia (PwD), mobile eye tracking was applied for non-obtrusive sensing and daily monitoring of dementia profiles. An anti-saccade measuring paradigm was used for eye movements captured during playing the Tablet PC serious game. It is known to detect impulse control problems as they occur in executive function related neurode-generative diseases [7]. The results gained from the experiments demonstrate that the serious game attentional diagnostic toolbox offers affordances for entertaining and analysis of behavioral parameters for longitudinal studies.

# 2 Playful Training and Mental Health

## 2.1 Related Work

Current technical assistance for PwD exclusively focus on applications with cognitive training and omit important training aspects that are beneficial in multi-component interventions. Playful cognitive stimulation for elderly (Lumosity, Cogmed, Cognifit) and with particular consideration of people with dementia (eMotiva, Onto D'mentia, memofit) has been largely exploited. European projects, such as, AALJP M3 W, CCE, ROSETTA, GAMEUP CAREBOX and ALFA have investigated means of monitoring and estimating the status of mental processes, motivating users for cognitive and physical activities in various ways. [8] provides a thorough overview on a plethora of serious games for dementia (SG4D) for physical, cognitive, psychosocial [9] and social-emotional health functions with various therapeutic achievements. [8] proposed a taxonomy on SG4D, concluding that assessment games are still highly underrepresented in the domain.

One of very rare studies on play experiences of people with Alzheimer's Disease (AD; [11]) emphasizes that games should be tailor-made getting suitable for different personalities with AD. Serious games, adapted to people with dementia, may constitute an important tool to maintain autonomy. Obviously, current products lack this flexibility that most obviously is required to adjust to appropriate modes and from this enable truly long lasting motivation and to enable to maintain training at their homes.

Executive dysfunction is characteristic in Alzheimer's disease [12], in particular, referring to inhibition abilities and the capacity to co-ordinate simultaneously storage and processing of information. [13, 14] found clear evidence for emotion-induced positive enhancement in executive control.

The project PLAYTIME[1] aims at optimal exploitation of the positive impact of emotion and motivation on executive performance, psychosocial contexts and persistent behavior change through the engagement of people with dementia, to make efficient use of the monitoring of consequences in daily life over long periods of time. The key objective is to increase quality of life of dementia patients but also of caregivers, getting capable to stay active at home for a longer time.

## 2.2 Playful Training with amicasa

A substantial innovation in the playful training suite of the product *amicasa*[2] is represented via the integrated, multimodal training unit concept. Tasks with the purpose to stimulate cognitive processes are not separated from the tasks that excite physical activities but are in a functional context for the end user. The global task with cognitive, auditive, visual, social and sensomotoric aspects is within the focus and integrated through the serious game framework, i.e., the motivation to gain rewarding and motivating game points through repeated training.

---

[1] http://www.aal-playtime.eu/.
[2] http://www.amicasa.com/.

*amicasa* is an interaction platform with an already very high number of task units (200) that is continuously increasing through additional themes that incorporate an exciting database for knowledge and exercises. The game character of the training engages the player and motivates for "knowledge acquisition and physical activities". The following multimodal unit categories are currently already in the pool of units:

- Training of memory and remembrance
- Visual memory
- Completing gaps in texts
- Interactive associations (pictures, form, color, content)
- Search games (visual comparison)
- Physical activities
- Playful cognitive test

Figure 2 depicts a typical training situation where (a) a formal caregiver assists the PwD in the game, and where (b) a memory game is played in a multi-user configuration, for example, in a residential care-home for the elderly.

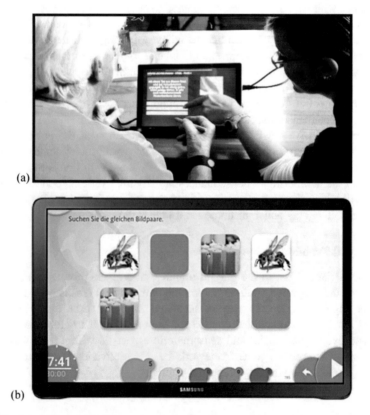

(a)

(b)

**Fig. 2.** Playful multimodal training using the serious game *amicasa* with a tablet PC with eye tracking device for executive functions diagnostics.

# 3 Diagnostics Using Eye Movement Features

## 3.1 Impairment of Inhibitory Functionality

Progressive neurological diseases, such as, Alzheimer, Parkinson, Huntington or Wilson, are well known for the decrease in eye movement behavior [15, 16]. The characteristics of the impairment support clinicians to localise brain lesions as well as to determine diagnostics about the trajectory of the diseases [15]. Dysfunctionality in the continuous tracking of stimuli was already associated with Alzheimer dementia by [17]. [7] has identified the important indication that Alzheimer patients are characterised with a significant impairment of their inhibitory functionality of eye movements, due to neurodegeneration of fronal and prefrontal lobes which are responsible for inhibitory effects [17]. In early stages of Alzheimer disease, the anti-saccade task is known to identify Alzheimer. This task requires from the test person a voluntary turning away from an actual stimulus and analyses the eye movement behavior further [18]. Figure 3a depicts a test person during the task with the amicasa serious game. Figure 3b depicts the case of position tracking of a test person's correct anti-saccade behavior (red) for a stimulus to the right (blue), and Fig. 3c shows incorrect behavior by following the position of the stimulus instead of turning away.

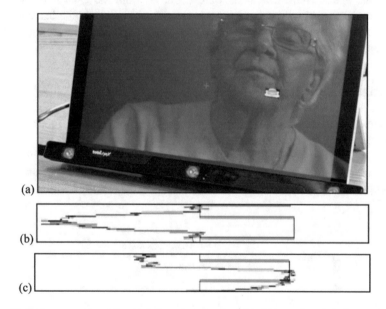

**Fig. 3.** Cognitive control test for Alzheimer impairment of inhibitory functionality (a) in which a voluntary turn away from a stimulus is required [19]. (b) Tracking of a test person's anti-saccade correct behavior (red) for stimulus (blue), (c) Incorrect behavior, i.e., the person follows the stimulus.

The anti-saccade test error is characterised by a large correlation with the MMSE test [19]. However, a direct classification of Alzheimer patients in early stages is not straight forward because the results were extracted from a statistic group comparisons and the individual trajectory can be rather different [19, 20].

Further investigations on the 'Visual Paired Comparison' (VPC) Test with evaluation of eye movements in a visuo-spatial cognitive control task [21] indicate that the behavior of persons with mild cognitive impairment is significantly different from dementia-free persons. [22] demonstrated that a classifier can be extracted from existing patient data using machine learning techniques with a classification rate of 87%.

### 3.2    Pervasive Measurement Approach

Our approach to the evaluation of the anti-saccadic test procedure is characterized through a pervasive measurement paradigm. The PwD is performing the training and serious game units at home, not in a laboratory environment. Consequently, the input data have to be filtered in order to gain the maximum quality for further processing and evaluation. Usually, a measurement frequency of about 5 Hz was applied as threshold to sort out meaningful data from noise prone data.

Various eye movement features were extracted from the data. Areas of interest (AOI) were designed with respect to pro-saccadic and anti-saccadic behavior. Errors were determined from the violation of the anti-saccade condition, i.e., turning attention on the opposite site of the visual stimulus.

## 4    Experimental Results

The amicasa training suite was configured on a Microsoft Surface Tablet with USB-connected Tobii EyeX mobile tracking technology, providing a 60 Hz sampling of gaze towards the display of the Tablet PC after a 5-point calibration procedure (Fig. 5).

There were two studies performed to evaluate the pervasive measurement technology.

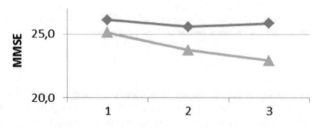

**Fig. 4.** MMSE measured in a 6-months period (Sect. 4.2; 1 = month 1, 2 = month 3, 3 = month 6) for the intervention group using the *amicasa* training (blue) and for the control group without *amicasa* training (green).

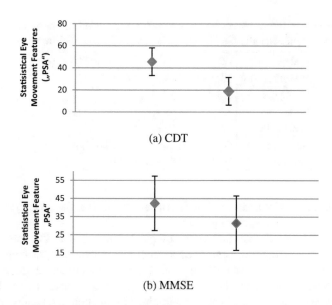

(a) CDT

(b) MMSE

**Fig. 5.** In a 6-months period study (Sect. 4.2) with 12 participants the error in the anti-saccadic - i.e., generating a kind of pro-saccadic, ('PSA') - feature was significantly predictive for the CDT, discriminating PwD (blue; M, S) from PDf (red; M, S).

## 4.1   1-Month Study

In the first study, 8 participants being clinically classified with Alzheimer disease were using the mobile tracking unit within a period of 4 weeks. After a quality filtering test and sorting out data with less than 5 Hz 60 training unit sessions with the anti-saccadic test were applied for data analysis.

Table 1 demonstrates that 4 persons with mild dementia performed the study starting with a MMSE of M = 25.8, S = 4.6 and a Clock Drawing Test of M = 5.5, S = 1.3 while the other 4 persons where starting with MMSE = 30 and CDT = 7 (dementia-free). The error feature showed a very good Pearson correlation $\rho = -0.632$ with the MMSE ranking which was reflected by a very discriminative level of the eye movement feature for PwD (M = 43.2, S = 20.0) and PDf (M = 7.7). Furthermore, both anti-saccadic and pro-saccadic features demonstrated discriminative levels between PwD and PDf conditions in order to enable classification for Alzheimer disease.

## 4.2   6-Months Study

An overall intervention long-term study was performed over a 6 months period. Figure 4 demonstrates the benefit of using the *amicasa* training suite, comparing the performance of an intervention group (N = 25, predominantly females) that used the *amicasa* training suite including MAS training in comparison with a control group (N = 25, predominantly females) without any specific training. The MMSE was measured in a 6-months period (month 1, 3, 6) for the intervention group that was using the *amicasa* training (blue) and for the control group without *amicasa* (green). While

**Table 1.** Features of the anti-saccadic test on inhibitory function of voluntary eye movement control (PDf = person dementia free, PwD = person with dementia), 1-month study (Sect. 4.1)

| Feature | PDf | PwD | Correlation ($\rho$) |
|---|---|---|---|
| MMSE [1, 30] | 30.0 ±0 | **25.8** ± 4.6 | |
| CDT [1, 7] | 7.0 ± 0 | 5.5 ± 1.3 | |
| Errors [%] | 7.7 | **43.2** ± 20.0 | **−0.632**, p = 0.09 |
| Success [%] | 30.7 ± 25 | 10.8 | |
| Anti-sacc. [%] | 46.3 ± 20 | 24.9 | **0.574**, p = 1.30 |
| Pro-sacc. [%] | 19.2 | **44.4** ± 16.3 | |

the control group performed in a typical Alzheimer decline, the group using *amicasa* did not decline (M values) substantially.

12 out of 25 participants that were equipped with a Tablet PC (see above) and applied the *amicasa* training suite used as well the mobile eye tracking units for a period of 6 months. After a data filtering with a removal of any unit training data with a mean data logging frequency larger than 4.5 Hz, and a removal of sessions where center positions were not fixated after a stimulus presentation, eventually 422 training unit sessions remained for analyses. Monthly measurements were aggregated into average measurement values.

Eye movement features were extracted and it turned out that the pro-saccadic feature was predictive with respect to CDT and MMSE. The error in the anti-saccadic - i.e., generating a kind of pro-saccadic ('PSA') - feature was significantly predictive with M = 45.7 (S = 12.5) for PwD (CDT < 5) and M = 19.0 (S = 12.8) for the PDf (CDT $\geq$ 5). Furthermore, the error like pro-saccadic feature PSA was as well predictive with M = 43.1 (S = 12.4) for PwD (MMSE < 26) and M = 31.8 (S = 13.3) for the PDf (MMSE $\geq$ 26).

The long-term study demonstrates the discriminative power of eye movement features in reference to classification of Alzheimer status. Consequently, a support vector machine (SVM) network was tuned with 5-fold cross validation on all available data and achieved a classification accuracy of 75% for MMSE (>26) and 100% for CT (>5).

# 5  Conclusions and Future Work

We conclude that eye movement features can be successfully applied to provide indicators for Alzheimer diagnostics, considering two independent studies that both showed the discriminative power to classify into dementia and non-dementia participants exclusively from gaze data. Future work will involve larger number of participants in field trials to get more robust and statistically significant estimators for Alzheimer classification. Furthermore, multiple eye movement features will be used for estimation and classification. In addition, multimodal sensing should even lead into better estimates, for example, by incorporating features from movement studies as planned in the PLAYTIME project.

**Acknowledgments.** The research leading to these results has received funding from the project PLAYTIME of the AAL Programme of the European Union, by the Austrian BMVIT/FFG (No. 857334), ZonMW, the VLAIO, and the Austrian BMVIT/FFG, by project AMIGO.

# References

1. Sabine, S., Iris, H., Reiner, K.: Wie sich die Regionen in Deutschland, Österreich und der Schweiz auf die Alterung der Gesellschaft vorbereiten können. Berlin-Institut für Bevölkerung und Entwicklung, Demenz-Report, Berlin (2011)
2. Burns, A., Iliffe, S.: Dementia, BMJ (Clinical research ed.) 338 (2009)
3. Forbes, D., et al.: Exercise programs for people with dementia. Cochrane Datab. Syst. Rev. **12**, CD006489 (2013)
4. Norton, S., et al.: Potential for primary prevention of Alzheimer's disease: an analysis of population-based data. Lancet Neurol. **13**, 788–794 (2014)
5. Graessel, E., et al.: Non-pharmacological, multicomponent group therapy in patients with degenerative dementia: a 12-month randomizied, controlled trial. BMC Med. **9**, 129 (2011)
6. Korczak, D., et al.: Wirksamkeit von Ergotherapie bei mittlerer bis schwerer Demenz. HTA-Bericht 129, Köln (2013)
7. Crawford, T.J., Higham, S., Renvoize, T., Patel, J., Dale, M., Suriya, A., et al.: Inhibitory control of saccadic eye movements and cognitive impairment in Alzheimer's Disease. Biol. Psychiatry **57**, 1052–1060 (2005)
8. McCallum, S., Boletsis, C.: Dementia games: a literature review of dementia-related serious games. In: Ma, M., Oliveira, M.F., Petersen, S., Hauge, J.B. (eds.) SGDA 2013. LNCS, vol. 8101, pp. 15–27. Springer, Heidelberg (2013). https://doi.org/10.1007/978-3-642-40790-1_2
9. Kasl-Godley, J., Gatz, M.: Psychosocial interventions for individuals with dementia: an integration of theory, therapy, and understanding dementia (2000)
10. Cerejeira, J., Lagarto, L., Mukaetova-Ladinska, E.B.: Behavioral and psychological symptoms of dementia. Front. Neurol. **3**, 73 (2012)
11. Anderiesen, H., et al.: Play experiences for people with Alzheimer's disease. Int. J. Des. **9** (2), 155–165 (2015)
12. Collette, F., et al.: Phonological loop and central executive functioning in Alzheimer's disease. Neuropsychologia **37**, 905–918 (1999)
13. Kanske, P., Kotz, S.A.: Hum. Brain Mapp. **32**(2), 198–208 (2011)
14. Kuskowski, M.A.: Eye movements in progressive cerebral neurological disease. In: Hillsdale, N.J., Johnston, C.W., Pirozzolo, F.J. (eds.) Neuropsychology of Eye Movements, pp. 146–176 (1988)
15. White, O.B., Saint-Cyr, J.A., Tomlinson, R.D., Sharpe, J.A.: Ocular motor deficits in Parkinson's disease. Brain **106**, 571–587 (1983)
16. Fletcher, W.A., Sharpe, J.A.: Smooth pursuit dysfunction in Alzheimer's disease. Neurology **38**, 272 (1988)
17. Kaufman, L.D., et al.: Antisaccades: a probe into the dorsolateral prefrontal cortex in Alzheimer's disease. A critical review. J. Alzheimer's Dis. **19**, 781–793 (2010)
18. Simpkins, L. K.: Antisaccades: A probe into the dorsolateral prefrontal cortex in Alzheimer's disease, Master's thesis, University of Toronto (2008)
19. Shafiq-Antonacci, R., Maruff, P., Masters, C., Currie, J.: Spectrum of saccade system function in Alzheimer disease. Arch. Neurol. **60**(9), 1272–1278 (2003)

20. Crutcher, M.D., et al.: Eye tracking during a visual paired comparison task as a predictor of early dementia. Am. J. Alzh. Dis. Other Dem. **24**, 258–266 (2009)
21. Lagun, D., Manzanares, C., Zola, S.M., Buffalo, E.A., Agichtein, E.: Detecting cognitive impairments by eye movement analysis using automatic classification algorithms. J. Neurosci. Methods **201**(1), 196–203 (2011)

# Smart Skin Flap Postsurgical Pre-warning Mobile App Design

Shihui Wang[1(✉)], Weihong Huang[1], Lingli Peng[1], Ding Pan[1],
Nvtong Huang[1], Jianzhong Hu[1], and Yonghong Peng[2]

[1] Mobile Health Ministry of Education-China Mobile Joint Laboratory,
Xiangya Hospital Central South University,
87 Xiangya Road, Changsha 410008, Hunan, People's Republic of China
sophiawang1005@qq.com, whuangcn@qq.com,
lingli.peng1980@qq.com, panding1980@qq.com,
nvtong1980@qq.com, jianzhonghu@hotmail.com
[2] University of Sunderland, Sunderland, UK
Yonghong.Peng@sunderland.ac.uk

**Abstract.** Skin flap transplantation surgery has been widely applied in repairing wound surface in clinical medicine. However, blood vessel crisis takes place easily after surgery, leading to failure of postoperative recovery. Thus, effective microcirculation observation of skin flap plays an important role in postsurgical care. For standard and convenient skin flap status monitoring and pre-warning, a smart mobile application is badly needed by both doctors and nurses. Since last August, contextual inquiry and in-depth interview of medical personnel have been conducted in the Department of Orthopedics in Xiangya Hospital Central South University, to clarify skin flap pre-warning clinical problems, requirements and application context. Feasible solution fits in clinical practice is proposed through user participated design of doctors, nurses, and technologists. UI feature list are created and UI design are prioritized by cognitive walkthrough of doctors and nurses, providing a good foundation for application development and promotion in hospital.

**Keywords:** Skin flap postsurgical pre-warning · Microcirculation observations
User participatory design

## 1 Introduction

Skin flap transplantation surgery has been widely applied in repairing wound surface, recipient site shape, and physiological function in clinical medicine. However, blood vessel crisis takes place easily after surgery, bringing re-transplantation or even amputation risks to patients [1–3].

For effective blood vessel crisis pre-warning and handling, postsurgical monitoring and early recognition of transplanted skin flap ischemia or congestion play an important role in postsurgical care [4].

However, current postsurgical pre-warning practice is short of standardization and convenience. With the advancement of the recent smartphone technology, a smart

© Springer International Publishing AG, part of Springer Nature 2019
N. J. Lightner (Ed.): AHFE 2018, AISC 779, pp. 119–129, 2019.
https://doi.org/10.1007/978-3-319-94373-2_13

mobile application to standardize and prioritize the postsurgical skin flap blood vessel crisis pre-warning practice is badly needed by both doctors and nurses.

Therefore, how to capture, analyze, monitor and keep record of the skin flap status for blood vessel crisis pre-warning, present an urgent research and design topic in the field of smart clinical care of special disease.

## 2 Literature Review

### 2.1 Smart Skin Flap Postsurgical Pre-warning Application

In the field of smart medical care in China, compared to the well-developed chronic disease management system solution, the special disease management solution is on the threshold, especially for smart skin flap postsurgical monitoring and pre-warning, related research and design applied in clinical practice just starts up.

In 1975, Creech and Miller described the attributes of the ideal monitoring device for free tissue transplantation: harmlessness to patients and flaps, rapid responsiveness, accuracy, reliability and applicability to all types of transplanted tissues [5].

Up to now, a series of technology solutions have been applied in a small number of cases of skin flap postsurgical monitoring and pre-warning experimentally, such as microendoscopy, microdialysis, ultrasound, plethysmography, tissue pH, surface temperature measurement, pulse oximetry and spectrometry. However, these cases have not been demonstrated effective for salvage rates [6–9].

Other devices and techniques, such as implantable Doppler probe (Cook-Swartz Doppler Flow Monitoring System), transcutaneous Doppler probe, tissue oxygenation monitors (O2C, ViOptix, and Licox), and reflectance photoplethysmography, despite their effectiveness, are relatively expensive and require for special training to operate, thus have been rarely applicable in resource-limited settings [10, 11].

In 2015, Kidakorn developed an easy to use Android mobile application, SlipaRamanitor for postoperative monitoring of free flap. Photos of transplanted free flap are taken and compared for color differences to detect for partial venous occlusion or partial arterial occlusion. This new mobile application has been proved effective in clinical test among 42 subjects, with 93% accuracy for venous occlusion, 95% for arterial occlusion, 6% for false-negative and 1% for false positive [11].

The clinical effectiveness of SlipaRamanitor application points out a way for medical solution by smart mobile phone technology.

However, the SlipaRamanitor application has limitation in clinical practice. The light control box design applied in the application is only suitable for certain type of skin flap, not covering skin flap of different sizes, shapes, and multiple curved surface in medical cases.

Therefore, a clinical reliable and easy to use smart skin flap postsurgical monitoring and pre-warning mobile application, are of great value and need to design and develop in clinical medicine.

## 2.2    User Participated Design Framework

Similar to application in specific area, there have been inevitable big knowledge and cognition gap between target users, technologists and designers in the field of smart medical care. How to involve medical professionals effectively to enable the final design output fit in clinical practice and context, presents an important issue to solve at the beginning of this research.

In 2005, Clay proposed user participatory design framework "explore, design and evaluate" to clarify user needs and design solutions of technology feasibility and usability. It involves target users, technology staff, and key stakeholders effectively into the product design and development process [12].

Up to now, user participated design has been applied in many cases, clarifying user needs and generating user friendly user interface [13–15].

However, as the smart medical care design case involves very professional clinical knowledge and complicated clinical use cases to clarify, it requires much quicker and iterative "explore, design and evaluate" user participated design and development process, see Fig. 1.

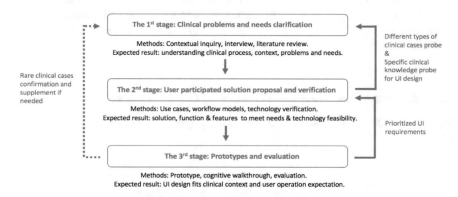

**Fig. 1.** User participated design process customized for clinical application case

Based on the above customized design framework, this research intends to clarify the current clinical problems and needs of the postsurgical skin flap monitoring and pre-warning process, through contextual inquiry and in-depth interview of doctor and nurses in the Department of Orthopedics, Xiangya Hospital Central South University.

It later attempts to propose an innovative smart skin flap postsurgical pre-warning mobile application solution based on image recognition and OCR technology by involving doctors, nurses and technologists. Different main use cases, functions, UI features and work flow model in the solution are enriched to fit in clinical practice through iterative loop among contextual probe, design and review.

Then, it tries to design and prioritize UI flow, layout and visuals through cognitive walkthrough of doctors and nurses on prototypes to meet user's operation expectation.

Finally, it plans to confirm and supplement some special medical cases in clinical practice for application version update.

# 3  Field Survey

## 3.1  Skin Flap Postsurgical Pre-warning Clinical Practice

The mainstay of flap pre-warning in hospital is clinical observation by experienced clinical care professionals [16]. It includes vital sign monitoring of the whole body and micro-circulation observation of the transplanted skin flap status, such as flap color, surface temperature, capillary refill, and skin turgor complemented by pinprick test if needed, observation area, pain, wound drainage and etc. [6, 17–19]. Among these clinical parameters, flap color is recognized to be the most reliable clinical indicator of flap viability [20].

In the year of 2016, based on the above clinical methods, Orthopedics Department of Xiangya Hospital Central South University proposed an 8-color card and 9 grid view design for blood vessel crisis recognition and location identification. It has effectively reduced the flap observation false-negative and false positive and increase the skin flap salvage rates.

However, in current clinical skin flap monitoring, recording and pre-warning practice, there exists some touchpoint to improve for standardization and convenience.

Starting from August in 2007, in-depth interview and contextual inquiry have been conducted in the Department of Orthopedics in Xiangya Hospital Central South University to clarify current skin flap post-surgical pre-warning process, problems and needs.

## 3.2  Skin Flap Monitoring and Pre-warning Clinical Process

The current skin flap post-surgical pre-warning process is clarified as follows, see Fig. 2.

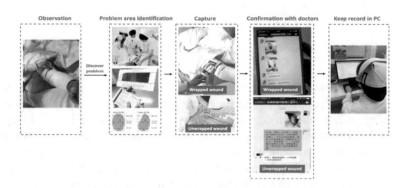

**Fig. 2.** Skin flap monitoring and pre-warning clinical process

It includes 5 steps: Regular observation, problematic area identification, capture skin flap status, confirm with doctors, and keep record on PC.

1. Regular observation: After skin flap surgery, observations are carried out during postsurgical risky period, at a frequency of 1 time every hour in the first 1–3 days and 1 time every 4 h from 4th to 7th day. The observation contents include vital sign of the whole body and microcirculation observation of the transplanted skin flap.
2. Problematic area identification: By referring to 9-grid view, 8-colors card, international swelling standards [21], surface temperature, capillary refill, and skin turgor complemented by pinprick test if needed, the problematic area of the skin flap is identified by nurse in the ward.
3. Capture flap status: The problematic skin flap status is then captured by nurse in photos or videos if needed.
4. Confirm with doctors: The nurse shares photos or video clips of flap status, and observation description with doctors in WeChat group communication for pre-warning confirmation and handlings afterwards.
5. Keep record on PC: The nurse writes down observation parameters and recognition result on notebook and later keeps record in the medical history system on PC at nursing station.

### 3.3 Current Skin Flap Monitoring and Pre-warning Problems

The current skin flap pre-warning process, although is clinical effective, lacks capture and communication standards for pre-warning, bringing much inconvenience and potential risk in current clinical practice, see Fig. 3.

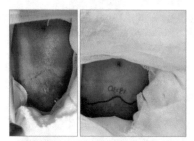 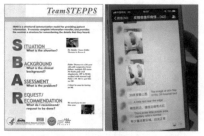

Lack of capture standardization and consistency          Lack of monitoring communication standardization

**Fig. 3.** Skin flap monitoring and pre-warning problems and needs

1. Lack of capture standardization: Due to different environment light, distance and angels in each capture, the doctor's judgement might be influenced to some extent while reviewing photos shared in WeChat group communication. In some cases, nurses are required to capture qualified photos repeatedly for proper recognition by doctors.
2. Color recognition inconsistency: For different mobile devices hold by doctors and nurses, the camera, screen, and pre-settings of mobile phone display bring some color differences in photo capturing and reviewing, leading to color recognition inconsistency.

3. Lack of communication standard: The communication among doctors and nurses of the patient skin flap status should include overall standard information, such as patient identity, situation, background, assessment result, and recommendation [22].

Besides the above problems, doctors and nurses referred to the following requirements for the smart skin flap pre-warning mobile application in clinical practice.

1. Sufficient image references for problem identification: Donor site image before surgery, recipient site after surgery, and every post-surgery skin flap monitoring images are required to capture and record for sufficient references of monitoring and pre-warning in postsurgical period.
2. Consistent capture standard: Every skin flap monitoring image captured by nurse are required to be in the same distance and angle with the captured recipient image by doctors after surgery for consistent comparison.
3. Dynamic monitoring parameter curve graph: A dynamic monitor parameter curve graph for skin flap status overview and access to images are required.
4. Video recording: Video recording, uploading and analyzing are required for reviewing capillary refill and skin turgor complemented by pinprick test.

## 4 Smart Mobile Application Solution Design

Based on the above clarified clinical requirements, main skin flap use cases to cover in this smart mobile application is defined and decided by key stakeholders. It targets to include regular and irregular skin flap shape of different sizes.

By involving doctors, nurses and technologists, the smart skin flap postsurgical monitoring and pre-warning mobile application solution is proposed, see Fig. 4.

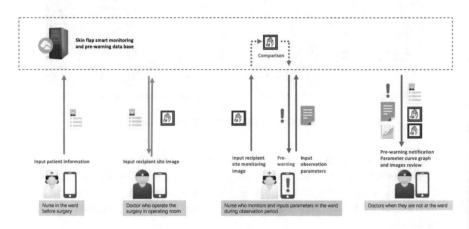

**Fig. 4.** Smart skin flap postsurgical pre-warning mobile solution

Before the surgery, the nurse captures donor site image in the ward and inputs basic information of the patient who is about to take the skin flap surgery in a few days.

After surgery, the doctor captures the recipient site image of this patient in the operating room in proper distance and angles, which will act as reference image for later monitoring capture and pre-warning recognition in the ward.

During the postsurgical monitoring period in the ward, the nurse captures the recipient site monitoring image by referring to the doctor previously captured image at a required frequency.

To reduce various environment light influence, the color card, as a reference object, is required to be captured together with the recipient area in the image.

Every time when the monitoring image is captured, comparison and analyzing are operated simultaneously in the skin flap smart pre-warning data server by referring to donor site and previously recipient images.

If problematic skin color or swelling is detected, indicating early phase of blood vessel crisis, there will be an immediate pre-warning feedback on the captured image of the nurse phone.

Then, the nurse records the microcirculation observation parameters of the problematic zone of the skin flap, such as color, swelling degree, temperature, and upload videos of capillary refill and skin turgor complemented by pinprick test if needed.

After the nurse uploads the recordings to the server, the doctor receives a pre-warning notification on his mobile phone, for pre-warning confirmation and recommendation of proper measures afterwards.

# 5 Smart Mobile Application UI Design

## 5.1 UI Function and Features Design

Based on user participated smart mobile application solution, UI functions, main UI screens and UI features of regular and irregular skin flap use cases are created.

Through doctors and nurses reviewing the above design, more detailed clinical requirements for UI features and flow are clarified with relevant clinical knowledge applying in UI design, see Fig. 5.

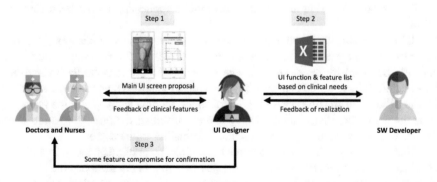

**Fig. 5.** App function and UI feature list generation process

By the iterative loop between probe, design and review, UI feature list and flow model is enriched to fit in clinical practice.

Later, this feature list is reviewed by developers for software development feasibility.

Finally, a few UI features are comprised for feasibility, with confirmation with doctors and nurses for no critical operation problem in clinical practice.

## 5.2   UI Design Prototypes and Cognitive Walkthrough

Based on the confirmed UI functions, features list, main UI screens and work flow model, UI blueprint specification has been created. Later, iterative cognitive walkthrough of UI blueprint specification by doctors and nurses is conducted for UI specification confirmation and prioritization, see Fig. 6.

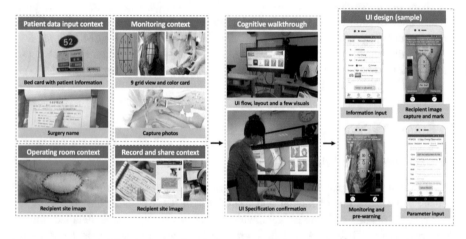

**Fig. 6.**   Interactive design and cognitive walkthrough

The overall smart skin flap postsurgical mobile application UI has been confirmed as follows.

Before the surgery, in the patient adding screen of this application, the basic information of the patient could be filled by the nurse in the ward through scanning the patient's bed card by her cellphone. The OCR technology extracts the patient basic information written on the bed card, such as name, medical ID, gender, age and etc. to fill the patient information page in the application automatically. Then the nurse captures the donor site image, adds surgery name and remarks. After information check, the nurse uploads the newly added patient information to the server.

After the surgery, the doctor captures the recipient site of this patient, in a distance of 35 cm to 50 cm parallel to the skin flap, by referring to the ideal capture hint in the view finder. After capture, the doctor marks 9-grid view, zone number, near /far end, and vascular pedicles location on the captured image of the skin flap for later monitoring and pre-warning references. For irregular skin flap shape, the vacant zone in the 9-grid view of the skin flap is marked with zone number plus 0.

After the patient is sent back to the ward from operating room, the nurse monitors and captures the recipient site image at a required frequency.

Every time when the nurse captures the recipient site image, the doctor previously captured image references, marked 9-grid view, near /far end, and vascular pedicles location will display in the view-finder for consistent capture references.

After monitoring capture, if a problem is detected by comparison and analysis in the server, there will be pre-warning on the captured images of the nurse's phone. The detected problematic zone area is highlighted in the 9-grid view of the skin flap.

After the nurse confirms the system pre-warning by micro-circulation observation, she records the observation parameters of each problematic zone on relevant pages in the application.

When the recorded observation parameters are uploaded to the server, the doctor in charge of this patient will receive pre-warning heads-up notification on his mobile phone. By clicking the notification, he could review photos and observation parameters curve graph for pre-warning confirmation and measure recommendation.

# 6    Conclusion

From the above research and UI design, this paper could draw the following conclusions:

1. It clarified clinical problems and needs in current clinical skin flap pre-warning process in Orthopedics Department of Xiangya hospital, as lack of consistent capture and communication standard, insufficient image references and color recognition inconsistency influence.
2. It proposed the smart skin flap postsurgical pre-warning mobile application solution through user participated design involving doctors, nurses and technologists to fit in clinical practice and technology feasibility.
3. It enriched feasible UI feature list based on iterative loop among probe, design and review by doctors, nurses and developers.
4. It generated and confirmed UI blueprint specification to fit in clinical practice by iterative cognitive walkthrough of doctors and nurses.
5. It provided a smart medical care mobile application UI design process model for academic research and development practice references.

Based on the current ongoing work, for better promotion and application in hospital, the plan for this application design and development in the near future is as follows:

1. Cover more skin flap types use cases: The current design work covers skin flap of regular and irregular shape in Orthopedics Department. It plans to cover use cases of joint skin flap and skin flap over 180°.

2. Cover wound wrapping use cases: Due to different medical philosophy of doctors and post-surgical situation, some skin flaps are partly wrapped after surgery, which requires future probe and confirmation with medical experts.

**Acknowledgements.** This research is partly supported by Grant No. 2017YFC0909900 from the National Key R&D Program of China and Grant No. 2017SK2013 from the Key R&D Program of Hunan Province China.

# References

1. Zhang, C., Sun, J., Zhu, H., et al.: Microsurgical free flap reconstructions of the head and neck region: Shanghai experience of 34 years and 4640 flaps. Int. J. Oral Maxillofac. Surg. **44**(6), 675–684 (2015)
2. Whitaker, I.S., Jessop, Z.M., Grinsell, D.: Experience of 592 free tissue transfers: the case for clinical assessment alone to monitor free flaps. Eur. J. Plast. Surg. **38**(2), 123–126 (2015)
3. Whitaker, I.S., Rozen, W.M., Chubb, D., et al.: Postoperative monitoring of free flaps in autologous breast reconstruction: a multicenter comparison of 398 flaps using clinical monitoring, microdialysis, and the implantable Doppler probe. J. Reconstr. Microsurg. **26**(6), 409–416 (2010)
4. Cervenka, B., Bewley, A.F.: Free flap monitoring: a review of the recent literature. J. Curr. Opin. Otolaryngol. Head Neck Surg. **23**(5), 393–398 (2015)
5. Creech, B.J.M.S., Miller, S.: Evaluation of Circulation in Skin Flaps. Skin Flaps, vol. 21. Little, Brown, Boston (1975)
6. Jallali, N., Ridha, H., Butler, P.E.: Postoperative monitoring of free flaps in UK plastic surgery units. J. Microsurg. **25**(6), 469–472 (2005)
7. Pratt, G.F., et al.: Modern adjuncts and technologies in microsurgery: an historical and evidence-based review. J. Microsurg. **30**(8), 657–666 (2010)
8. Whitaker, I.S., et al.: Variations in the postoperative management of free tissue transfers to the head and neck in the United Kingdom. Br. J. Oral Maxillofac. Surg. **45**(1), 16–18 (2007)
9. Luu, Q., Farwell, D.G.: Advances in free flap monitoring: have we gone too far? J. Curr. Opin. Otolaryngol. Head Neck Surg. **17**(4), 267–269 (2009)
10. Engel, H., et al.: Remote real-time monitoring of free flaps via smartphone photography and 3G wireless internet: a prospective study evidencing diagnostic accuracy. J. Microsurg. **31**(8), 589–595 (2011)
11. Kiranantawat, K., et al.: The first smartphone application for microsurgery monitoring: SilpaRamanitor. J. Plast. Reconstr. Surg. **134**(1), 130–139 (2014)
12. Spinuzzi, C.: The methodology of participatory design. J. Tech. Commun. **52**(2), 163–174 (2005)
13. Schuler, D., Namioka, A. (eds.): Participatory Design: Principles and Practices. CRC Press, Boca Raton (1993)
14. Asaro, P.M.: Transforming society by transforming technology: the science and politics of participatory design. J. Acc. Manag. Inf. Technol. **10**(4), 257–290 (2000)
15. Falcão, T.P., et al.: Participatory methodologies to promote student engagement in the development of educational digital games. J. Comput. Educ. **116**, 161–175 (2018)
16. Kreidstein, M.L., Levine, R.H., Knowlton, R.J., Pang, C.Y.: Serial fluorometric assessments of skin perfusion in isolated perfused human skin flaps. Br. J. Plast. Surg. **48**, 288–293 (1995)

17. Haddock, N.T., Gobble, R.M., Levine, J.P.: More consistent postoperative care and monitoring can reduce costs following microvascular free flap reconstruction. J. Reconstr. Microsurg. **26**(07), 435–439 (2010)
18. Smit, J.M., et al.: Advancements in free flap monitoring in the last decade: a critical review. J. Plast. Reconstr. Surg. **125**(1), 177–185 (2010)
19. Salgado, C.J., Moran, S.L., Mardini, S.: Flap monitoring and patient management. J Plast. Reconstr. Surg. **124**(6S), 295–302 (2009)
20. Hentz, V.R., Mathes, S.J.: Plastic Surgery. Saunders, Philadelphia (2005)
21. Chunlin, H.: Skin Flap Surgery. Shanghai Science and Technology Publisher, Shanghai (2013)
22. Martin, H.A., Ciurzynski, S.M.: Situation, background, assessment, and recommendation - Guided huddles improve communication and teamwork in the emergency department. J. Emerg. Nurs. **41**(6), 484–488 (2015)

# Delineation of Hemorrhagic Mass from CT Volume

Manas K. Nag[1](✉), Anusha Vupputuri[2](✉), Saunak Chatterjee[1],
Anup K. Sadhu[3], Jyotirmoy Chatterjee[1], and Nirmalya Ghosh[2]

[1] School of Medical Science and Technology,
Indian Institute of Technology, Kharagpur, India
manasnag481@gmail.com
[2] Department of Electrical Engineering,
Indian Institute of Technology, Kharagpur, India
[3] EKO Diagnostics, Medical College and Hospital Campus, Kolkata, India

**Abstract.** Computed tomography (CT) is the preferred imaging modality for diagnosis of hemorrhage. The hematoma appears as hyper intense mass in the image. Computer aided diagnosis assists clinicians for making a better prediction and helps in surgery planning. Computer assistive method based on random walker is proposed for detection and delineation of hemorrhagic mass or hematoma from Computed Tomography (CT) volumes. 20 patients affected by hemorrhage is considered for this study. Each subject's image has a size of $512 \times 512 \times 96$. Every case has 96 images. In a CT volume each case has 96 slices. Each slice is of $512 \times 512$. The slice, which contains hematoma mass or ischemic lesion, is selected using one layer autoencoder. 60% of the patient volume is used for training and 40% of the patient volume is used for testing. The training accuracy of auto encoder was 100%, and testing accuracy was 99.5%. After the slices are classified as healthy and non-healthy, k-means clustering was applied on non-healthy slices for localization of hematoma. Random walker algorithm was applied on the localized lesion for delineation of hematoma from CT images. The computer generated output is compared with the manually delineated output with the help of similarity indices. The Dice similarity index and Jaccard coefficient was calculated as $0.768 \pm 0.101$ and $0.634 \pm 0.128$ respectively. The proposed algorithm suggests an alternate method for detection of hematoma using CT images.

**Keywords:** CT · Hemorrhagic mass · Random walker · Dice similarity index

## 1   Introduction

Stroke is the third leading cause of death and prime cause of disability in industrialized countries [1]. Stroke occurs when the supply of oxygenated blood is limited in our body. When the blood supply is limited due to the presence of clot it gives rise to ischemic stroke and when it is limited due to the rupture of blood vessel it leads to hemorrhagic stroke.

M. K. Nag and A. Vupputuri—Equally contributed

© Springer International Publishing AG, part of Springer Nature 2019
N. J. Lightner (Ed.): AHFE 2018, AISC 779, pp. 130–138, 2019.
https://doi.org/10.1007/978-3-319-94373-2_14

Manual segmentation of lesion and hematoma is considered as gold standard, but suffers from intra- as well as inter- observer variability and moreover, the method is time consuming and tiring. A computer assisted method can reduce the drawback of manual delineation to some extent.

Various research groups have attempted for computer assistive delineation of ischemic lesion as well as hematoma from CT or magnetic resonance imaging (MRI) volumes or slices. Matesin et al. [2] proposed the use of symmetry and seeded region growing for detection of stroke lesion. Maldjian et al. [3] proposed atlas based segmentation for detection of middle cerebral artery (MCA) stroke lesion. Usniskas et al. [4] proposed segmentation of stroke lesion on the basis of mean and standard deviation. Chan et al. [5] developed a knowledge based system for detection of hemorrhagic mass from CT slices. Bardera et al. [6] proposed the application of semi-automated region growing for segmentation of necrosis and edema from CT images. Chawla et al. [7] proposed histogram based classification of stroke and mid line symmetry axis approach for detecting abnormal slices. Tang et al. [8] proposed a computer based diagnosis by computing several texture features, the features were calculated by extracting circular adaptive region of interest (CAROI). Li et al. [9] proposed the usage of trained Bayesian network for detection of subarachnoid hemorrhage from brain CT images. Prakash et al. [10] proposed segmentation of intra-cerebral hemorrhage and intra-ventricular hemorrhage from CT images using regularized level set function. Celine et al. [11] proposed voxel based outlier detection for segmenting the stroke lesion.

There has been very little approach for delineation of stroke lesion in CT images. Ischemic stroke is very less addressed as the boundary of ischemic stroke is not marked properly. Auto-encoder based slice selection and random walker is proposed in this manuscript for detection of hematoma and ischemic stroke lesion.

## 2    Materials and Methods

### 2.1    Imaging of Brain

The brain volume was captured using 16 slicer Brivo series 385 CT scanner manufactured by GE (Brivo CT385 series, Waukesha, USA). The window width and center is 100 and 40 HU respectively. The size of each volume is $512 \times 512 \times 96$. The raw data were collected and converted in neuroimaging informatics technology initiative (NifTI) format. In total 36 patients' data were involved in this study which includes 20 cases of hemorrhagic stroke which includes 5 cases of intra-cerebral hemorrhage (ICH), 9 cases of intra-ventricular hemorrhage, 3 cases of subarachnoid hemorrhage (SAH) and 3 cases of epidural hemorrhage (EPH).

### 2.2    Pre-processing of CT Volume

The skull is removed from each CT volume, as it has no role to play in this study. As skull contains the highest CT number, it is removed with the help of simple thresholding. The remains of skull still exist which is later removed with the help of better outlier removal. As the CT brain volume is heterogeneous in nature, Gaussian smoothing with kernel size $(11 \times 11 \times 11)$ were used.

## 2.3     Selection of Slices

Auto-encoder was used for selection of abnormal slices containing hematoma. 60% of all the resized volumes were used for testing and remaining 40% were used for testing. A single layer auto-encoder (16384 node input and 100 node encoder) was trained along with a binary softmax classifier for classification of normal (healthy slices) and abnormal (contains lesions or hematoma) slices. Rectified linear unit (ReLU) was used as an activation function for the encoder layer (Fig. 1).

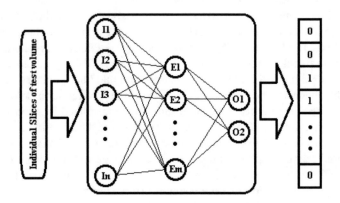

**Fig. 1.** Demonstration on selection of slices

## 2.4     Selection of Foreground Seed

Foreground seed selection is a crucial stage of segmentation. If seed selection is not properly performed, then delineation results will be affected. The localization of lesion or hematoma was done with the application of k-means clustering. The number of clusters in case of hemorrhage was three. Four foreground seeds were taken from the clusters with highest HU. The seeds from particular clusters were selected via an interactive method.

## 2.5     Selection of Background Seed

The leftover clusters were selected for background seed in both of the stroke cases. The seeds were selected randomly from the leftover clusters. Three seeds were initialized as background. Background seed is also selected with the help of interactive method.

## 2.6     Detection of Hematoma

Total four foreground and three background seeds were used for initialization. $S$ is the one of the slice containing hematoma having size $512 \times 512$. $S_i$ is the intensity value at location $i$, the region of interest (ROI) is the hematoma. The hematoma region is termed as $S_{Hema}$ and the rest of the region is termed as $S_{WM}$ (as the rest of the region contains white matter). Hence, $S_{hema} \cap S_{WM} = 0$. If the graphical representation of slice is $G$, then $I$ will be the node, i.e. $i \in I$. Posterior probability of class for the node $i$ was calculated for the delineation of hematoma, i.e. probability of specific node I was marked as hematoma. Maximum a posteriori (MAP) was calculated for marking node $i$.

$$\arg \max \{p(hematoma \mid i, s), p(white\ matter \mid i, s)\tag{1}$$

Random walker [12] was applied for calculating the probability for each node at graph $G$. Four seed points from hematoma and three from white matter, in total seven seed points(SP) were considered, were marked on $G$.

$$SP \subseteq \{(SP \in S_{hema}) \cup (SP \in S_{WM})\}\tag{2}$$

In random walker algorithm an entire image can be represented as a unidirectional graph $G(V,E)$, with edges $e$ and vertices $v$ (pixels in case of images), where $e \in E$ and $v \in V$. Edge e, between two pixels is considered to be a Gaussian weighted function of intensity differences between the two nodes. Edge weight $EW_{i,j}$ between nodes i and j is given by Eq. 3. where, is free parameter and $I_i$ and $I_j$ are the intensities values at the pixel $i$ and $j$.

$$EW_{i,j} = \begin{cases} exp\left(-\lambda |I_i - I_j|^2\right), & if\ i\ and\ j\ are\ adjacent \\ 0, & Otherwise \end{cases}\tag{3}$$

LM is defined as the Laplacian combinational matrix and $V_i$ and $V_j$ are any two edges in the neighborhood vertex. Then the elements of the matrix LM are defined by adjacency of any two vertices and $d_i$ represents the degree of vertex at $i$.

$$LM_{i,j} = \begin{cases} d_i, & if\ i = j \\ -EW_{i,j}, & if\ v_i\ and\ v_j\ are\ adjacent\ nodes \\ 0, & Otherwise \end{cases}\tag{4}$$

$$d_i = \sum EW_{i,j} \forall V_i\tag{5}$$

Probability of a random walker standing at any of the unmarked seed points ($x_{um}$) to reach the marked seed points ($x_m$) is given by differentiating the dirichlet integral D [x] in Eq. 6. with $x_{um}$ where

$$D[x] = \frac{1}{2} x^T L x$$
$$= \frac{1}{2} [x_m x_{um}] \begin{bmatrix} L_m & B \\ B^T & L_{um} \end{bmatrix} \begin{bmatrix} x_m \\ x_{um} \end{bmatrix}\tag{6}$$

$$L_{um} x = -B^T M\tag{7}$$

M is the label column matrix of seed points in which every seed point corresponding to its column is labelled 1 at its respective position and other elements of the column vector are zero.

## 2.7   Performance Measurement

Two raters have independently marked the hematoma. The common overlapping areas of both the raters were used for comparison with the computer generated outputs. If $M_1$ is manually segmented output by $1^{st}$ expert and $M_2$ is the manually segmented output by $2^{nd}$ expert. $M_1 \cap M_2 = M$ .

$M$ is used for comparison of computer generated output along with $M$. Four similarity measures such as sensitivity, positive predictive value ($PPV$), jaccard coefficient ($JC$) and dice similarity index ($DSI$). When the segmented volume is 1 and ground truth is also 1, it is true positive, when ground truth is 0 and segmented volume is also 0, it is true negative, when ground truth is 0 and segmented volume is 1, it is false positive and when ground truth is 1 and segmented volume is 0, it is false negative.

$$sensitivity = \frac{True\ positive\ (TP)}{TP\ +\ False\ negative\ (FN)} \tag{8}$$

$$PPV = \frac{TP}{(TP\ +\ False\ positive\ (FP))} \tag{9}$$

$$DSI = \frac{2.TP}{(2TP\ +\ FP\ +\ FN)} \tag{10}$$

$$JC = \frac{TP}{TP\ +\ FP\ +\ FN} \tag{11}$$

## 3   Results and Discussions

Please check that the lines in line drawings are not interrupted and have a constant The combination of proposed algorithms was used for segmentation of hematoma from CT volume. While localizing the hematoma, it was noticed that hematoma is detected along with the white matter as it share close HU values. In the following Table 1, the performance of the proposed algorithm is compared with other existing state of art.

In order to check the robustness of the proposed algorithm, it was implemented on ischemic stroke CT volume for detection of ischemic stroke lesion. In case of ischemic stroke lesion the boundary of lesion is not well marked, which often confuses the clinicians. The approach made for foreground was modified as the physical appearance of ischemic stroke lesion differs from that of hematoma. The ischemic stroke lesion is hypo-intense with respect to surrounding tissues. The seed selection for foreground was done from the cluster which possess second lowest HU value, as the cluster containing background and lateral ventricle contains the least HU value. In Table 2, performance of proposed algorithm is compared with other state of art methods for delineation of ischemic stroke lesion.

**Table 1.** Comparison of the proposed method with existing state of art in hematoma detection

| Authors | State of art | Performance measures |
|---|---|---|
| Li et al. (2011) [#] | Bayesian decision theory (only SAH) | DSI: 0.76 ± 0.09 |
| Celine et al. (2013) [#] | Voxel based outlier detection | DSI minimum: 0.58<br>DSI maximum: 0.65 |
| Proposed | Auto encoder and random walker | Sensitivity: 0.694 ± 0.133<br>PPV = 0.878 ± 0.077<br>JC = 0.634 ± 0.128<br>DSI = 0.768 ± 0.101 |

**Table 2.** Comparison of proposed method with existing state of art in case of ischemic stroke

| Authors | State of art | Performance measures |
|---|---|---|
| Chawla et al. (2009) | Histogram based classification | Accuracy: 90% |
| Tang et al. (2011) | CAROI (circular adaptive region of interest) | Sensitivity: 93.3%<br>Specificity: 90.3% |
| Proposed | Auto encoder and random walker | Sensitivity: 0.687 ± 0.228<br>PPV = 0.516 ± 0.267<br>JC = 0.412 ± 0.267<br>DSI = 0.551 ± 0.212 |

The training accuracy of auto encoder in both the cases (hemorrhage and ischemic) was 100%, and testing accuracy in case of hemorrhage and ischemic stroke was 99.5% and 50% respectively. As the edge of ischemic stroke is not distinct with the surrounding tissues. The accuracy in case of ischemic was not satisfactory; hence the directions of clinicians were followed for selection of seeds slice wise. The results are not satisfactory, in case of ischemic stroke the proposed methodology needs refinement.

Example automated results are shown for hemorrhagic stroke (Fig. 2) and ischemic stroke (Fig. 3) in comparison to respective ground truth results from two independent raters.

It can be concluded form Table 1 that the proposed algorithm outperforms the existing state of art. In Table 1, DSI of Li et al. is equivalent to ours, but they have considered only the case of SAH. In Table 2, both Chawla et al. and Li et al. have performed their results on 2D-slices which might suffer from outliers that can be removed by 3D connectivity-based cleaning. The results reported in Table 2, is the delineation of ischemic stroke lesion, the proposed algorithm needs more refinement for obtaining better results.

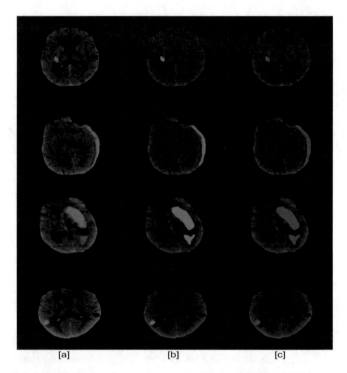

**Fig. 2.** [a]: Original representation of various hemorrhagic slices (ICH, EPH, IVH, And SAH), [b] Intersection of ground truths generated by two raters, [c] Computer generated outputs.

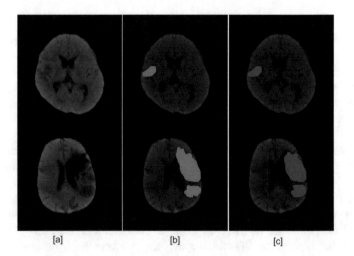

**Fig. 3.** [a]: Original representation of ischemic lesion slices, [b] Intersection of ground truths generated by two raters, [c] Computer generated outputs.

# 4   Conclusion

A new approach for the delineation of hematoma is proposed. Proposed algorithm has the potential to overcome the iso-intense white matter and hematoma and segments the hematoma with a satisfactory performance. The probability mask of hematoma has been calculated by random walk. In present work, seed selection was done slice wise, it would be better if in future the selection is made from whole volume. In case of ischemic stroke slice selection, single layer auto encoder's performance was not found satisfactory. In future, it could be made deep networks for better result.

**Acknowledgements.** MK Nag would like to acknowledge Council of Scientific and Industrial Research, New Delhi, Senior research fellowship grant (No: 9/81(1296)/17) for financial assistance. All the authors would like to acknowledge EKO diagnostics for clinical inputs and providing the data for accomplishing this study.

# References

1. van Swieten, J.C., Koudstaal, P.J., Visser, M.C., Schouten, H.J., van Gijn, J.: Interobserver agreement for the assessment of handicap in stroke patients. Stroke **19**(5), 604–607 (1988)
2. Matesin, M., Loncaric, S., Petravic, D.: A rule-based approach to stroke lesion analysis from CT brain images. In: Proceedings of the 2nd International Symposium on Image and Signal Processing and Analysis ISPA 2001, pp. 219–223 (2001)
3. Maldjian, J.A., Chalela, J., Kasner, S.E., Liebeskind, D., Detre, J.A.: Automated CT segmentation and analysis for acute middle cerebral artery stroke. Am. J. Neuroradiol. **22**(6), 1050–1055 (2001)
4. Usinskas, A., Pranckeviciene, E., Wittenberg, T., Hastreiter, P., Tomandl, B.F.: Automatic ischemic stroke segmentation using various techniques BT - neural networks and soft computing, pp. 498–503 (2003)
5. Chan, T.: Computer aided detection of small acute intracranial hemorrhage on computer tomography of brain. Comput. Med. Imaging Graph. **31**(4), 285–298 (2007)
6. Bardera, A., et al.: Semi-automated method for brain hematoma and edema quantification using computed tomography. Comput. Med. Imaging Graph. **33**(4), 304–311 (2009)
7. Chawla, M., Sharma, S., Sivaswamy, J., Kishore, L.T.: A method for automatic detection and classification of stroke from brain CT images. In: Annual International Conference of the IEEE Engineering in Medicine and Biology Society EMBC 2009, pp. 3581–3584 (2009)
8. Tang, F., Ng, D.K.S., Chow, D.H.K.: An image feature approach for computer-aided detection of ischemic stroke. Comput. Biol. Med. **41**(7), 529–536 (2011)
9. Li, Y.H., Zhang, L., Hu, Q.M., Li, H.W., Jia, F.C., Wu, J.H.: Automatic subarachnoid space segmentation and hemorrhage detection in clinical head CT scans. Int. J. Comput. Assist. Radiol. Surg. **7**(4), 507–516 (2012)
10. Prakash, K.N.B., Zhou, S., Morgan, T.C., Hanley, D.F., Nowinski, W.L.: Segmentation and quantification of intra-ventricular/cerebral hemorrhage in CT scans by modified distance regularized level set evolution technique. Int. J. Comput. Assist. Radiol. Surg. **7**(5), 785–798 (2012)

11. Gillebert, C.R., Humphreys, G.W., Mantini, D.: Automated delineation of stroke lesions using brain CT images. NeuroImage Clin. **4**, 540–548 (2014)
12. Grady, L.: Random walks for image segmentation. Pattern Anal. Mach. Intell. IEEE Trans. **28**(11), 1768–1783 (2006)

# Most Effective Enforced Exercise Time for Aerobic Exercise to Burn Body Fat

Tamaki Mitsuno[1(✉)] and Yuko Shinohara[2]

[1] Faculty of Education, Shinshu University, 6-ro, Nishinagano, Nagano, Japan
mitsuno@shinshu-u.ac.jp
[2] Former Faculty of Education, Shinshu University,
6-ro, Nishinagano, Nagano, Japan
9e1616j@shinshu-u.ac.jp

**Abstract.** Physical exercise is important to limit fat mass and prevent obesity. Of four studied exercise times, aerobic exercise before lunch (4 h after breakfast) was most effective in reducing body fat. This reduced the rate of body fat 1.20 times more than exercise after breakfast, 1.63 times more than after lunch, and 1.30 times more than before dinner (P < 0.01). Exercise before lunch used the most blood sugar, thereby consuming body fat. The difference between exercise before lunch and before diner might be explained by the metabolic efficiency of the body rhythm. This study used four stages of exercise intensity. At any of the four exercise times, the mildest intensity exercise (20% increased heart rate) was effective in reducing body fat. For women who do not exercise regularly, continuous slow movement on an empty stomach may reduce body fat.

**Keywords:** Body fat · Lipid consumption · Energy consumption
Carbohydrate consumption · Respiratory metabolism · Aerobic exercise
Japanese young adult female · Oxygen intake · Heart rate

## 1 Introduction

In Japan, the main cause of illness-related death since World War II has been geriatric diseases including cancer, heart disease, and cerebrovascular disease from infectious diseases (e.g., tuberculosis or pneumonia). The onset and progression of geriatric diseases has been attributed to aging; however, it has become clear that lifestyle is a major contributing factor [1]. In addition, symptoms of these geriatric diseases have increased in children because of lifestyle factors [2]. Therefore, the Ministry of Health, Labour and Welfare changed "geriatric diseases" to "lifestyle-related diseases" in 1996. Obesity is a major cause of lifestyle-related diseases, and approximately 90% of obesity is defined as simple obesity. Obesity [3, 4] is considered a contributing factor to diseases later in life, including diabetes [5], high blood pressure [6], dyslipidemia [7], myocardial infarction [8, 9], and cerebral infarction [10]. To prevent obesity and live a healthy life, it is important to be mindful of eating habits and participate in regular exercise. In addition, it is necessary to keep body fat at an appropriate level. Excessive caloric intake [11] and lack of exercise contribute to reduced fitness and possibly long-term illness. However, vigorous exercise places considerable demand on people

© Springer International Publishing AG, part of Springer Nature 2019
N. J. Lightner (Ed.): AHFE 2018, AISC 779, pp. 139–148, 2019.
https://doi.org/10.1007/978-3-319-94373-2_15

unaccustomed to such activity. Mersy et al. [12] noted that aerobic exercise benefits health, which in turn affects lipoprotein metabolism in sedentary healthy young women [13]. Therefore, in this study, we used aerobic exercise measured with an ergometer as a simple way to assess work performed during exercise. This study aimed to identify easily achievable conditions that enhance body fat metabolism during aerobic exercise by assigning moderate exercise in combination with normal eating habits, based on a prescribed diet [14–16].

# 2    Method

## 2.1    Participants and Experimental Schedule

Study participants were nine healthy Japanese females aged in their twenties who did not normally participate in regular exercise. Table 1 presents participants' physical characteristics and intensity of exercise loads. Participants were non-smokers, with no history of systemic disease, and were not engaged in physical training or dietary programs. Respiratory metabolism was measured in the follicular phases of participants' menstrual cycles [17] in winter [18, 19]. Figure 1 illustrates the four experimental schedules used in this study: Experiment I enforced exercise 2 h after breakfast, Experiment II enforced exercise before lunch (4 h after breakfast), Experiment III enforced exercise 2 h after lunch, and experiment IV enforced exercise before supper (4 h after lunch). Participants woke at 06:00 after 7 h of sleep, and consumed a prescribed diet (the same breakfast and lunch menus) at 07:30 and 12:30.

**Table 1.** Participants' physical characteristics

| Item | Age | Height | Weight | BMI | Girth (cm) | | | Exercise intensity (W) | | | | |
|------|-----|--------|--------|-----|------------|------|-----|--------|--------|--------|--------|--------|
| | (year) | (m) | (kg) | (kg/m$^2$) | Top bust | Waist | Hip | Step 1 | Step 2 | Step 3 | Step 4 | Step 1' |
| Mean | 21.3 | 1.54 | 52.5 | 21.2 | 86.5 | 70.8 | 93.6 | 23.9 | 40.6 | 54.4 | 67.8 | 23.9 |
| SD | 1.1 | 0.11 | 8.0 | 2.9 | 3.2 | 5.7 | 5.4 | 4.2 | 3.9 | 4.6 | 3.6 | 4.2 |

Table 2 shows the breakfast menu, which is typical for youth. They then entered a climate-controlled room (environmental temperature 24.5 ± 0.3° C; relative humidity 50.3% ± 2.5%; luminance 827 ± 27 lx; and air current 8.0 ± 0.1 cm/s) 2 h before the experiments. Participants were seated at rest for 1 h while wearing a short-sleeved 100% cotton t-shirt and 100% polyester running pants. Their respiratory metabolism levels were measured with a Vmax-229 (Sensormedics, CA, USA) [20], using the breath-by-breath method for 40 min starting at 9:00. Body fat percentage, muscle, and basal metabolic rate were measured using an electric bioelectrical impedance analysis scale [21] (BC-520, TANITA, Tokyo, Japan). Body weight was measured with a platform scale (IPS-150 K, Shimazu, Kyoto, Japan). Metabolism of body fat was assessed by measuring respiratory metabolism before, during, and after aerobic exercise. The device used measured the amount of inhaled oxygen (L/min) and exhaled

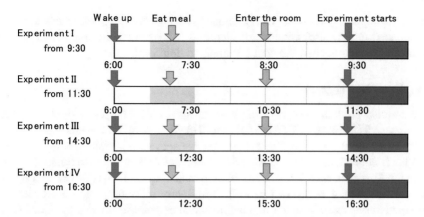

**Fig. 1.** Four enforced exercise times for measuring respiratory metabolism.

**Table 2.** Prescribed diet (breakfast)

| Food (Unit) | Weight (g) | Energy (kcal) | Water (g) | Protein (g) | Lipid (g) | Carbohydrate (g) | Ash (g) |
|---|---|---|---|---|---|---|---|
| Bread | 67.0 | 176.9 | 25.5 | 6.2 | 2.9 | 31.3 | 1.1 |
| Strawberry jam | 10.0 | 19.7 | 5.1 | 0.1 | 0.0 | 4.8 | 0.0 |
| Butter | 5.0 | 37.3 | 0.8 | 0.0 | 4.1 | 0.0 | 0.1 |
| Instant coffee (Decaf) | 5.0 | 14.4 | 0.2 | 0.7 | 0.0 | 2.8 | 0.4 |
| Milk | 50.0 | 33.5 | 43.7 | 1.7 | 1.9 | 2.4 | 0.4 |
| Total | 137.0 | 281.7 | 75.2 | 8.7 | 8.9 | 41.4 | 2.0 |

carbon dioxide (L/min) for every lungful of air. Energy consumption (EC) per one liter of oxygen (kcal/$O_2 l$) was calculated by obtaining the respiratory quotient (RQ) [22, 23] using a Zunts-Schumberg-Lusk table [24], which shows analysis of the oxidation of mixtures of carbohydrate and fat. EC was calculated using the following equation.

$$EC = 1.22RQ + 3.83 \text{(the unit: kcal}/O_2 l) \tag{1}$$

This was used to determine the EC ratio supplied from carbohydrate versus lipid metabolism. The carbohydrate ratio Z for EC was determined using the equation:

$$Z = 3.1714RQ - 221.81 \tag{2}$$

The lipid ratio X was calculated as:

$$X = 100 - Z \tag{3}$$

Therefore, the amount of energy consumed (kcal/O2 $l$) during respiration was divided into the relative EC (kcal/min) supplied by carbohydrate consumption (CC) or lipid consumption (LC) using oxygen intake (L/min). Next, carbohydrates and lipids metabolized during respiration were calculated using the relationship of 4.1 kcal per gram of carbohydrate and 9.3 kcal per gram of lipid [25].

## 2.2  Exercise Program

The exercise program was performed using an exercise bicycle (Aerobic Exercise Ergometer, STB-1400, NIHONKHODEN, Tokyo, Japan) The exercise load of the exercise bicycle is shown in Fig. 2. Participants engaged in 30 min of aerobic exercise with loads equivalent to 25%, 40%, 55%, 70%, and 25% of their maximum heart rate using the Karvonen equation [16, 25], in sequential 6-minute intervals (the second 25% interval served as a cool-down period). Respiratory metabolism and heart rate were measured during exercise and 5 min before and after exercise as a control. EC, LC, and CC were calculated from RQs [25].

## 2.3  Lipid and Carbohydrate Metabolism

Figure 3 shows a typical example of the relationship between oxygen intake and carbon dioxide output using the breath-by-breath method, with dots representing the number of breaths. No points were detected that exceeded the anaerobic threshold, confirming that the exercise was aerobic. According to Rennie et al. [26], heavy and long-term exercise resulted in the consumption of body protein in men. The RQs in the present study were regarded as "non-protein RQs," as the exercise was carried out at light loads for a relatively short (30-min) exercise duration. Further, participants' diets did not include a lot of protein [27] (see Table 2). CC and LC were then calculated according to the fix rule [28, 29], and compared for each exercise load (stage) [25].

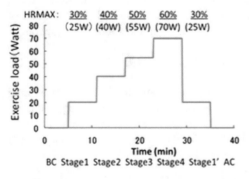

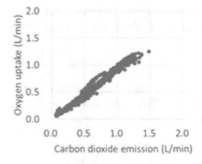

**Fig. 2.** Exercise load of the exercise cycle for 30 min.

**Fig. 3.** Relationship between oxygen and carbon dioxide emission

**2.4    Statistics**

Average EC, CC, LC, and $O_2$ intake were calculated every 10 s from the respiration metabolism determined by the breath-by-breath method. Changes in EC, CC, LC, and $O_2$ intake among the exercise times were confirmed for each time using one-way analysis of variance, and significant differences examined using Tukey's method. LC values were focused, and recalculated as relative LC based on before control values at rest. LC was compared among exercise times using paired t-tests with consideration of individual differences. Furthermore, the LC from each exercise stage was compared using paired t-tests with consideration of individual differences.

# 3    Results and Discussion

A typical example of EC, CC, and LC every 10 s is shown in Fig. 4 (participant 1). Variation in CC resembled that in EC (which changed by exercise stage), but differed from the variation in LC. Therefore, these data were distributed and compared across each exercise time. The comparison of EC, CC, LC, and $O_2$ intake values for each exercise time are shown in Fig. 5. EC and $O_2$ intake did not change with each exercise time (Tukey's method). CC was higher at 9:30 and 14:30 than at 11:30, and LC was higher at 11:30 than at 14:30. Therefore, LC significantly increased during aerobic exercise at 11:30. LC values for each participant are shown in Fig. 6. These values changed each day for each participant. LC values were recalculated as relative LC based on before control values at rest, and were compared among exercise times using paired t-tests with consideration of individual differences. Significant findings by exercise time are shown at the right side of Fig. 7. The value at 11:30 was the highest; therefore, exercise before lunch was the best time to burn body fat.

Significant correlations between EC and CC were found, but there were no significant correlations between EC and LC. The 9:30 and 14:30 exercise times were 2 h after a meal, when the body has more access to carbohydrate from foods that are easier to burn than lipids. However, exercise at 11:30 (4 h after breakfast), the amount of carbohydrate in blood available to burn had decreased, meaning lipids in blood or muscle were easier to burn than after meal, thus secretion of insulin was controlled and lipase was activated [29]. The results for exercise at 16:30 (the same condition as at 11:30 in terms of being 4 h after a meal) showed higher values than at 14:30, but not than at 9:30. The circadian rhythm of lipid metabolism may be related to this result [30], and should be considered in future studies. The relative LC at each stage is shown on the right side of Fig. 7. The result for stage 1 was greater than stages 3 and 4, indicating the effective intensity of burning body fat was stage 1 or the lightest intensity exercise [25] (20% increased heart rate). This shows that the most efficient way to burn body fat was 30 min of aerobic exercise at an intensity of 20% more than participants' resting heart rate.

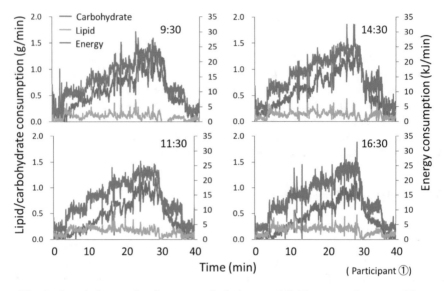

**Fig. 4.**  A typical example of energy, carbohydrate, and lipid consumption every 10 s.

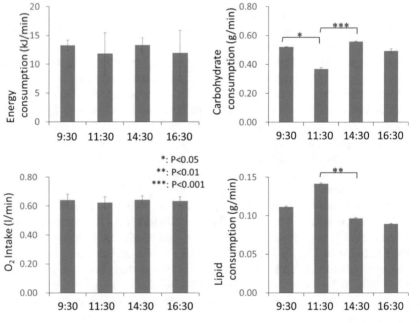

**Fig. 5.**  Energy, carbohydrate, and lipid consumption, and $O_2$ intake values for each exercise time.

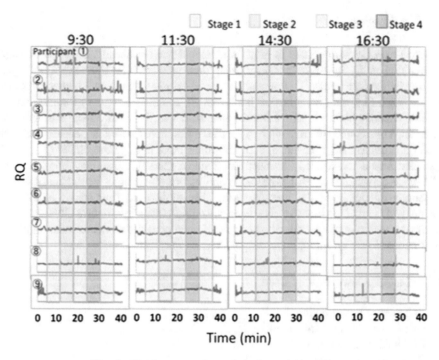

**Fig. 6.** Lipid consumption values for each participant.

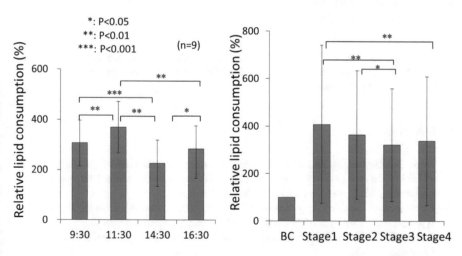

**Fig. 7.** Relative lipid consumption at each exercise time and stage. Exercise time is shown on the left, and stage on the right.

# 4   Conclusion

Physical exercise is important to limit fat mass and prevent obesity. Study participants were nine healthy Japanese females aged in their twenties who did not normally participate in regular exercise. Of four studied exercise times when were 2 h after breakfast, before lunch (4 h after breakfast), 2 h after lunch, and before supper (4 h after lunch), aerobic exercise before lunch (4 h after breakfast) was the most effective in reducing body fat. This reduced the rate of body fat 1.20 times more than exercise after breakfast, 1.63 times more than after lunch, and 1.30 times more than before dinner ($P < 0.01$). Exercise before lunch used the most blood sugar, thereby consuming body fat. The difference between exercise before lunch and before diner might be explained by the metabolic efficiency of the body rhythm. This study used four stages of exercise intensity. At any of the four exercise times, the mildest intensity exercise (20% increased heart rate) was effective in reducing body fat. For women who do not exercise regularly, continuous slow movement on an empty stomach may reduce body fat.

## 4.1   List of Abbreviations Used

- EC: energy consumption
- CC: carbohydrate consumption
- LC: lipid consumption
- BMR: basal metabolic rate
- OI: oxygen intake
- RHR: relative heart rate
- $VO_2$ max: VdotO$_2$ max

**Acknowledgments.** A part of this work was supported by JSPS Kakenhi (grant number 17H01954). We thank Audrey Holmes, MA, from Edanz Group (www.edanzediting.com/ac) for editing a draft of this manuscript.

# References

1. Japan Ministry of Health Labour and Welfare: Basic directionality of the illness measure esthat focused its attention on a lifestyle (Verdict of the concrete opinion). http://www.mhlw.go.jp/index.shtml. Accessed 17 Dec 1996. (in Japanese)
2. Department of Epidemiology and Health Policy: Infant lifestyle-related disease (geriatric-type disease of children). http://www.med.u-toyama.c.jp/healpro/meeting.html. (in Japanese)
3. Bouchard, C.: Physical Activity and Obesity, pp. 1–389. Human Kinetic Publishers Inc., Champaign (2000)
4. Galgani, J., Ravussin, E.: REVIEW: Energy metabolism, fuel selection and body weight regulation. Int. J. Obes. **2**, S109–S119 (2008)
5. Fujioka, K., Seaton, T.B., Rowe, E., Jelinek, C.A., Raskin, P., Lebovitz, H.E., Weinstein, S. P.: The Sibutramin/diabetes clinical study group: weight loss with sibutramine improves control and other metabolic parameters in obese patients with type 2 diabetes mellitus. Diabetes Obes. Metab. **2**, 175–187 (2000)

6. Whyte, H.M., Phil, D.: Blood pressure and obesity. Circulation **XIX**, 511–516 (1959)
7. Carr, M.C., Brunzell, J.D.: Abdominal obesity and dyslipidemia in the metabolic syndrome: importance of type 2 diabetes and familial combined hyperlipidemia in coronary artery disease risk. J. Clin. Endocrinol. Metab. **89**, 2601–2607 (2004)
8. Yusuf, S., Hawken, S., Ounpuu, S., Bautista, L., Frnzosi, M.G., Commerford, P., Lang, C. C., Rumboldt, Z., Ones, C.L., Lisheng, L., Tanomsup, S., Wangai, P., Razak, F., Sharma, A. M., Anand, S.S.: Obesity and the risk of myocardial infarction in 27 000 participants from 52 countries: a case-control study. Lancet **366**, 1640–1649 (2005)
9. Aoyagi, K., Kusano, Y., Takamura, N., Abe, Y., Osaki, M., Une, H.: Obesity and cardiovascular risk factors among men and women aged 40 years and older in a rural area of Japan. J Physiol. Anthoropol. **25**, 371–375 (2006). http://www.jstage.jst.go.jp/browse/jpa2. https://doi.org/10.2114/jpa2.25.371
10. Xiaodong, Y., Shujuan, W., Yaru, X., Jing, L.: A clinical follow-up study on the risk of cerebral infarction in Chinese aging overweight and obese population. Obes. Res. Clin. Pract. **5**, e1–e78 (2011). https://doi.org/10.1016/j.orcp.2010.09.251
11. Rogge, M.M.: The role of impaired mitochondrial lipid oxidation in obesity. Biol. Res. Nurs. **10**, 356–373 (2009)
12. Mersy, D.J.: Health benefits of aerobic exercise. Postgrad. Med. **90**, 103–110 (1991)
13. Ootani, K., Hashimoto, S., Hayashi, S., Kimura, T., Naito, M.: Effects of aerobic exercise training on lipoprotein metabolism and antioxidant status in sedentary but otherwise healthy young women. J. Integr. Study Diet. Habits **22**, 114–120 (2011)
14. Carstens, M.T., Goedecke, J.H., Dugas, L., Evans, J., Kroff, J., Levitt, N.S., Lambert, E.V.: Fasting substrate oxidation in relation to habitual dietary fat intake and insulin resistance in nondiabetic women: a case for metabolic flexibility? Nutr. Metab. **10**, 8 (2013). http://www. nutritionandmetabolism.com/content/10/1/8
15. Mitsuno, T., Hibino, A.: Which support pants are the most effective for burning body fat? JFBI **9**, 1–13 (2016)
16. ACSM Certified Personal Trainer SM: The Heart Rate Debate. http://www.acsm.org/ publicinformation/articles/2016/10/07/the-heart-rate-debate
17. Lamina, S., Hanif, S., Muhammed, H.: Influence of menstrual cycle on maximal aerobic power of young female adults. AJPARS **3**, 36–41 (2011)
18. Tsumura, Y., Makonakwkeyoon, L., Limtrakul, P., Hirota, N., Sone, Y.: Seasonal variation in amount of unabsorbed dietary carbohydrate from the intestine after breakfast in young female Thai participant: comparison with that of Japanese participant. J. Physiol. Anthropol. **29**, 141–147 (2010)
19. Morinaka, T., Wozniewicz, M., Jeszjka, J., Bajerska, J., limtrakul, P., Makonkawkeyoon, L., Hirota, N., Kumagai, S., Sone, Y.: Comparison of seasonal variation in the fasting respiratory quotient of young Japanese, Polish and Thai women in relation to seasonal change in their percent body fat. J. Physiol. Anthropol. **31**, 1–12 (2012). http://www. jphysiolanthropol.com/content/31/1/10
20. Okura, M., Nakaya, H., Yamamoto, S., Ojima, Y., Sakai, S., Sakanoue, N.: The validity of the estimated maximal oxygen up take by different indirect methods. Bull. Kochi Rehabil. Inst. **1**, 5–24 (1999)
21. TANITA HP: Electric bioelectrical impedance analysis. http://www.tanita.co.jp/support/faq. htr. (in Japanese)
22. Rennie, M.J., Edwrds, R.H.T., Krywawch, S., Davies, C.T.M., Hallday, D., Waterlow, J.C., Millward, D.J.: Effect of exercise on protein turnover in man. Clin. Sci. **61**, 627–639 (1981)
23. Du Bois, E.F.: Clinical calorimetry: thirty-fifth paper. a graphic representation of the respiratory quotient and the percentage of calories from protein fat and carbohydrate. J. Biol. Chem. **59**, 43–49 (1924)

24. Lusk, G.: Animal calorimetry: twenty-fourth paper. analysis of the oxidation of mixtures of carbohydrate and fat. J. Biol. Chem. **59**, 41–42 (1924)
25. Mitsuno, T., Nagayasu, M., Shinohara, Y., Maruyama, A.Y.: Most effective exercise load for burning body fat with aerobic exercise in young Japanese women. In: Advances in Human Factors and Ergonomics in Healthcare and Medical Device. Advances Intelligent Systems and Computing, vol. 590. https://doi.org/10.1007/978-3-319-60483-1_21
26. Robert, D.A.: Introduction to Nutrition and metabolism, 5th edn. CRC Press, New York (2014)
27. Ferrannin, A.: The theoretical bases of indirect calorimetry: a review. Metabolism **37**, 287–301 (1988)
28. Sugimoto, A.: The measurement of physical activity—a review of recent progress. Rehabil. Med. **37**, 53–61 (2007). (English abstract and Japanese text)
29. Frayn, K.N.: Adipose tissue as a buffer for daily lipid flux. Diabetologia **45**, 1201–1210 (2002). https://doi.org/10.1007/s00125-002-0873-y
30. Gooley, J.J., Chua, E.C.: Diurnal regulation of lipid metabolism and applications of circadian lipidomics. J. Genet. Genomics **41**, 231–250 (2014)

# Factors Building Commitment of Healthcare Workers

Anna Stankiewicz-Mróz[(✉)]

Department of Management Systems and Innovation,
Lodz University of Technology, Piotrkowska 266, 90-924 Lodz, Poland
anna.stankiewicz-mroz@p.lodz.pl

**Abstract.** This paper presents the result of research on organizational commitment in the sector of health protection. 150 doctors and nurses employed in three hospitals in Lodz and in two Sanitary and Epidemiological Stations located in Lodz participated in the research. Gallupa Test (G12) was used to measure the engagement together with in-depth structured individual interviews (IDI). The research showed a problem of the lack of balance of resources and work demands, which results in the decrease of the affective commitment and causes the danger of professional burnout of medical staff. The engagement in the group of respondents increased with age but in none of the age categories both among doctors and nurses exceeded the level of 37%.

**Keywords:** Factors of organizational commitment · Health protection
JD-R theory

## 1 Introduction

The shortage of medical personnel is becoming more and more visible in Poland. Hospital managers report difficulties in recruiting and retaining both the doctors and the personnel of the medium level. Therefore, the understanding of the conditions for building and maintaining the organizational engagement of healthcare workers and a creation of such a working environment that strengthens this attitude is one of the most important issues. The aim of this paper is to analyze the factors which create commitment of healthcare workers with an emphasis put on their connection with the selected features of the respondents and the identification of the risk in this area. In the presented research the perspective of an employee was deliberately used. For the sake of theoretical coherence, the implementation of the goal was embedded within the framework of the theory of requirements and work resources of Schaufeli and Bakker [1] and a three-factor model of the attachment to the organization proposed by Meyer and Allen [2].

## 2 Literature Review

Contemporary organizations need committed employees who work with enthusiasm, who show initiative and who devotedly strive for the quality and efficiency of work. The commitment is defined as an "emotional result for an employee created on the

© Springer International Publishing AG, part of Springer Nature 2019
N. J. Lightner (Ed.): AHFE 2018, AISC 779, pp. 149–158, 2019.
https://doi.org/10.1007/978-3-319-94373-2_16

basis of the most important elements of the working place" [3], "a positive mutual relation between an employee and their organization, in which both parties respect their mutual needs and support each other to satisfy them. Thanks to it the employees and organizations obtain additional profits [4]. The commitment is therefore a measurer of the strength of relation between the employee and the company. Meyer and Allen built a three-dimensional model of organizational commitment taking the different motives creating commitment into consideration. They distinguish: emotional commitment (affective) which is measured by the employee's identification with the organization, its values and internalization of organizational norms. The work is connected with positive emotion. This kind of commitment is described by the attitude: "I work here because I want". The normative commitment results from a perceptible commitment of an employee for the organization. This kind of commitment might be associated with a moral duty described by the statement: "I work here because I should". The commitment of duration is visible in the attitude "I work here because I have no other choice". Bragg [5] underlines that some employees consider that they are "trapped" in the company. They would like to go away but they do not have where to go or are connected with the place of work by health connection, family connections or the time until the end of the professional life.

A similar approach to the issues of commitment is presented by Harter, Schmidt and Keyes [6] pointing at passive commitment and active commitment. The passive commitment is expressed in the attachment to the executed work whereas the active one includes also the passive commitment but it also means an active inclusion of an employee in the problems of the company concentrating on its development and the identification with the aims and values of the company.

Maslach [7] notices that the engagement in work is in reality the lack of the professional burn out and emotional exhaustion visible in depersonalization, cynism and negative feeling towards work. Building and maintaining a long-term commitment of employees is very important in case of these sectors and organizations in which employees are most threatened with the syndrome of a professional burn-out. This threat refers first of all to the employees of social service sector (health protection, education, social help). Kahn [8] perceives the commitment as an engagement of an employee to the professional role and the identification with it which results in investing the emotional, cognitive and emotional resources of the employee in the professional position. The commitment is sometimes identified with the feeling of responsibility for the executed work [9], a conviction that the way of executing it and a quality are particularly important. Schaufeli and Bakker [1] pay attention to the differentiation between commitment and job satisfaction, which results from the evaluation done in reference to work; it refers more to what one thinks about own job than how one feels while working. The organizational commitment should be distinguished from commitment. Andrew and Sofian [10] underlines that commitment refers only to emotional and motivational state connected with work whereas attachment refers to a strength of employee's identification with the organization, its aims and values.

Shuck and others [11] notice that the majority of researchers perceive the commitment as a kind of cognitive, behavioral and emotional energy directed on the achievement of the positive effects of work. The commitment therefore has tangible effects for the organization. The research show that committed employees less often quite jobs [12], are in a better physical and psychological condition [13], which in turn influences a lower level of sick leaves. The higher level of the executed work [14] and a bigger creativity of engaged employees are also underlined.

The process of work commitment can be explained on the basis of the assumptions of *Job Demands-Resources Theory* (JD-R) [15]. The job demands are the factors with social, emotional or cognitive character which an employee must overcome and with which must fight while executing a job. The resources are the aspects of work or the features of the employee which decrease the level of stress and enable the achievement of professional goals stimulating the personal development. The work resources can take the form of: interpersonal relations with colleagues which allow to struggle with everyday requirements [16]. The positive interpersonal relations between employees allow for failing and making mistakes without being afraid of criticism, create a feeling of safety and lead to a bigger engagement of employees into the executed work [8]. If the resources possessed by the employee and present at work are sufficient to fulfill the requirements than the area to develop commitment exists. If there is a lack of resources and the requirements are high than the emotional exhaustion and professional burn-out may happen.

The resources favor the development of engagement, especially when work requirements are high. The presence of big resources with low requirements is not beneficial, it leads to a lack of interest in work and tiredness [1].

# 3   Deficits in Health Care Sector in Poland

The health care system in Poland has many deficits resulting first of all from the low financial expenses on health care at 6.30% GDP [17]. The insufficient number of medical staff and its bad age structure are one of the key problems. In 2016 in Poland 145 000 doctors had a right to practice the profession together with 288 000 of nurses and 37000 of midwives [18]. Unfortunately Poland has the lowest number of doctors per 1000 inhabitants in the EU, which in Poland is 2, 3 (the average for the EU countries is 3, 5 doctors) [18]. Additionally, the tendencies in the age structure are frightening. In 2016, just as it was the case in the previous years, there was an increase of the number of people belonging to the oldest age group- 65 + both in the group of the doctors and nurses. In case of the last group in 2016 this increase was significant- more than 6000 (21000 people belonged to this category). A similar situation was in the age group of 55–64, where the number of nurses increased by more than 2000 [19]. The number of doctors per the number of patients is a very important factor which influences the time devoted to patients and in turn their satisfaction from the contact with the doctor and the opinion on them. The situation in Poland is not favorable as far as the time dedicated to patients for consultations is concerned. The data included in the report Health at a Glance Europe (2016) show that only 60% of respondents considered this time as sufficient whereas the average for the EU countries (EU 11) is 82.8% and the best result (97.5%) belongs to Belgians and Czechs (97.2%). A high number of consultations per doctor in Poland and a feeling of a short time of the visit or consultation may lead to worse opinions of the work of doctors by the Polish patients than is the case in other countries) [20]. Despite the aforementioned deficits, the trust for medical professions, as shown by the research "Trust for professions 2016" remains high and quite stable.

However, the doctors are the professional group from the higher half of the ranking to which the trust has decreased the most. In the same research from two years earlier 8 out of 10 respondents trusted the doctors. Today the trust indicator is a few percent lower and is 74% [21]. One tries to solve the problems with the lack of staff by expanding the number of employees of health sector who work on the basis of contractual agreements. The contractual agreements allow for a more flexible organization of work and are a trial to cope with the lack of doctors and nurses. The contractual agreements allow to bypass a right to 11-h rest directly after a duty. In case of contractual agreements the limits and the opt-out clause are not binding[1].

Unfortunately, the current legal status which allows for uninterrupted long hours of work of doctors and nurses may cause that fatigue on duty will pose a risk to the safety of patients and the staff themselves.

The biggest problems with weekly or monthly working time is how much it is for a doctor or a nurse employed on the basis of a contractual agreement in total in all the places where they work on not only in the given hospital (employed on the basis of the civil contract). It is quite common that doctors and nurses have a few places of work and their employers due to the lack of the staff are in the difficult situation. During the research, both the doctors and nurses paid attention to the fact that very often the managers of hospitals "force" them to sign an opt-out clause expecting them to work "beyond measure"- as noticed by ono of the respondents.

# 4    Research Methodology

The analysis of the research results is a part of a wider research project conducted from 2015 until 2017. 150 employees of healthcare sector employed in three hospitals in Lodz and in two Sanitary and Epidemiological Stations (Epidemiological surveillance departments) located in Lodz participated in the research. The respondents were employed as doctors and nurses. The structure of respondents is presented in Table 1.

**Table 1.** The structure of respondents as for the place of work, position, age and sex

| | Age | | | | | Sex | |
|---|---|---|---|---|---|---|---|
| Place of work/position | Less than 28 | 28–40 | 41–53 | 54–65 | Over 65 | Female | Male |
| Hospitals | | | | | | | |
| Doctor | 0 | 26 | 34 | 12 | 6 | 32 | 46 |
| Nurse | 8 | 14 | 24 | 14 | – | 60 | – |
| Sanitary and Epidemiologiacl Stations | | | | | | | |
| Doctor | | 1 | 8 | 3 | – | 11 | 1 |

---

[1] The opt-out clause is a written statement of a person on duty (most often a physician) about giving consent to work in excess of 48 h per week in the adopted settlement period. Signing this clause is very often a problem in determining the actual working time of a given doctor. The opt-out directive stipulates that the physician may or may not, individually, voluntarily agree to extend the working time beyond 48 h during a week and the employer is not allowed to discriminate or draw consequences against an employee who does not give such consent.

The selection of the sample was purposeful. It was conducted with the usage of snowball sampling. In the research two techniques were used: to evaluate resources and work demands in-depth structured individual interviews (IDI) were used. Additionally to measure the commitment Gallup Test (G12) was used. The research was supposed to provide the answer to the following research questions: Rq1: Which factors do really create the engagement of employees and is there a relation between these factors and the demographic features of healthcare employees such as age and sex and Rq 2: what are the limitations for the affective engagement in healthcare centers during the presence and what changes should take place in the analyzed area.

During the research the analysis of the factors connected with the commitment of employees according to the assumptions of the theory of JD-R Schaufeli and Bakker [1] was done. These are work resources which constitute the opportunities and threats for an employee. They should be considered be employees as sufficient to fulfill work requirements. At the stage of conceptualization of research it was considered that the commitment factors enumerated in Gallup test (G12) are the work resources (Table 2).

**Table 2.** Job demands and work resources in health care sector, evaluated by doctors and nurses

| Job demands | Work resources |
|---|---|
| • requiring contacts with patients,<br>• complexity of work,<br>• risk, threats, stressful work environment<br>• work time,<br>• emotional requirements,<br>• physical requirements,<br>• work overload,<br>• high responsibility,<br>• work-home conflict,<br>• "obstacles" (e.g. bureaucracy, shortages of tools and equipment) | • sense of importance of the work performed,<br>• the possibility of professional development,<br>• social support,<br>• autonomy at work,<br>• feedback on the results of work,<br>• knowledge of the expectations of the superior,<br>• award as an expression of appreciation,<br>• company mission showing how the work is done is important,<br>• involvement of co-workers in the work performed,<br>• social relations in the workplace,<br>• feeling of being important |

The evaluation of work resources is presented in Table 3. It was connected with a position, age and sex of respondents.

Respondents' responses were ranked by number of indications.

The research showed a low evaluation of resources in the group of doctors. It refers to such elements as: awards as a sign of appreciation (11%) or a formulation of the mission of the company showing how the work of this professional group is important (17%).

**Table 3.** Evaluation of work resources versus age and sex of doctors examined by means of Gallup Test (G12)

| Work resources | Age categories | | | | Sex | | Total |
|---|---|---|---|---|---|---|---|
| | 28–40 (N = 27) | 41–53 (N = 42) | 54–65 (N = 15) | Over65 (N = 6) | Women (N = 43) | Men (N = 47) | |
| Social relations in the work place | 14 | 32 | 11 | 4 | 32 | 29 | 61 |
| Social support | 8 | 32 | 8 | 1 | 25 | 24 | 49 |
| Autonomy at work | 6 | 22 | 12 | 3 | 20 | 23 | 43 |
| Engagement of colleagues in work | 12 | 16 | 6 | 4 | 14 | 24 | 38 |
| Possibility of a professional development | 8 | 21 | 7 | 1 | 14 | 23 | 37 |
| Feeling of being important | 6 | 18 | 6 | 2 | 12 | 20 | 32 |
| The possibility to do what the employee can do best | 6 | 14 | 5 | 4 | 13 | 16 | 29 |
| Feedback on work results | 3 | 12 | 5 | 2 | 10 | 12 | 22 |
| Knowledge of the expectations of superior | 4 | 7 | 5 | 4 | 8 | 12 | 20 |
| Mission of the company showing how the executed work is important | 4 | 6 | 1 | 4 | 7 | 8 | 15 |
| Award as a sign of appreciation | 3 | 3 | 3 | 1 | 4 | 6 | 10 |

The respondents in the group of the doctors considered the competencies of their superiors as very low while giving feedback on their work (24%) and clear information on expectations (22%). The results of the evaluation of work resources by the nurses is presented in the Table 4.

**Table 4.** Evaluation of job resources versus the age of nurses questioned with the usage of Gallup Test (G12).

| Work resources-categories of answers | Age categories | | | | Total |
|---|---|---|---|---|---|
| | Less than 28 (N = 8) | 28–40 (N = 15) | 41–53 (N = 24) | 54–65 (N = 13) | |
| Social relations in the work place | 6 | 10 | 16 | 10 | 42 |
| Social support | 6 | 10 | 12 | 9 | 37 |
| Autonomy at work | 5 | 9 | 11 | 8 | 33 |
| Engagement of colleagues in work | 5 | 11 | 10 | 9 | 29 |
| Possibility of a professional development | 4 | 9 | 8 | 8 | 29 |
| Feeling of being important | 3 | 8 | 7 | 10 | 28 |
| The possibility to do what the employee can do best | 3 | 8 | 7 | 10 | 28 |
| Feedback on work results | 4 | 5 | 8 | 8 | 25 |
| Knowledge of the expectations of superior | 3 | 9 | 7 | 9 | 23 |
| Mission of the company showing how the executed work is important | 5 | 6 | 7 | 5 | 23 |
| Award as a sign of appreciation | 3 | 5 | 6 | 3 | 17 |

The research showed, just as it was the case in the group of the doctors a low evaluation of the work resources such as: knowledge of the expectation of the superiors (38%), feedback of the work results (38%). The biggest problem is, just as in case of the doctors, the lack of awards as a sign of appreciation (28%). The higher evaluation of the work resources which can lead to a higher level of affective commitment took place only among the elder employees.

They declare a higher level of resources such as: well-established professional position, a higher remuneration, a bigger feeling of safety. This regularity refers both to the doctors and to the nurses. The similar result was obtained in the research of Mathiew and Zając [22], Ahmad and Baker [23] and Khan and Zafar [8], but for the different sectors. The influence of social relations on the commitment of employees is more visible than in case of other factors. 68% of respondents in the group of doctors and 61% in the group of nurses pointed at this factor. This relationship was also confirmed in the different research [24, 25].

The perception of job demands is the second important element important for the issues of identification of commitment. This identification was done by means of individual deepened interview (IDI).

The research showed a lack of balance between the demands and human resources in the health care sector. This problem results first of all from a long-term, excessive demand for work, resulting from the lack of doctors and nurses, which leads to the prolonged working hours and as a consequence, brings a risk of overload leading to an energetic exhaustion. One of the respondents during the interview described it in the following way: *"There was such a moment in my life when I worked even 520 h per month so I only had slightly more than 200 h for the private life and resting. Many of my friends work in the hospital, then in the ambulatory and later they come back to the hospital to have a duty on Hospital Emergency Department. In Poland the doctor is obliged to finish a duty and go home but if the doctor works on the contractual agreement, this does not refer to them"* Even 42 doctors working in the hospitals have pointed at the issues of a permanent tiredness and a feeling of exhaustion resulting from "work beyond measure". This problem did not occur among the doctors employed in Sanitary-Epidemiological Stations.

The bureaucracy was a considerable problem pointed both by the doctors and the nurses.

*"A necessity to create a large documentation concerning the patient and the lack of IT support leads to the situation when instead of taking care of the patients we fill in the papers, which makes our work very difficult- underlined one of the respondents"*. The so called "technical conditions of work" caused also many emotions. In one of the hospitals located in Lodz, one of the younger doctors participating in the research stated: "In *the doctor's office when we work with the patients, we also change our clothes, keep our personal belongings; there is also a computer on which we check the results of medical tests before going to operating block"*.

The excessive workload leads to the distortion of work-life balance underlined by the respondents. One of the respondents during the interview described it in the following: "Currently *I spend with my seven-year old daughter about five to six hours besides weekends. Sometime I do not see my wife who is also a doctor 3–4 days per week. The worst is that I do not have time and I do not see a way out. I would like to live outside work…"*

The commitment is often identified with the feeling of responsibility for the executed work [26], a conviction that they way of executing it is particularly important. In the research both the doctors and the nurses pointed at permanent stress connected with the responsibility for health and life of patients which is additionally deepened by an excessive work.

The respondents paid also attention to the lack of managerial skills of their superiors, mainly in the field of motivating and solving conflicts, resulting first of all from the divisions between the different employees in the health sector. The respondents paid also attention to the problems resulting from the practices of autocratic management and as noticed by one of the respondents "vague authority" of the superiors. Additionally, almost 60% of the doctors and almost 65% of nurses paid attention to the "lack of sufficient support from the superiors in the difficult situations (e.g. unjustified complaint of patients). The research showed that a lack of coherent motivational systems and a lack of resources for motivational activities are important factors limiting the commitment of employees. A very big stratification of wages cause a feeling of discouragement among the employees who earn considerably less. Cultural conditions are a significant limitation to the feeling of engagement (hierarchical structures of health care facilities with "feudal" dependencies). One of the surveyed doctors summarized this a in the following way: "the main problem in our profession is this immense disparity. So, the enormity of work, effort and sacrifice that you put into this profession versus what you get in return".

# 5   Conclusions

The problems of health protection which are the consequence of the insufficient financing of this sector, lack of the staff and wrong age structure of the medical staff have their implications for the management of the employees' commitment. The building of the system which will result in a long-term commitment of medical staff becomes a real challenge in the current conditions.

In the research the attention was drawn according to the assumptions of JD-R theory to the analysis of the factors which influence the level of employees' commitment.

The research results clearly show a lack of balance between job demands and its resources, which in the consequence lead to a decrease of the affective commitment and causes a danger of a burn-out.

The low level of commitment of young doctors is particularly frightening as they are already disappointed with their work at the beginning of their career.

In this professional group the highest level of commitment is declared by the respondents between 41 and 53, more often men than women.

The identified differences between the selected groups of employees point at a necessity to take into consideration the differences in commitment management. In the context of the presented threats it must be underlined that first of all the model of specialist education should be changed as well as its organization and the way of financing. It is necessary to increase the number of places of organizing specialization conducted in the better conditions, with no need for volunteering and taking up additional jobs. The young doctors underline a lack of the feeling of safety and a possibility to plan a professional development.

Despite the popularity of the research on commitment there are little research in reference to health-care sector. The comparative research which allow for the analysis of commitment in health-care in the international perspective, mainly the research conducted in the countries of Central and Easter Europe which would allow to state whether it is reasonable to transfer the practices related to this area from the United States are also missing.

# References

1. Schaufeli, W.B., Bakker, A.B.: The conceptualization and measurement of work engagement'. In: Bakker, A.B., Leiter, M.P. (eds.) Work Engagement: A Handbook of Essential Theory and Research, pp. 10–24. Psychology Press, New York (2010)
2. Meyer, J.P., Allen, N.J.: A tree-component conceptualization on organizational commitment. Hum. Res. Manage. Rev. **1** (1991)
3. McCashland, C.R.: Core components of the service climate: linkages to customer satisfaction and profitability. Dissertation Abstracts International US: Univ. Microfilms International **60**(12-A), 89 (1999)
4. Daniel: Engagement policies boost pre-tax profits at Nationwide, pp. 1–7. Personnel Today (2004)
5. Bragg, T.: Improve employee commitment "industrial management" **44**, 18–19 (2002)
6. Harter, J.K., Schmidt, F.L., Keyes, C.L.: Well-being in the workplace and its relationship to business outcomes: a review of Gallup studies. In: Keyes, C.L. (ed.) Flourishing: The Positive Person and The Good Life. American Association Hay Group, Washington (2003)
7. Maslach, C.A: Multidimensional theory of burnout. In: Cooper C.L. (ed.) Theories of Organizational Stress. Oxford University Press, New York (1998)
8. Khan, F., Zafar S.: An empirical study of affective commitment across demographic groups in the banking sector of Pakistan. Pak. J. Commer. Soc. Sci. **7**(3), 555–563 (2013)
9. Britt, T.W., Castro, C.A., Adler, A.B.: Self-engagement, stressors, and health: a longitudinal study. Pers. Soc. Psychol. Bull. **31**(11), 1475–1486 (2005)
10. Andrew, O.C., Sofian, S.: Individual factors and work outcomes of employee engagement. Procedia – Soc. Behav. Sci. **40**, 498–508 (2012)
11. Shuck, B., Ghosh, R., Zigarmi, D., Nimon, K.: The jingle jangle of employee engagement: further exploration of the emerging construct and implications for workplace learning and performance. Hum. Res. Dev. Rev. **12**(1), 11–35 (2012)
12. Yalabik, Y.Z., Popaitoon, P., Chowne, J.A., Rayton, B.A.: Work engagement as a mediator between employee attitudes and outcomes. Int. J. Hum. Res. Manage. **24**, 2799–2823 (2013)
13. Leijten, F.R., van den Heuvel, S.G., Ybema, J.F., van der Beek, A.J., Robroek, S.J., Burdorf, A.: The influence of chronic health problems on work ability and productivity at work: a longitudinal study among older employees. Scand. J. Work Environ. Health. **40**(5), 473–482 (2014). https://doi.org/10.5271/sjweh.3444
14. Shimazu, A., Schaufeli, W.B., Kamiyama, K., Kawakami, N.: Workaholism vs. work engagement: the two different predictors of future well-being and performance. Int. J. Behav. Med. **22**(1), 18–23 (2015)

15. Schaufeli, W.B, Taris, T.W.: A critical review of the job demands-resources model: implications for improving work and health. In: Bauer, G.,F., Hämmig, O. (ed.), Bridging Occupational, Organizational and Public Health: A Transdisciplinary Approach, pp. 43–68. Springer Science + Business, Media, Dordrecht (2014)
16. Bakker, A.,B., Bal, P.M.: Weekly work engagement and performance: a study among starting teachers'. J. Occup. Organ. Psychol. **83,** pp. 189–206 (2010)
17. OECD Statistics 2017 (2017). http://www.oecd.org/els/health-systems/health-data.htm
18. Health at a Glance Europe 2016 (2016). http://www.oecd.org/health/health-at-a-glance-europe-23056088.htm
19. Zdrowie i ochrona zdrowia w 2016 roku, GUS, Warszawa (2017)
20. Lekarze w badaniach opinii społecznej 2016, Ośrodek Studiów, Analiz i Informacji Naczelnej Izby Lekarskiej, Warszawa (2016)
21. Raport "Zaufanie do zawodów". GKF, Warszawa (2016)
22. Mathieu, J., Zajac, D.: A review of meta-analyses of the antecedents, correlates and consequences of organizational commitment. Psychol. Bull. **108**(2), 171–194 (1990)
23. Ahmad, K.Z., Abu Bakar, R.: The association between training and organizational commitment among white-collar workers in Malaysia. In: Int. J. Train. Dev. **7,** 166–185 (2003)
24. Chew, I., Putti, J.: Relationship on work-related values of Singaporean and Japanese managers in Singapore. Hum. Relat. **48**(10), 1149–1170 (1995)
25. Bochner, S., Hesketh, B.: Power distance, individualism/collectivism, and job-related attitudes in a culturally diverse work group. J. Cross-Cult. Psychol. **25**(2), 233–257 (1994)

# Construction and Analysis of Database for Outer Packaging of Identical Medicine

Michiko Ohkura[1]([✉]), Yusuke Tanitsu[1], Masaomi Kimura[1],
and Fumito Tsuchiya[2]

[1] Department of Computer Science and Engineering,
Shibaura Institute of Technology, 3-7-5, Toyosu, Koto-ku, Tokyo, Japan
ohkura@sic.shibaura-it.ac.jp, {mal5055,
masaomi}@shibaura-it.ac.jp
[2] International University of Health and Welfare,
2600-1, Kitakanemaru, Ohtawara, Tochigi, Japan
tsuchiya@jshp.or.jp

**Abstract.** The objective of this research is to reduce the burden on medical staff related to the outer packaging and wrappings of medicine. Currently, generic medicines are being sold and there are multiple outer packaging kinds even for the identical medicine. For such outer packaging, various sizes and displays are adopted. The reasons why a large number of outer packaging exists among medicine are not only the variety of dosage forms and amounts but also many manufacturers and distributors of generic products. However, no research has compared the forms and the positions of the information display of the outer packaging of identical medicine. Therefore, we constructed a database of outer packaging that contains generic products of the same medicine and analyzed them by focusing on size and display. This paper describes the research results on its target medicine: Amlodipine Tablet 5 mg.

**Keywords:** Medical staff · Generic medicine · Outer packaging
Amlodipine · Size · Display

## 1 Introduction

Generic medicines are being sold worldwide in many different kinds of outer packaging even for the same medicine [1]. Various sizes and displays have been adopted for these outer packaging. That is, the reason why so many differences are found in the outer packaging for the same medicine is not only the variety of dosage forms and amount but also that there are many manufacturers and distributors of generic products.

Regarding the outer packaging of medicines, we previously constructed a database that addressed various kinds of medicines and compared their operability, resealing capability, and disposability of the packaging [2]. However, no research has compared the size and display of the outer packaging of identical medicine. Therefore, we constructed a database of such packaging that contains generic products of identical medicine and analyzed them by focusing on size and display.

This paper reports our research results with our target medicine: Amlodipine Tablet 5 mg [3].

© Springer International Publishing AG, part of Springer Nature 2019
N. J. Lightner (Ed.): AHFE 2018, AISC 779, pp. 159–167, 2019.
https://doi.org/10.1007/978-3-319-94373-2_17

# 2 Construction of a Database on Outer Packaging for Amlodipine Tablet 5 mg

## 2.1 Defining Attributes

Since no outer case database on the outer packaging of "amlodipine tablet 5 mg" exists that includes its original and generic products, we defined its attributes by referencing

**Table 1.** Attributes related to information on outer package's surface.

| # | Attribute | Explanation |
|---|---|---|
| 1 | Name of medicine | Name of medicine |
| 2 | Manufacturer | Name of manufacturer |
| 3 | Distributor | Name of distributor |
| 4 | Dosage form | Dosage form |
| 5 | Content | Content of medicine |
| 6 | Amount | Medicine amount |
| 7 | JAN code | Japanese Article Number Code |
| 8 | HOT 9 | HOT 9 number |
| 9 | HOT 13 | HOT 13 number |
| 10 | GS-1 | GS-1 number |
| 11 | Size (shortest) | The shortest literal length of outer package |
| 12 | Size (middle) | The second shortest length of outer package |
| 13 | Size (longest) | The longest length of outer package |
| 14 | Name position (front) | Position of medicine's name on largest front surface |
| 15 | Name position (back) | Position of medicine's name on largest back surface |
| 16 | Number of surfaces with name | Number of surfaces on which name is displayed |
| 17 | Content position (front) | Content position on largest front surface |
| 18 | Content position (back) | Content position on largest back surface |
| 19 | Number of surfaces with content | Number of surfaces on which content is displayed |
| 20 | Amount position (front) | Position of amount on largest front surface |
| 21 | Amount position (back) | Position of amount on largest back surface |
| 22 | Packaging unit | Packaging unit displayed on surface |
| 23 | Explanation of GS-1 | Explanation of GS-1 |
| 24 | Surfaces of expiration date and bar code | Whether the expiration date and bar code are displayed on the same surface |
| 25 | Surfaces of English only | Whether name is displayed in English |
| 26 | Powerful warning in English | Whether the warning powerful is displayed in English |
| 27 | Information that vanishes after opened | Whether information vanishes after package is opened in its intended way |
| 28 | Background color of expiration date | Background color of expiration date |
| 29–34 | Pictures | Picture of each surface |
| 35 | Surface of JAN code | Surface on which JAN code is displayed |
| 36 | Surface of GS-1 code | Surface on which GS-1 code is displayed |
| 37 | Kind of GS-1 code | Kind of GS-1 code |
| 38 | Surface of expiration date | Surface on which expiration code is displayed |
| 54 | Position of powerful warning | Display position of the warning powerful in a surface |
| 55 | Frame of powerful warning | Form of display frame of the warning powerful |

our previously constructed database [2]. The attributes we defined were divided into the following three groups:

A. Attributes related to the information on the surface of the outer packaging (40 items);
B. Attributes related to ease of opening (9 items);
C. Attributes related to ease of resealing the package and its disposal (6 items).

Tables 1, 2 and 3 show those attributes.

**Table 2.** Attributes related to ease of opening.

| # | Attribute | Explanation |
|---|---|---|
| 39 | Intended opening method | Opening method intended by pharmaceutical company |
| 40 | Number of steps | Number of steps needed to open in intended method |
| 41 | Sign to indicate the opening place | With/without a sign to indicate opening place |
| 42 | Arrow to indicate opening place | With/without an arrow to indicate opening place |
| 43 | With/without fragments | With/without fragments after package is opened in intended method |
| 44 | Surface to be opened | Surface on which to start opening |
| 45 | Side to be opened | Intended surface when a package is opened in intended method |
| 46 | Shape to be pushed | Point to be pushed |
| 47 | Versatility on dominant arm | With/without versatility based on dominant arm of user |

**Table 3.** Attributes related to ease of resealing and disposal.

| # | Attribute | Explanation |
|---|---|---|
| 48 | Capability to be resealed | With/without artifice to reseal a package |
| 49 | Device to reseal | Device to reseal a package |
| 50 | Disposability | With/without device to dispose of package |
| 51 | Device to dispose | Type of device to dispose of package |
| 52 | Device after being resealed | Device after resealed to reopen |
| 53 | Tamper-proof | With/without device to determine whether package has been opened or is unopened |

## 2.2   Construction of Database

Based on the attributes defined above, we constructed a database of the outer packaging of our target with 113 records, including the original products, Amlodin and Norvasc, and generic products as follows:

- Amlodin tablet 5 mg (2) [4]
- Amlodin OD tablet 5 mg (2) [4]
- Norvasc tablet 5 mg (2) [5]
- Norvasc OD tablet (2) [5]
- Amlodipine tablet 5 mg (57)
- Amlodipine OD tablet (48)

Each original product is distributed in sheets of 10 and 14 tablets. OD tablets are orally disintegrating pills that are taken without water.

# 3   Database Analysis

## 3.1   Size

Figures 1, 2, 3 and 4 show the following histograms: 11: size (shortest), 12: size (middle), 13: size (longest), and volume calculated from the three sizes. Figures 2 and 4 suggest that the outer packages should be divided into two groups. Based on the clustering analysis results (Ward method [6]), the outer packages were divided by 6: amount of packaging under 280 tablets and above 500 tablets. Because 100 was the most frequent amount under 280 tablets, we made a histogram for outer packaging for only 100 tablets (Fig. 5). Because 700 was the most frequent amount above 500, we made a histogram for outer packaging for only for 700 tablets (Fig. 6). In both the histograms of Figs. 5 and 6, the largest outer packaging is more than twice as big as the smallest ones. These histograms suggest that varieties of outer packaging exist for only one amount of the same medicine, which increases the time required time to deal with by medical staff.

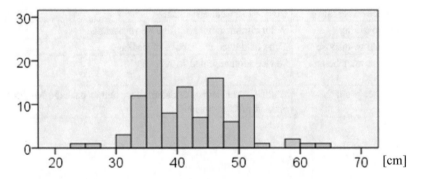

**Fig. 1.** Histogram of 11: size (shortest).

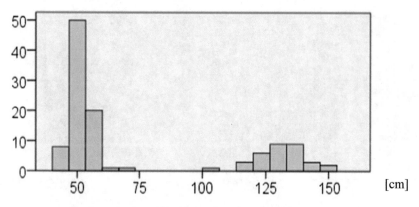

**Fig. 2.** Histogram of 12: size (middle).

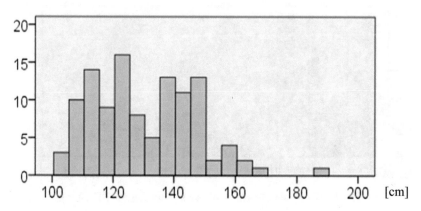

**Fig. 3.** Histogram of 13: size (longest).

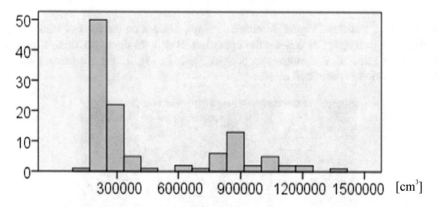

**Fig. 4.** Histogram of volume.

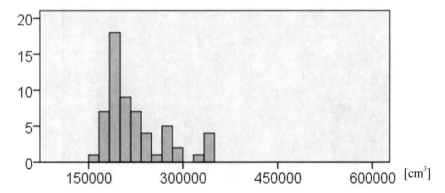

**Fig. 5.** Histogram of volume of outer packaging for 100 tablets

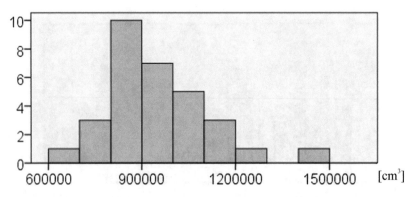

**Fig. 6.** Histogram of volume of outer packaging for 700 tablets

## 3.2 Display Position

**Definition of Position.** Figure 7 defines display positions on the front or back surface of the outer packaging. A denotes the upper left, B denotes the upper right, C denotes the bottom left and D denotes the bottom right. In Fig. 7, the medicine's name's display position is described as AB.

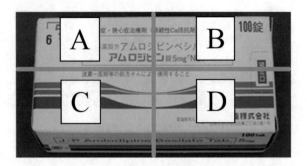

**Fig. 7.** Definitions of display positions

**Table 4.** Frequency distribution of name position.

| Position | Frequency |
|---|---|
| No display | 23 |
| A | 11 |
| B | 2 |
| C | 8 |
| AB | 109 |
| AC | 10 |
| CD | 24 |
| ABCD | 29 |
| Total | 226 |

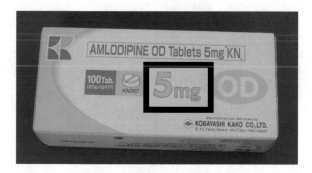

**Fig. 8.** Example of content display

**Table 5.** Frequency distribution of content display.

| Position | Frequency |
|---|---|
| No display | 17 |
| A | 23 |
| B | 26 |
| C | 58 |
| D | 70 |
| AC | 7 |
| BD | 13 |
| CD | 11 |
| ABCD | 1 |
| Total | 226 |

**Display Position of Name.** Table 4 shows the frequency distribution of positions of the front and back surfaces calculated from 14: name position (front) and 15: name position (back). AB (upper) is the most frequent position for the name display. However, the ratio of AB is less than 50% and varieties of display positions of names are recognized. Because the medicine's name is the most vital piece of information, such a variety of display position heavily burdens medical staff.

**Display Position of Content.** Figure 8 shows an example of content display. Table 5 shows the frequency distribution of the positions for the front and back surfaces calculated from 17: content position (front) and 18: content position (back). A display in one area (A, B, C, or D) is more frequent than in a combination of areas such as AB and AC. D is the most common position, and C is second.

**Display Position of Amount.** Table 6 shows the frequency distribution of the positions for the front and back surfaces calculated from 20: amount position (front) and 21: amount position (back). B (upper right) is the most frequent position for the display of amount.

**Table 6.** Frequency distribution of position of amount.

| Position | Frequency |
|------------|-----------|
| No display | 16 |
| A | 32 |
| B | 139 |
| C | 11 |
| D | 12 |
| AB | 2 |
| AC | 3 |
| BD | 3 |
| CD | 2 |
| Total | 226 |

**Combination of Display Positions.** From a crosstab of the information (name, content, and amount) and display positions, the number of combinations was 58. The frequency combinations are shown in Table 7.

**Table 7.** Frequency combinations of information positions.

| Order | Name position | Content position | Amount position | Frequency |
|-------|---------------|------------------|-----------------|-----------|
| 1 | Upper (AB) | D | B | 28 |
| 2 | Bottom (CD) | D | B | 18 |
| 3 | Upper (AB) | C | B | 16 |
| 4 | Center (ABCD) | D | B | 13 |

## 4   Discussion

From our analysis of the size results, we found various sizes of outer packaging even for the same amount of our target medicine. Such different forms of outer packaging increase the burden on pharmacists. From our analysis of the display position results of the information, we identified 58 display combinations only for the medicine. Such a variety of information displays of outer packaging also increases the burden on pharmacists.

As the use of generic medicines continues to rise pharmacists must deal with many more types of medicines. We employed "Amlodipine Tablet 5 mg" as our research target because it has many generic products in Japan. Its outer packaging has over 100 different forms as well as various positions of information display. Japanese industrial products are standardized by Japanese Industrial Standards (JIS). However, there are no standards for medicine, even those made in factories. Amlodipine tablets are sometimes found in databases of medical incidents. The meaningless variety of the outer packaging of this medicine increases the burden on pharmacists and causes medical incidents. For both our target medicine and other medicines, we argue for the standardization of the forms and the information display in outer packaging to reduce the burden on pharmacists, lower medical costs, and increase safety for patients.

## 5   Conclusion

We constructed a database of outer packaging that contains the generic products of identical medicine and analyzed it by size and display. From our analysis results, we found many kinds of outer packaging of various sizes and different display positions of information even for the same amount of a medicine. We believe that the meaningless variety of outer packaging increases the burden on pharmacists and might cause medical incidents. We strongly propose standardization of the forms and the positions of the information displayed on outer packaging to reduce the burden on pharmacists, lower medical expenses, and increase safety for patients.

## References

1. Generic Drugs Saving in the U.S. http://www.gphaonline.org/media/wysiwyg/PDF/GPhA_Savings_Report_2015.pdf
2. Yoshimi, H., Muraoka, H., Izumiya, A., Kimura, M., Ohkura, M., Tsuchiya, F.: Construction and analysis of database on outer cases of medicines. In: Jacko, J.A. (ed.) Human-Computer Interaction -Design and Development Approaches-. LNCS, vol. 6761, pp. 226–234. Springer, Heidelberg (2011)
3. Amlodipine Besylate. https://www.webmd.com/drugs/2/drug-5891/amlodipine-oral/details
4. Amlodin Guide. (in Japanese). http://kanja.ds-pharma.jp/products/pdf/amlodin_tab_guide.pdf
5. Norvasc. https://www.rxlist.com/norvasc-drug.htm
6. Ward Jr., J.H.: Hierarchical grouping to optimize an objective function. J. Am. Stat. Assoc. **58** (301), 236–244 (1963)

# Ergonomics Risk Assessment of Musculoskeletal Disorders (MSD) During Simulated Endotracheal Intubation in Hospital Universiti Sains Malaysia (HUSM)

Shaik Farid Abdull Wahab[1(✉)], Mohamad Hamzi Mohd Noor[1], and Rohayu Othman[2]

[1] School of Medical Sciences, Universiti Sains Malaysia,
Kubang Kerian, 15160 Kota Bharu, Kelantan, Malaysia
drsfarid@usm.my, yutaka_mejie@yahoo.co.uk
[2] Universiti Malaysia Kelantan,
Locked Bag 01, 16300 Bachok, Kelantan, Malaysia
Aiman_shaik@yahoo.com

**Abstract.** Endotracheal intubation is an important procedure in emergency medicine. This procedure is done as a method to secure the airway of patient during cardiac arrest. Body posture during intubation may cause musculoskeletal disorders, but doctor do not have awareness about effect of ergonomic factors on their health. There is a rise in prevalence of work related musculoskeletal disorder (MSD) in medical personnel performing any procedure due to lack of physical ergonomic. There is little evidence on optimum bed level for intubation in association with ergonomic body posture. This study was performed to evaluate the effect of different bed level during endotracheal intubation on ergonomic risk using REBA methods and to find optimum level for intubation with less risk of MSD. This cross sectional study was performed among 30 emergency residents using REBA methods. This study has been carried out at red zone of accident and emergency department Hospital Universiti Sains Malaysia, Kota Bharu, Kelantan. During this study, 30 doctors were asked to performed endotracheal intubation using a mannequin at 3 different bed levels: supra pubic, umbilical and sub-xyphoid level. At each level, their body posture was recorded and score were given based on REBA. We compared mean REBA score for each level. This study showed that high risk and very high risk for MSD when intubation was performed at the level of supra-pubic and umbilical. However, the score for sub-xyphoid was low risk for MSD. As a conclusion, we should advise the medical personnel to intubate patient at a sub-xyphoid level.

**Keywords:** Endotracheal intubation · Ergonomics · REBA
Musculoskeletal disorders

© Springer International Publishing AG, part of Springer Nature 2019
N. J. Lightner (Ed.): AHFE 2018, AISC 779, pp. 168–174, 2019.
https://doi.org/10.1007/978-3-319-94373-2_18

# 1 Introduction

The respiratory system consists of the lung and a series of the airways that connects the lung to the external environment. Airway can be divided into upper airways and lower airways. Upper airways consist of the nasal cavity, pharynx and the larynx. The lower airway tracts consist of the trachea, bronchi, and lung.

In an emergency setting, maintaining airway patency takes priority over the management of all other conditions. The Inadequate airway will cause reduced oxygen delivery to vital organs like the brain, heart, and kidneys. Irreversible brain damage will occur within 4 min without oxygen. Inadequate airway is usually caused by soft tissue obstruction, foreign body, and laryngospasm. There are few methods of opening and maintaining the airways patency. First by manual maneuvers like jaw thrust and chin lift. Second is by using airway adjunct like oropharyngeal or nasopharyngeal airway. Lastly is by definitive airway. Definitive airway can be divided into endotracheal intubation and surgical airway.

Definitive airway means a tube is placed in the trachea with cuff inflated below the vocal cords. The tube connected to some oxygen enriched assisted ventilation and the airway is secure in place with tape. The criteria for establishing a definitive airway are based on clinical findings which included (a) an airway problem in which there is inability to maintain a patent airway by other techniques such as jaw thrust and oropharyngeal airway, with impending or potential airway compromise in conditions like facial fractures, following inhalational injury and retropharyngeal hematoma, (b) patient had breathing problems such as the inability to maintain adequate oxygenation by face mask supplementation and presence of apnea, failure oxygenation like severe pulmonary edema and failure to ventilation such as status asthmatics, (c) disability problems such as presence of closed head injury Glasgow coma scale 8 or less requiring assisted ventilation, need to protect the lower airways from aspiration of blood or vomitus or sustained seizures activity.

Once it has been decided that the patient requires intubation based on the above mentioned 3 indications, endotracheal intubation is the most reliable way to ensure oxygenation, ventilation, and prevention of aspiration during emergency airway management. The urgency of the situation and the circumstances indicating the need for airway intervention dictate the specific route and method to be used, whether crash intubation or rapid sequence intubation (RSI). Crash intubation is considered when the patient intubated without pre-treatment, induction or paralysis instituted. Usually patients who present cardiorespiratory arrest or are in extremis with agonal efforts, the airway needs to be secured immediately. RSI is the administration, after pre-oxygenate, of potent induction agent followed by a rapidly neuromuscular blocking agent to induce unconsciousness and motor paralysis for endotracheal intubation. In the absence of an identified crash or difficult intubation, RSI is the method of choice for managing the emergency airway.

In the adult male, endotracheal tube (ETT) size is usually 8–9 mm internal diameter and the female 7–8 mm. Endotracheal intubation is usually performed in resuscitation zone, with the patient in the supine position, the clinician used their left hand to hold laryngoscope. Insert it into the right side of the patient mouth and displace the tongue to the left. Follow the base of the tongue until epiglottis is visualized, lift the laryngoscope upwards and forward without using wrist movement. This maneuver should bring the epiglottis into view. Gently insert the ETT through the vocal cord into tracheas. Inflate the cuff until expiratory leak just disappears. Check the placement of ETT and continue bag valve mask tube ventilation. Secure the ETT once intubation had been successfully performed and position confirmed. Proceed with post-intubation management. A failed intubation is defined as 2 failed attempts by experienced physician. It is not a procedure without complication, the most common complication is failed intubation, airways trauma, tube malposition and aspiration gastric content or blood. Endotracheal intubation is a common lifesaving procedure done in an emergency setting, typically performed by a medical assistant, nurse, and doctor. Competency in endotracheal intubation requires significant training and clinical experience. Failure to establish airways patency associated with morbidity and mortality. There is a rise in prevalence of work-related musculoskeletal disorder (MSD) in medical personnel performing any procedure due to lack of physical ergonomic [1]. Ergonomics is an applied science concerned with designing and arranging things people use so that the people and things interact most efficiently and safely, also called biotechnology, human engineering, human factors [2, 3]. Currently, insufficient data is available to describe the physical ergonomic with the effect of patient position (hospital bed level) for successful intubation [4]. Textbooks usually describe how to position of head and neck of the patient and how to insert laryngoscope, but do not provide the best patient position for endotracheal intubation. Improper patient positioning (bed level) forces the health personnel to have awkward body postures while doing the procedure during intubation [5]. The objective of this study is to suggest the optimum bed level for intubation that can reduce the risk of musculoskeletal disorder among healthcare personnel at the emergency department. The Musculoskeletal disorder can be assessed using Rapid Entire Body Assessment (REBA).

## 2   Research Methodology

This cross-sectional study was performed among 30 emergency residents using REBA methods. This study has been carried out at red zone of accident and emergency department Hospital Universiti Sains Malaysia, Kota Bharu, Kelantan. 30 emergency residents voluntarily participated in this study. Each participant require intubate the trachea of a mannequin using a size 3 Macintosh blade and endotracheal tube (ETT) size 8 with styled inside. The mannequin was placed over adjustable hospital bed. Participant is required to perform a procedure at 3 difference bed level which is supra-pubic, umbilical and sub-xyphoid. The researcher started the video recording and assisted the participant by passing the devices required. A trial is finish when the cuff of the ETT was inflated, the laryngoscope is removed. Video recording is put on left sided due to laryngoscope is always hold with the left hand, upper arm and wrist measurement always refer to the left side of a participant. All filming is using canon camcorder placed on tripod in a standard position. A video image is capture at the moment of intubation and the images put as anonymous and coded. From the images capture, the worse body posture is taken for each level. From that posture selected, the degrees of joint flexion (angles) is measure using protractor from the line perpendicular to the long axis of the arm, neck, lower back and leg and scores it into REBA work sheet. At each level, their body posture was recorded and score were given based on REBA. We calculate mean REBA score for each level and compared it to find the optimum bed level associated with ergonomic body posture.

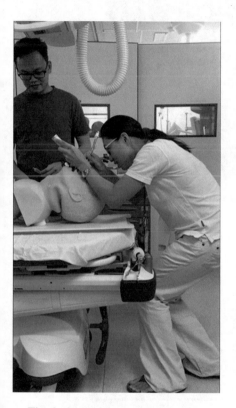
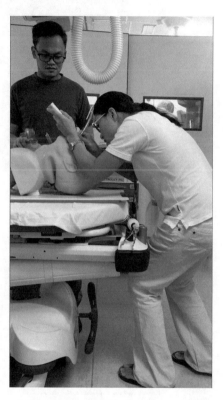

**Fig. 1.** Intubation at supra-pubic level        **Fig. 2.** Intubation at umbilical level

# 3   Result

The aim of the present study was to compare the effects on body posture angles in intubating person at 3 difference bed level. The body posture angles were calculated by using REBA score system. During the study, REBA scores were calculated and recorded on REBA worksheet for each of the participants at 3 difference level. Table below showed REBA scores for each of the participant for each level (Figs. 1, 2 and 3).

Table 1 shows result of REBA score for 30 participants for each level. There were a significant mean difference of REBA between groups with the p-value < 0.001. The mean of REBA for supra-pubic level was highest with 10.60(0.89) of mean and standard deviation respectively. The mean of REBA for sub-xyphoid was 3.17 and 8.33 for umbilical level. The intubation at sub-xyphoid level resulted in smaller deflection

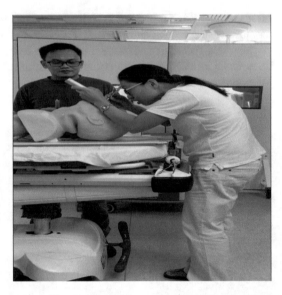

**Fig. 3.** Intubation at sub-xyphoid level

**Table 1.** REBA scores for the emergency residents performing endotracheal intubation

| Participants | Supra-pubic level | Umbilical level | Sub-xyphoid level |
|---|---|---|---|
| 1 | 12 | 10 | 4 |
| 2 | 11 | 10 | 4 |
| 3 | 11 | 9 | 4 |
| 4 | 11 | 8 | 2 |
| 5 | 10 | 8 | 3 |
| 6 | 11 | 10 | 4 |
| 7 | 9 | 7 | 5 |
| 8 | 10 | 9 | 4 |
| 9 | 8 | 6 | 2 |
| 10 | 9 | 8 | 3 |
| 11 | 11 | 9 | 3 |
| 12 | 11 | 9 | 1 |
| 13 | 11 | 8 | 1 |
| 14 | 12 | 10 | 3 |
| 15 | 11 | 9 | 4 |
| 16 | 11 | 8 | 4 |
| 17 | 11 | 9 | 3 |
| 18 | 11 | 8 | 4 |
| 19 | 11 | 8 | 3 |
| 20 | 11 | 8 | 4 |
| 21 | 11 | 8 | 4 |

(*continued*)

**Table 1.** (*continued*)

| Participants | Supra-pubic level | Umbilical level | Sub-xyphoid level |
|---|---|---|---|
| 22 | 11 | 8 | 4 |
| 23 | 9 | 7 | 3 |
| 24 | 11 | 10 | 3 |
| 25 | 10 | 7 | 1 |
| 26 | 10 | 9 | 5 |
| 27 | 11 | 5 | 1 |
| 28 | 11 | 8 | 4 |
| 29 | 11 | 10 | 2 |
| 30 | 10 | 7 | 3 |

for all 6 posture angles compared to the others level. In particular, less flexion of the trunk and neck result more erect position; less flexion of the knees, lower arm and wrist resulted in a significantly lower REBA score (MEAN 3.17) (see figure c). This gave a rounded score of 3 (Table 3) for intubation at sub-xyphoid level which indicate low risk. Additional analysis revealed intubation at supra-pubic and umbilical level caused participant to twist the neck, bend of the trunk and flexed the legs resulted higher REBA score. Mean REBA scores for supra-pubic and umbilical level were high risk for musculoskeletal disorder. From an ergonomic point of view, intubation at level of sub-xyphoid should be preferred over umbilical and supra-pubic level (Table 2).

**Table 2.** Comparisons mean REBA score and standard deviation for 3 difference level:

| Variables | Supra-pubic Mean (SD) | Umbilical Mean (SD) | Sub-xyphoid Mean (SD) | F-test (df) | p-value |
|---|---|---|---|---|---|
| Reba | 10.60(0.89) | 8.33(1.24) | 3.17(1.15) | 357.27 (2,87) | <0.001 |

**Table 3.** REBA scoring

| 1 | Negligible risk |
|---|---|
| 2–3 | Low risk, change may be needed |
| 4–7 | Medium risk. Further investigate. Change soon |
| 8–10 | High risk. Investigate and implement change |
| 11+ | Very high risk. Implement change |

# 4  Discussion

Tracheal intubation is the most frequent procedures performed for management of airways in the emergency department. There is a lot of thing need to consider when performing endotracheal intubation, we might consider anatomical difficult airway, physiological difficult airway and psychological of the person performing the procedure. This study concerned with the obstacle of bed height. Experts have recommended that bed level heights be adjusted so the patient's head level at the lower portion of the performer sternum [2]. However, there are no scientific data to support this suggestion. Aiming to improve the body posture during tracheal intubation, we compared the effect of bed level and body postures angles and assessed using the REBA postural assessment tool. As expected, intubation at sub-xyphoid level associated a more ergonomic body posture and lower REBA scores. One limitation of the study is that, we are using simulated setting and there are differences between human airways and manikin airways.

# 5  Conclusion

In this study, we more accurately tested the differences in bed height on ergonomic body postures. The result showed more ergonomic body posture when intubating at sub-xyphoid level. Applications of this finding could contribute to the improvement of endotracheal intubation training within medical students [6].

# References

1. De Laveaga, A., Wadman, M.C., Wirth, L., Hallbeck, M.S.: Ergonomics of novices and experts during simulated endotracheal intubation. Work 41(Supplement 1), 4692–4698 (2012)
2. Lee, H.C., Yun, M.J., Hwang, J.W., Na, H.S., Kim, D.H., Park, J.Y.: Higher operating tables provide better laryngeal views for tracheal intubation. BJA: Br. J. Anaesth. 112(4), 749–755 (2014)
3. Hignett, S., McAtamney, L.: Rapid entire body assessment (REBA). Appl. Ergon. 31(2), 201–205 (2000)
4. Oh, J.H.: Effects of bed height on the performance of endotracheal intubation and bag mask ventilation. Signa vitae: J. Intensive Care Emerg. Med. 12(1), 47–51 (2016)
5. Matthews, A.J., Johnson, C.J.H., Goodman, N.W.: Body posture during simulated tracheal intubation. Anaesthesia 53(4), 331–334 (1998)
6. Caldiroli, D.F.M., Sommariva, A., Frittoli, S., Guanziroli, E., Cortellazzi, P., Orena, E.F.: Upper limb muscular activity and perceived workload during laryngoscopy: comparison of Glidescopew and Macintosh laryngoscopy in manikin: an observational study. Br. J. Anaesthesia 112(3), 563–569 (2014)

# Risk of Musculoskeletal Disorders (MSD) in Rescuer Performing CPR at Kneeling, Standing and Step-on-Stool Position

Shaik Farid Abdull Wahab[1]([✉]), Nurul Husna Abdul Ghani[1], and Rohayu Othman[2]

[1] School of Medical Sciences, Universiti Sains Malaysia, Kubang Kerian, 16150 Kota Bharu, Kelantan, Malaysia
drsfarid@usm.my, nanurul85@gmail.com
[2] Kolej Kemahiran Tinggi MARA, Lubok Jong, 1700 Pasir Mas, Kelantan, Malaysia
aiman_shaik@yahoo.com

**Abstract.** CPR is a live-saving procedure commonly performed in emergency department. Chest compression is a crucial component of CPR requires the rescuer to provide large force at certain rate. Emergency medical staff frequently needs to perform CPR in uncomfortable and awkward position such as kneeling on the floor or stretcher, standing in moving ambulance and standing on step-stool. Musculoskeletal pain and fatigue are often reported among rescuer after performing. The study aimed to assess the ergonomic risk factor of musculoskeletal disorders in rescuer performing chest compression at 3 different positions: kneeling, standing and step-on-stool. A cross-sectional study involving 30 participants consist of emergency doctors, nurses and paramedic was carried out in Emergency and Trauma Department of Hospital Universiti Sains Malaysia, Kelantan. All participants were required to perform chest compression on mannequin each at kneeling, standing and step-on-stool position. Participants are video graphed while performing high-quality CPR. Ergonomic risk score is assessed by using Rapid Entire Body Assessment (REBA) tool. This study showed that the highest mean REBA score recorded at kneeling position, followed by standing position and step-on-stool position. Mean REBA score at all 3 positions belongs to high risk group and it is necessary to further investigate and implement change as soon as possible.

**Keywords:** CPR · Ergonomics · REBA · Musculoskeletal disorders

## 1 Introduction

Emergency department is known as one of the hectic area in a hospital as it constantly receives patients all day long. Emergency doctors and paramedics work under constant stress with increasing number of visits to emergency room. Prolonged physical stress has contributed to burnout among emergency healthcare workers [1], thus necessitate further action to provide ergonomic working environment to avoid bad implication on the emergency medical services.

© Springer International Publishing AG, part of Springer Nature 2019
N. J. Lightner (Ed.): AHFE 2018, AISC 779, pp. 175–182, 2019.
https://doi.org/10.1007/978-3-319-94373-2_19

Cardiopulmonary resuscitation is a basic life saving procedure commonly performed in emergency department. It is recognized as one of the highest physically demanding task to perform [2]. Due to unpredictable nature of cases encountered, paramedics often need to perform CPR at various position including kneeling on the floor or stretcher, standing on moving ambulance and standing on step-stool to accommodate person managing the airway of patient. Component of CPR comprises of repetitive movement of joint in awkward position to deliver adequate force to produce chest deflection.

Combination of above mentioned factors has raised concern regarding the effect of CPR on emergency healthcare workers particularly risk of developing work-related musculoskeletal disorder (WMSD). There are many studies carried out aiming to improve quality of CPR delivered to the patient, however little is known about the effect of CPR on the rescuer. With increase of workload, ageing of workforce and economic impact of work-related musculoskeletal disorder (WMSD), it is crucial to explore the ergonomics of emergency healthcare to reduce the mismatch.

This study will look into the ergonomic risk of developing MSD using REBA score in 3 most frequent position of rescuer during CPR to recognize the best position for CPR and worse position for CPR to avoid compromising healthcare worker safety and health.

## 2   Research Methodology

This cross-sectional study has been carried out in Emergency and Trauma Department of Hospital Universiti Sains Malaysia, Kelantan involving 30 participants comprises of medical officers, paramedics and staff nurse. Each participant are required to perform 2 min continous chest compression on mannequin at kneeling, standing and on step-stool position. CPR at kneeling position requires participant to kneel on right side of mannequin which was put on the floor while performing CPR. CPR at standing position requires participant to stand on right side of mannequin which located on bed with height of 54 cm (lowest height of bed in resuscitation area). CPR on step-stool position requires participant to stand on step-stool with height of 34 cm which is placed beside the bed. Participants were videographed while performing high-quality CPR as per recommendation by American Heart Association (AHA) in Basic Life Support 2015. REBA score was used to evaluate the risk of MSD for each participant. REBA score was choosen as it is a universal ergonomic assessment tool that was designed for easy use and evaluator does not require advanced degree in ergonomic to do the scoring [3].

## 3   Result

Table 1 shows demographic details of study participants. The age of participants ranged from 20–39 years (mean = 28.3 years, SD = 5.762). Mean BMI was 22.58 (SD = 3.94, range = 16.4–35.0). 19 males (63.3%) and 11 females (36.7%) involved in this study. The mean weight and height of participants were 62.22 kg (SD = 12.57) and 1.66 m (SD = 0.09) respectively. 56.7% of participants were medical officers, 40% were paramedic and 3.3% was staff nurse. 43.3% of all participants have working experience of more than 5 years.

**Table 1.** Demographic details of participant (n = 30)

| Variables | | |
|---|---|---|
| Gender (n %) | Male | 19 (63.3) |
| | Female | 11 (36.7) |
| Age (years) | Mean (SD) | 28.3 (5.76) |
| | Range | 20–39 |
| Height (m) | Mean (SD) | 1.66 (0.09) |
| | Range | 148–180 |
| Weight (kg) | Mean (SD) | 62.22 (12.57) |
| | Range | 37–90 |
| BMI (kg/m2) | Mean (SD) | 22.58 (3.94) |
| | Range | 16.4–35 |
| Designation (n %) | MO | 17 (56.7) |
| | Paramedic | 12 (40.0) |
| | Staff nurse | 1 (3.3) |
| Working experience | <2 years | 13 (43.3) |
| | 2–5 years | 4 (13.3) |
| | >5 years | 13 (43.3) |

Highest mean REBA score is recorded at kneeling position (9.6, SD = 1.10), followed by standing position (9.33, SD = 0.96) and step-stool position (8.33, SD = 1.54). Figures 1, 2 and 3 show positions of rescuer at kneeling, standing and step-stool while performing CPR.

At kneeling position, all participants scored 3 for trunk position indicating flexion of trunk in range between 20–60°. For legs they scored 3 due to flexion of both knee more than 60°. This factor contributed to highest mean A score compared to other position which is 7.3 (SD = 0.54). For upper arm position, majority of participant (66.7%) score 3; flexion of shoulder at 45–90° (+3) with shoulder raise (+1) which is deducted by 1 as participants were seen leaning during compression. Table 2 shows distribution of REBA score according to body parts at kneeling position.

At standing position, majority of participants scored 2+ for neck position (63.3%) indication flexion of neck >20° which contributed to highest mean score of neck position compared to other position (1.97, SD = 0.61). 53.3% participants scored 4+ for upper arm position contributed by flexion of shoulder between 45–90% with addition of +1 score due to raised shoulder. No leaning noted in all participants and majority had to tiptoe in order to keep upper limb perpendicular to mannequin's chest wall which lead to highest mean score B of 5.50 (SD = 0.51). Table 3 shows distribution of REBA score according to body parts at standing position.

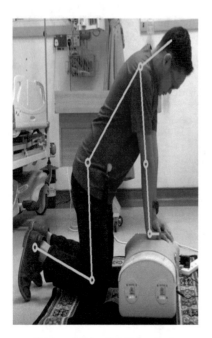

**Fig. 1.** CPR at kneeling position

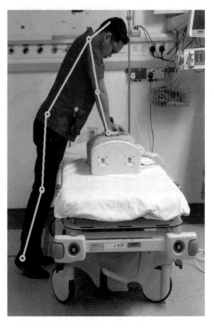

**Fig. 2.** CPR at standing position

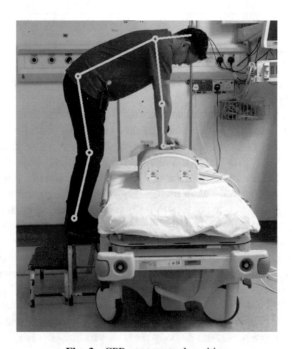

**Fig. 3.** CPR at step-stool position

**Table 2.** Distribution of REBA score for participant at kneeling

| | REBA score | | | | | | | | | | | | Mean |
|---|---|---|---|---|---|---|---|---|---|---|---|---|---|
| | 1 n (%) | 2 n (%) | 3 n (%) | 4 n (%) | 5 n (%) | 6 n (%) | 7 n (%) | 8 n (%) | 9 n (%) | 10 n (%) | 11 n (%) | 12 n (%) | (SD) |
| Neck | 22 (73.3) | 7 (23.3) | 1 (3.3) | | | | | | | | | | 1.3 (0.54) |
| Trunk | | | 30 (100) | | | | | | | | | | 3 (0.0) |
| Leg | | | 30 (100) | | | | | | | | | | 3 (0.0) |
| Upper arm | 10 (33.3) | 20 (66.7) | | | | | | | | | | | 2.67 (0.48) |
| Lower arm | 30 (100) | | | | | | | | | | | | 2 (0.0) |
| Wrist | 30 (100) | | | | | | | | | | | | 2 (0.0) |
| A score | | | | | | 22 (73.3) | 7 (23.3) | 1 (3.3) | | | | | 7.3 (0.54) |
| B score | | | 10 (33.3) | | 20 (66.7) | | | | | | | | 4.33 (0.96) |
| Grand score | | | | | | | | 8 (26.7) | 2 (6.7) | 14 (46.7) | 6 (20) | | 9.60 (1.10) |

**Table 3.** Distribution of REBA score at standing position

| | REBA score | | | | | | | | | | | | Mean |
|---|---|---|---|---|---|---|---|---|---|---|---|---|---|
| | 1 n (%) | 2 n (%) | 3 n (%) | 4 n (%) | 5 n (%) | 6 n (%) | 7 n (%) | 8 n (%) | 9 n (%) | 10 n (%) | 11 n (%) | 12 n (%) | (SD) |
| Neck | 6 (20.0) | 19 (63.3) | 5 (16.7) | | | | | | | | | | 1.97 (0.61) |
| Trunk | | | 30 (100) | | | | | | | | | | 3.0 (0.0) |
| Leg | 15 (50.0) | 15 (50.0) | | | | | | | | | | | 1.50 (0.51) |
| Upper arm | | | 14 (46.7) | 16 (53.3) | | | | | | | | | 3.53 (0.51) |
| Lower arm | | 30 (100) | | | | | | | | | | | 2.0 (0.0) |
| Wrist | 1 (3.3) | 29 (96.7) | | | | | | | | | | | 1.97 (0.18) |
| A score | | | 2 (6.7) | | 14 (46.7) | 13 (43.3) | 1 (3.3) | | | | | | 6.37 (0.85) |
| B score | | | | 15 (50.0) | 15 (50.0) | | | | | | | | 5.50 (0.51) |
| Grand score | | | | | 1 (3.3) | 1 (3.3) | | 14 (46.7) | 13 (43.3) | 1 (3.3) | | | 9.33 (0.96) |

At step-stool position, 30% of participant score 4+ for trunk position which means flexion of trunk of >60% (mostly noted in taller participants). This has contributed to highest mean score of trunk position compared to other position (3.3, SD = 0.47). Mean A score is the lowest which is 6.07 (SD = 1.34) and mean B score is 4.53 (SD = 0.89). CPR at step-stool position has the lowest mean REBA score of 8.33 (1.54). Table 4 shows distribution of REBA score according to body parts at step-stool position.

**Table 4.** Distribution of REBA score at step-stool position

| | REBA score | | | | | | | | | | | | Mean |
|---|---|---|---|---|---|---|---|---|---|---|---|---|---|
| | 1 n (%) | 2 n (%) | 3 n (%) | 4 n (%) | 5 n (%) | 6 n (%) | 7 n (%) | 8 n (%) | 9 n (%) | 10 n (%) | 11 n (%) | 12 n (%) | (SD) |
| Neck | 21 (70.0) | 8 (26.7) | 1 (3.3) | | | | | | | | | | 1.33 (0.55) |
| Trunk | | | 21 (70.0) | 9 (30.0) | | | | | | | | | 3.30 (0.47) |
| Leg | 16 (53.3) | 6 (20.0) | 8 (26.7) | | | | | | | | | | 1.73 (0.87) |
| Upper arm | | 7 (23.3) | 23 (76.7) | | | | | | | | | | 2.77 (0.43) |
| Lower arm | | 30 (100) | | | | | | | | | | | 2.0 (0.0) |
| Wrist | | 29 (96.7) | 1 (3.3) | | | | | | | | | | 2.03 (0.18) |
| A score | | | | 6 (20.0) | 3 (10.0) | 8 (26.7) | 9 (30.0) | 4 (13.3) | | | | | 6.07 (1.34) |
| B score | 1 (3.3) | 5 (16.7) | 1 (3.3) | 23 (76.7) | | | | | | | | | 4.53 (0.89) |
| Grand score | | | | | | 6 (20.0) | 3 (10.0) | 4 (13.3) | 11 (36.7) | 4 (13.3) | 2 (6.7) | | 8.33 (1.54) |

# 4  Discussion

Study findings showed that CPR at kneeling, standing and step-stool position predisposed the rescuer to the risk of developing musculoskeletal disease (MSD) based on the REBA score. All 3 positions have mean REBA score which belong to high risk group that require investigation and changes as soon as possible. Heavy physical work, repetitive movement at awkward position with are the important elements contributing to WMSD [4]. According to Trowbridge 2009, in order to achieve adequate chest deflection, rescuer need to apply up to 530 N in which the force is transmitted across the wrist. CPR involves repeated lifting of trunk and upper body in order to deliver adequate force to produce compression across the chest wall. This exertion creates large force over L5-S1 vertebra which is the most vulnerable region for back injury [5].

CPR at kneeling position showed the least ergonomic position for the rescuer despite previous studies that favour kneeling in term of achieving good quality of chest compression [6–8]. It is commonly taught in CPR courses and training and frequently adapted by the paramedic in prehospital care. Further evaluation is needed in term of optimizing the safety for both parties: the patient and rescuer while performing CPR.

Limitation of this study is that it did not investigate the effectiveness of CPR at 3 different positions. However, Bonnes et al. in 2015 in a meta-analysis of non-randomized studies showed a benefit in favour of mechanical device in term of survival to admission compared to manual CPR [9]. Giving that all 3 positions of CPR showed high REBA score, inclusion of mechanical device in prehospital care thus seen as modality to improve outcome of patient and simultaneously improving the ergonomic aspect of the rescuer duty.

## 5 Conclusion

Although the sample size of the study is small, it managed to address the need of further exploration in improving emergency medical service from ergonomic point of view in order to maintain excellent care for the community. Poor ergonomic aspect of CPR should be looked as a crucial indicator for assimilation of mechanical device as advancement in medical technology in helping medical healthcare worker to provide better care for the people.

## References

1. Willem Stassen, B.V.N., Stein, C.: Burnout among advanced life support paramedics in Johannesburg, South Africa. Emerg. Med. J. **2013**(30), 331–333 (2012). https://doi.org/10.1136/emermed-2011-200920
2. Fischer, T.L., Renee, K.E.S., MacPhee, S.: The ottawa paramedic service (OPS) research team (2017). Identifying the critical physical demanding task of paramedic work: towards the development of a physical employment standard. Appl. Ergon. **65**, 233–239 (2017). https://doi.org/10.1016/j.apergo.2017.06.021
3. Dima Al Madani, A.D.: Rapid entire body assessment: a literature review. Am. J. Eng. Appl. Sci. **9**(1), 107–118 (2016)
4. da Costa, B.R., Vieira, E.R.: Risk factor for work-related musculoskeletal disorders: a systematic review of recent longitudinal studies. Am. J. Ind. Med. **58**, 285–323 (2010). https://doi.org/10.1002/ajim.20750
5. Jones, A.Y.M., Lee, R.Y.W.: Cardiopulmonary resuscitation and back injury in ambulance officers. Int. Arch. Occup. Environ. Health. **78**, 332–336 (2005). https://doi.org/10.1007/s00420-004-0577-3
6. Hong, C.K., Park, S.O., Jeong, H.H., Kim, J.H., Lee, N.K., Lee, Y., Lee, J.H., Hwang, S.Y.: The most effective rescuer's position for cardiopulmonary resuscitation provided to patients on beds: a randomized, controlled, crossover mannequin study. J. Emerg. Med. **46**(5), 643–649 (2014). https://doi.org/10.1016/j.jemermed.2013.08.085
7. Chi, C.H., Tsou, J.Y., Su, F.C.: Effects of rescuer position on the kinematics of cardiopulmonary resuscitation (CPR) and force of delivered compression. Resuscitation **76**, 69–75 (2007). https://doi.org/10.1016/j.resuscitation.2007.06.007

8. Yasuda, Y., Kato, Y., Sugimoto, K., Tanaka, S., Tsunoda, N., Kumagawa, D., Toyokuni, Y., Kubota, K., Inaba, H.: Muscle used for chest compression under static and transportation conditions. Prehospital Emerg. Care **17**(2), 162–169 (2013). https://doi.org/10.3109/10903127.2012.749964

9. Bonnes, J.L., Brouwer, M.A., Navarese, E.P., Verhaert, D.V., Verheugt, F.W., Smeets, J.L., de Boer, M.J.: Manual cardiopulmonary resuscitation versus CPR including a mechanical chest compression device in out-of-hospital cardiac arrect: a comprehensive meta-analysis from randomized and observational studies. Ann. Emerg. Med. **67**(3), 349–360 (2016). https://doi.org/10.1016/j.annemergmed.2015.09.023

# Nurse Station of Accident and Emergency Department, USM

Shaik Farid Abdull Wahab[1]([⊠]), Ahmad Rasdan Ismail[2],
and Rohayu Othman[3]

[1] School of Medical Science, Universiti Sains Malaysia,
Kubang Kerian, 16150 Kota Bharu, Kelantan, Malaysia
drsfarid@usm.my
[2] Faculty of Creative Technology and Heritage, Universiti Malaysia Kelantan,
Locked Bag 01, 16300 Bachok, Kelantan, Malaysia
arasdan@gmail.com
[3] Kolej Kemahiran Tinggi MARA Pasir Mas,
Lubok Jong, 17000 Pasir Mas, Kelantan, Malaysia
Aiman_shaik@yahoo.com

**Abstract.** Every ward at any departments in hospital will have a nurse counter. Nurse counter or nurse station is a determined place for nurses to do their deskwork. Urgent phone calls and note writing, are among common activities done at the station. Sometimes, discussions and short meeting are also done at the nurse station. Despite the name, this workstation is also used by medical officers, even specialist when they need to sit and write. A usual set of computer and printers, as well as stationeries and telephone are placed at this station. Chairs are also provided. Files and forms are also available at the station. Some stations have both sitting and standing counters for nurses or medical officers to do their works. This objective of this study is to evaluate the current condition of nurse station at Red Zone of Accident and Emergency Department, Hospital Universiti Sains Malaysia, Kubang Kerian, Kelantan, Malaysia. Measurement of the nurse station was taken during the evaluation. The body postures of personnel at the counter were observed. The lighting at the station was also recorded. This study is needed because nurse station is an important part at Accident and Emergency Department. The evaluation result shows, this area was not given a fair attention despite its important. This study justified how the current condition of nurse station has been overlooked and immediate attention should be given in order to ensure better working condition at the station.

**Keywords:** Accident and Emergency Department · Nurse station

## 1 Introduction

Healthcare industry is unique. Every department in the hospitals runs by various types of people, with different job specifications. From specialists, medical officers, nurses, medical assistants, attendants, and general workers, all have undeniable important duties of their own. Unlike certain professions like teachers, lawyers, or executives, workstation in healthcare industry can be considered unique. In healthcare, especially in the Accident

© Springer International Publishing AG, part of Springer Nature 2019
N. J. Lightner (Ed.): AHFE 2018, AISC 779, pp. 183–188, 2019.
https://doi.org/10.1007/978-3-319-94373-2_20

and Emergency Department, nurses counter is a place where almost all-administrative work such as, filling forms, documenting patient progress chart, making phone calls, printing relevant documents and many others.

The workstation is not only meant for nurses. Specialist and medical officers also used the nurse station for discussion. Some nurse stations are equipped with computers and printers. There is one study discussion about the right name to describe the work area, either nurses station or nursing station [1].

Some researchers have shown great interest in the ergonomic of the nurse station due to the growth of computer usage and information technology in healthcare [2]. Nowadays, information search for latest medication or articles can be done online, hence the usage of computer increase. Some hospitals even use database system to record their patients' details.

Poor furniture arrangement is not the only concern at nurse workstation. There is also issues about poor lighting at workplace that might cause health effect to the workers [3]. It is also a common practice at the hospital that nurse workstation is also equipped with computers and printers. Issue regarding visual display terminal (VDT) in healthcare has also been discussed by few researchers [4, 5].

## 2   Research Methodology

A safety walk-about and observation has been conducted at Accident and Emergency Department in order to observe the condition of nurse counter at Accident and Emergency Department. Layout of the nurse counter, arrangement of chairs, equipment available at the station was recorded. Body postures of both standing and sitting healthcare workers were recorded. Lighting at the nurse station was also evaluated using heavy duty data logging light meter, HD450.

For lighting assessment, the nurse counter (writing area) was divided into 4 equal areas and lux meter was placed in the middle of the areas. As for the computer section, both standing and sitting, two measurement points were taken at a distance 20 cm apart, and another two points at the top of the screen, at a distance 10 cm between the points. This method is adapted from Lighting Assessment in the workplace [6].

## 3   Result and Discussion

Finding from the safety walk-about and observation at the Accident and Emergency Department of Hospital University Sains Malaysia shows that, at this workstation, medical officers and nurse write notes, make calls to other departments and sometimes discussion was also made here. Some of the medical officers searched for information at this counter.

The counter consists of two parts, one is sitting and the other one is standing. The sitting part of the workstation is mainly used for clerical work such as writing notes and referral letter. The standing part of the workstation is equipped with monitor that is used to read and interpret x-ray films.

Figure 1 shows how the sitting posture of one of the healthcare workers. As shown in Fig. 1, the worker's shoulder was raised. This is due to the condition the chair. The height of the chair was not adjustable. Furthermore, the backrest was too inclined. The chair was not in a good condition. The overuse might cause the chair to be in that condition.

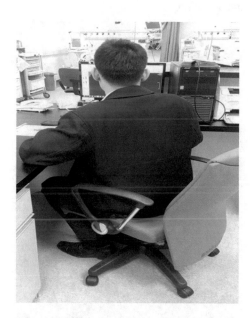

**Fig. 1.** Sitting postures at nurse work station

Figure 2 shows the posture of a heathcare, observing the xray while writing on paper. It is obvious that he need to turn side ways because the monitor was on his left, while writing on notes in front of him. As seen in Fig. 2, his right arm is not supported while he was writing.

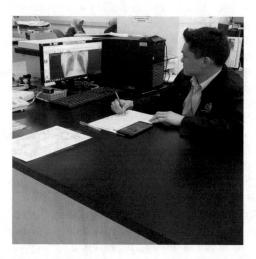

**Fig. 2.** Healthcare worker needs to turn his head while writing on notes.

As for Fig. 3, it was a common standing posture observed at the nurse station at the Accident and Emergency Department. It was obvious that the healthcare worker needs to bend his head due to the position of the monitor. The was no foot rest provided at the standing part of the nurse station.

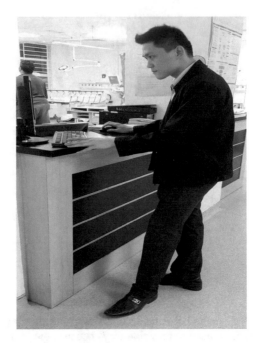

**Fig. 3.**  Standing posture at nurse work station

During the observation made, another finding seen at nurse workstation was the placement of the computer and usage of electrical extension. As shown in Fig. 4, the central processing unit was on the table top, together with the monitor and keyboard. This arrangement make the space for writing becomes limited.

The use of inappropriate electrical extension is another finding seen at the nurse station. It is not advisable to use electrical extension due to electrical hazard. Numbers of socket needed should be calculated and determined during the design phase to avoid this situation from happening.

The Accident and Emergency Department of Hospital Sains Malaysia used artificial lighting for the whole area. There was no window available in the area. Table 1 below shows the on – site measurement for the nurse workstation.

According to Guidelines on Occupational Safety Health In The Office [7], suggested suitable light levels are as below:

Comparing value from Tables 1 and 2, it is clearly shown that the current lux reading at the nurse workstation is lower than recommended by the guideline. Additional lamp need to be install in order to improve the lighting condition.

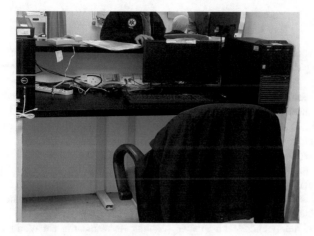

**Fig. 4.** Arrangement of computer and electrical socket at nurse station

**Table 1.** On-site measurement

| Parts of the nurse workstation | On site measurement-lux |
| --- | --- |
| Computer – sitting | 160.4 |
| Computer – standing | 85.3 |
| Desk area | 185 |

**Table 2.** Suitable light levels

| Task/area | Lux |
| --- | --- |
| General background | 200 |
| Routine office work | 400 |
| Work with poor contrast (Proof reading) | 600 |

# 4   Conclusion

The findings proved that the condition of nurse workstation is not conducive. The types of hazards found range from electrical hazards, ergonomics hazard and also physical hazard. The table used must be change, as well as the chair. Since the numbers of people working at the nurse workstation can be many and varies, the selection of furniture must be accordingly. Apart from reduce discomfort and increase the efficiencies of the workers, durability of the furniture must also be considered.

# References

1. Jarrell, A.D., Shattell, M.M., Shattell, M.M.: 'Nurses Station' or 'Nursing Station'? How to appropriately describe our work space in acute care? Issues Ment. Health Nurs. **31**, 237–238 (2010)
2. Hedge, A., James, T., Pavlovic-Veselinovic, S.: Ergonomics concerns and the impact of healthcare information technology. Int. J. Ind. Ergon. **41**(4), 345–351 (2011)
3. Reinhold, K., Tint, P.: Lighting of workplaces and health risks. Elektronika ir Elektrotechnika **2**(2) (2009)
4. Tziaferi, S.G., Sourtzi, P., Kalokairinou, A., Sgourou, E., Koumoulas, E., Velonakis, E.: Risk assessment of physical hazards in greek hospitals combining staff's perception, experts' evaluation and objective measurements. Saf. Health Work **2**(3), 260–272 (2011)
5. Hedge, A., James, T., Pavlovic-Veselinovic, S.: Ergonomics concerns and the impact of healthcare information technology. Int. J. Ind. Ergon. **41**, 345–351 (2011)
6. Occupational Safety and Health Branch: Lighting Assessment in the Workplace
7. Guidelines on Occupational Safety and Health for Working with Video Display Units (VDU's), 1st edn., June 2003 (2014)

# Lighting Assessment at Resuscitation Area of Accident and Emergency Department, Universiti Sains Malaysia

Shaik Farid Abdull Wahab[1](✉), Ahmad Rasdan Ismail[2],
and Rohayu Othman[3]

[1] School of Medical Sciences, Universiti Sains Malaysia,
Kubang Kerian, 16150 Kota Bharu, Kelantan, Malaysia
drsfarid@usm.my
[2] Faculty of Creative Technology and Heritage, Universiti Malaysia Kelantan,
Locked Bag 01, 16300 Bachok, Kelantan, Malaysia
arasdan@gmail.com
[3] Kolej Kemahiran Tinggi MARA Pasir Mas,
Lubok Jong, 17000 Pasir Mas, Kelantan, Malaysia
aiman_shaik@yahoo.com

**Abstract.** Lighting is one of the environment factors that are important. Good and adequate lighting ensure proper task can be done successfully. Properly designed lighting will allow workers to work better with less risk of occupational hazard. The important of natural lighting is undeniable. However, there are certain buildings that have to depend on artificial lights only. The purpose of this study is to evaluate the lighting at resuscitation area of Accident and Emergency Department. Resuscitation area is one of area at the Red Zone where all the patient resuscitation will take place. This study had been carried out at Resuscitation Area, Accident and Emergency Department of Hospital Universiti Sains Malaysia (HUSM), Kubang Kerian, Kelantan, Malaysia. The existing lightings were evaluated using a lux meter (light meter). The evaluation was a procedure-based approached and carried out on the beds at where procedures were done. Since procedures were done on bed, the bed area was divided into six (6) equal squares. The light sensor was placed at the center of each squares and reading were recorded. Measurement from floor to the bed surface was also measured. Data from the lux meter will be compared with the existing guideline. The findings revealed that lighting in this zone were not designed based on tasks requirements, thus justified the additional lights added later.

**Keywords:** Accident and Emergency Department · Lighting · Red Zone

## 1 Introduction

Healthcare industry involves with wide range of work activities, from precision works to gross works. Suturing, blood taking, central vein cannulation, are procedures that can be considered as precision works, while patient lifting, patient transferring, and patient or limb movement activities fall to the other category of non-precise work.

© Springer International Publishing AG, part of Springer Nature 2019
N. J. Lightner (Ed.): AHFE 2018, AISC 779, pp. 189–195, 2019.
https://doi.org/10.1007/978-3-319-94373-2_21

In Accident and Emergency Department, both types of works category existed throughout the days. Common procedures such as blood taking, intravenous cannulation and continuous bladder drainage are common precision works that requires adequate amount of lighting. Tasks such as patient lifting and patient transferring do not require much concentration. Previous study stated that, lighting is one of the element that have impact not only to patients, but to management as well as therapist [1]. The best of lighting at workplace might have balance between natural lighting and artificial lighting. Some workplaces used both types of lighting, but some might depend only on artificial lighting only. This might happened due to unknown constraints at design phase that do not allow the building to have windows or limited contact of natural lighting such as basement area.

Many researchers have agree that physical environment, including lighting plays an important roles in ensuring better workplace and do not induce stress to the worker [2]. Concern about adequate lighting increase especially when working in night shift in all departments in the hospital [3].

An interesting points by previous researcher mentioned that in order to create healing environment, with sense of calmness for everyone, from patients, healthcare workers and visitor, day lighting is important [4]. Inappropriate lighting has been identified as one of workplace stressors that cause poor health effects to the healthcare workers [2].

A significant relationship between health outcomes and environment conditions is not a myth, in fact this has been proved by research [5]. Growing evidence due to development of interest among researchers justified how poor physical environment lead to poor efficiency, productivity as well as satisfaction [5].

Poor and inadequate lighting has been proved as one of reason that cause musculoskeletal disorder among nurses [6]. One study that had been conducted before, tried to find the significant relationship between back accidents among nursing personnel, asked about adequate lighting in the patients' room in the study protocol [7]. Apart from the effect of poor lighting, there is study carried out to justify how proper lighting can have healing effect to the patient, including children [8]. Wears and Perry, in their studies emphasize the importance of having proper lighting in enhancing performance and increase safety at Accident and Emergency Department [9]. Previous researcher also agreed that poor lighting lead to increase of time off due to accident and injuries, absenteeism and finally will cause decrease in quality of work and productivity [10]. Poor environment condition (poor lighting) act as stressor that elevated stress and difficulty to cope with demanding tasks among nurses in public health services [11].

The interest in lighting is not limited to the Accident and Emergency Department only. Radiologist needs proper lighting to read radio images and lighting plays undeniably important role [12]. The importance of lighting together with color has led to an interesting research that determine to find solution for poor ambient hospital environment [13]. Lighting issues at workplace has become a discussion in various industries such as gas processing plant [14], construction industry [15] and garment industry [16].

In this study, certain area in the resuscitation zone being assessed for its lighting by measuring their luminance adequacy.

# 2   Research Methodology

Method used in this study has been adopted from Lighting Assessment in the Workplace, Occupational safety and Health Branch Labour Department [17]. According to the guideline, lighting assessment can be done by two approaches, which are lighting assessment by checklist and lighting assessment by measurement. This study proceeds by using lighting assessment by measurement.

The study process comprises of three parts, which are observation of the Red Zone, gridding the work area and data recording. The observation was made earlier before conducting the assessment in order to evaluate the real lighting condition at the zone. Then, data collection was made. During the observation, there real conditions in the Red Zone was observed. During this time, types of procedures commonly done at the Red Zone also been identified.

Illuminance is determined by a light meter. For this purpose, a data logging light meter, HD450 was used. It is a handy instrument with attached sensor. The sensor will detect the light. Measurement of illuminance can be in Lux or foot-candle. For this study, measurement in Lux was selected. Six measurements were made for each bed. Average value of recorded data was calculated and compared with the illumination recommended for the task.

Since tasks done at Red Zone are considered as visually – demanding, illuminance was measured at the task position, which is at the bed. Illuminance measurement should be taken at height of the work plane, and for this study, the work plane was the bed surface. In this study, the bed surface acts as the work plane, and also known as the horizontal plane. Imaginary grid lines of six equally divided areas were made on the patient's bed. The light sensor of the flux meter was placed at the centre of each area and data were recorded. Recording of the lux meter were taken in resuscitation area and bed area.

Meanwhile in Red Zone beds, reading for each bed were recorded for two conditions, one there was no curtains around the bed, and second, curtains were pulled to surround the bed area. Red zones are fitted with curtains for patient as for their privacy. Figure 1 shows the example of the bed division and the measuring grid area.

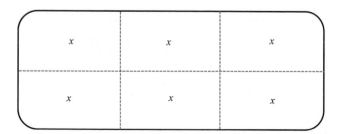

**Fig. 1.** Diagram of bed with imaginary line and illuminance reading site, *x*

During the assessment, the measurement point should not be too close to any obstruction such as wall or curtains that might affect the reading on light meter. Light meter must be allowed to settle for a few seconds until reading recorded were stable.

The imaginary area need to cover the whole bed because, procedures performed on the patient can be at the upper body, middle body part or lower body part. These imaginary areas also cover for both left and right part of the patient's body. Common procedure performed at upper body are suturing and central line insertion. Phlebotomy is commonly performed at middle body part (at arm), while as for lower body, continuous bladder drainage is a common procedure.

In this study, the factor of extreme temperature (too hot or too cold) is not considered. If the study needs to be carried out at extreme temperature conditions, this factor must be taken into consideration because it might have some affects to the light meter. The effects of extreme temperature can influence the data recorded by the light meter.

The light meter must be calibrated at least once a year. If the light meter is used frequently, it must be calibrated for every six months. The usage of measurement tool in this study was calibrated as per scheduled.

# 3   Result and Discussion

During the assessment, the height from floor to the bed surface and from bed surface to the ceiling were measured. The measurement of bed used in Red Zone of Accident and Emergency Department was 67 cm × 212 cm. The approximate height from floor to the bed surface is 73 cm and from ceiling to the bed surface was 207 cm. There are two areas involved in this study, which is Resuscitation Area and common bed area in the Red zone.

There are three beds in the resuscitation area. This area is meant for resuscitation cases only. In this area, there is an additional lighting hanging on the ceiling. However, data recorded in Table 1 shows reading of flux meter from the artificial lighting, not the additional lighting. For Resuscitation area, there is no natural lighting available. There are no windows in the room. All lighting comes from the artificial lighting by the lamp.

**Table 1.** On site measurement at Red Zone – Resuscitation area

| Bed | On – site measurement (lux) |
| --- | --- |
| B1 | 142.3 |
| B2 | 191.6 |
| B3 | 190.3 |

Table 2 shows lux reading at bed area in the Red Zone. Data was recorded based on two conditions, with curtain around the bed and without curtain around the bed. For the Red Zone, same material and same color of curtain was used. Similarly, with the resuscitation area, there is no natural lighting available. All areas were light using the artificial lamp. There is no window at this area also.

**Table 2.** Illuminance at Red Zone – Bed area

| Bed | Luminance – without curtain | Luminance – with curtain |
|-----|------------------------------|---------------------------|
| B4  | 163.1                        | 77.6                      |
| B5  | 303.15                       | 259.3                     |
| B6  | 216.5                        | 164.35                    |
| B7  | 128                          | 117.4                     |

During observation, it was noticed that beds B5 and B6 are two most used beds in the Red Zone. The result from lighting assessment supported the observation. Healthcare workers prefer to use these two beds due to the better lighting at these beds. B4 is the less preferred bed to be use.

For Red Zone of Accident and Emergency Department Hospital Universiti Sains Malaysia, all areas used artificial lighting. There are no windows in the building that can allow natural light enters the area. Thus, during daytime or nighttime, artificial lightings are used fully. Apart from that, Malaysia's climate is hot and humid throughout the year, with sunlight available throughout the year. Therefore, the time of day taken to measure the lighting is not relevant.

This study only considered lux reading from the lamps mounted on the ceiling. These lamps are installed during the design of the Red Zone by the building contarctors. Some bed areas need to be equipped with additional lamps. Guideline on Occupational Safety and Health in The Office by Department of Occupational Safety and Health Malaysia stated that, for general background, 200 lx is required and as for routine office work, 400 lx is needed [18]. Comparing data from Tables 1 and 2 with recommended lux level [19], the existing lights are not sufficient for the healthcare workers at Accident and Emergency Department to do their tasks.

Current Guidelines on Occupational Safety and Health For Lighting at Workplace 2018 stated that, for intensive care, general lighting should be 100 lx, simple examination 300 lx and 1000 lx is needed for further examination and treatment [20]. The guideline also explained the effects of poor lighting such as visual fatigue and poor and awkward postures. Healthcare workers need to bend closer when performing procedures due to inadequate lighting.

Based on Tables 1 and 2, the lux levels at resuscitation area and at bed area are below than the required reading for routine office work. As mentioned above, for Red Zone, tasks performed demand full concentration and require precise detail. Furthermore, the addition of additional lighting indicates that light provided by the ceiling mounted lamps are not adequate. It is important to note that, the additional light added after the building was built. Thus, additional cost was needed for this purpose. Therefore, it is important to design a red zone, with adequate lighting right at the design stage to avoid unnecessary cost addition. The application of new budget can be timely. This will cause the healthcare worker to work in unsafe environment. This will affect the healthcare workers' wellbeing, increase of human error and jeopardize patient's safety. As mention above, poor lighting may lead to risk factor of musculoskeletal disorder among the healthcare workers.

# 4  Conclusion

The findings proved that the condition of lighting is lower than the recommendation from the suggested source. This can be a starting point to make further investigation and improve the current condition at Accident and Emergency Department of Hospital Sains Malaysia, Kelantan. Selection of suitable lamp with adequate numbers of lamp, and placement of the lamp in the department should be given a priority. Also, in the future, the design of Accident and Emergency Department should be added with proper numbers of windows in order to allow natural lighting. Apart from saving electricity, natural lighting has been known as one of healing factors in the hospital. This move will make a better workplace for all the healthcare workers to work in a better environment. With better lighting, performance of the healthcare workers can be increase, thus productivity can also be increased and injuries can be reduced. In the future, the design of Accident and Emergency Department should incorporate experts from architecture, ergonomics and healthcare user itself in order to make sure the design will meet the demand and requirements of the end user.

# References

1. Fenety, A., Kumar, S.: An ergonomic survey of a hospital physical therapy department. Int. J. Ind. Ergon. (1992)
2. Mph, M.A., Dainty, K.N., Deber, R., Sibbald, W.J.B.: The intensive care unit work environment: Current challenges and recommendations for the future. J. Crit. Care 24(2), 243–248 (2009)
3. Tziaferi, S.G., Sourtzi, P., Kalokairinou, A., Sgourou, E., Koumoulas, E., Velonakis, E.: Risk assessment of physical hazards in greek hospitals combining staff's perception, experts' evaluation and objective measurements. Saf. Health Work 2(3), 260–272 (2011)
4. Edwards, L., Torcellini, P.: A literature review of the effects of natural light on building occupants (2002)
5. Mourshed, M., Zhao, Y.: Healthcare providers' perception of design factors related to physical environments in hospitals. J. Environ. Psychol. (2012)
6. Westgaard, R.H., Winkel, J.: Ergonomic intervention research for improved musculoskeletal health: a critical review. Int. J. Ind. Ergon. (1997)
7. Engkvist, I.L., Hagberg, M., Wigaeus-Hjelm, E., Menckel, E., Ekenvall, L.: Interview protocols and ergonomics checklist for analysing overexertion back accidents among nursing personnel. Appl. Ergon. 26(3), 213–220 (1995)
8. Abbas, M.Y., Ghazali, R.: Healing environment of pediatric wards. In: Procedia - Social and Behavioral Sciences (2010)
9. Wears, R.L., Perry, S.J.: Human factors and ergonomics in the emergency department. Ann. Emerg. Med. (2002)
10. Reinhold, K., Tint, P.: Lighting of workplaces and health risks 2(2) (2009)
11. Beh, L.: Job stress and coping mechanisms among nursing staff in public health services. Int. J. Acad. Res. Bus. Soc. Sci. 2(7), 131–176 (2012)
12. Leccese, F., Salvadori, G., Montagnani, C., Ciconi, A., Rocca, M.: Lighting assessment of ergonomic workstation for radio diagnostic reporting. Int. J. Ind. Ergon. 57, 42–54 (2017)
13. Dalke, H., Little, J., Niemann, E., Camgoz, N., Steadman, G., Hill, S., Stott, L.: Colour and lighting in hospital design. In: Optics and Laser Technology (2006)

14. Cordiner, L., Graves, R.J.: Ergonomic intervention during a gas processing plant refurbishment. J. Ind. Ergon. **19**, 457–470 (1997)
15. Jaffar, N., Abdul-Tharim, A.H., Mohd-Kamar, I.F., Lop, N.S.: A literature review of ergonomics risk factors in construction industry. Procedia Eng. **20**, 89–97 (2011)
16. Kaya, Ö.: Design of work place and ergonomics in garment enterprises. Procedia Manuf. **3** (Ahfe), 6437–6443 (2015)
17. Occupational Safety and Health Branch: Lighting Assessment in the Workplace
18. Ministry of Human Resources: Guidelines on occupational safety and health in the office, vol. 1 (1996)
19. Lux, R.: Required light levels, vol. 1000, pp. 13–17 (2000)
20. Guidelines on Occupational Safety and Health for Lighting at Workplace (2018)

# Characteristics of Competence Evaluation of Resilience in the Chronic Diseases Treatment: An Examination of Medical Engineers Who Conduct Hemodialysis

Yoshitaka Maeda[1](✉) and Satoshi Suzuki[2]

[1] Medical Simulation Center, Jichi Medical University,
Yakushiji, Shimotsuke-shi, Tochigi 3311-1, Japan
y-maeda@jichi.ac.jp
[2] Department of Clinical Engineering, Kanagawa Institute of Technology,
Shimo-ogino, Atsugi-shi, Kanagawa 1030, Japan
suzuki@cet.kanagawa-it.ac.jp

**Abstract.** Relevant societies have created guidelines on the tasks of medical engineers (ME) during hemodialysis (HD). However, patients differ in terms of characteristics such as physical features, and requests related to past treatment. Additionally, as the physical condition of each patient is always changing, MEs need to perform resiliently to respond to such situational changes. It is therefore important to evaluate the resilience competencies of ME novices. Most medical studies on competence evaluation have focused on the treatment of acute conditions (e.g., surgery) in which the medical staff have to respond to real-time changing situations. However, in HD, each patient's historical information, including past HD treatments, is a very important source for MEs' resilient behavior. Therefore, it is important to evaluate their competencies with reference to these characteristics. In the present study, based on Miller's pyramid, we classified the MEs' competencies and examined the characteristics of competence evaluation in HD.

**Keywords:** Resilience engineering · Expertise · Skill education
Hemodialysis

## 1 Introduction

**Hemodialysis.** There were more than 320,448 dialysis patients in Japan [1]. Hemodialysis, which involves removing waste materials and moisture that have accumulated in the body, due to renal failure, is a commonplace method for treating this malady. With hemodialysis, a needle is placed in the patient's arm, and extracorporeal circulation is affected to remove this waste [1, 2]. Patients in the maintenance phase receive treatment three times a week with each session lasting about four hours.

Hemodialysis operations are for the most part carried out by Medical Engineers (MEs), who are licensed by the national government. In accordance with a physician's orders, they utilize various types of medical equipment and also maintain this equipment. 16,582 such technicians work in dialysis facilities throughout Japan.

© Springer International Publishing AG, part of Springer Nature 2019
N. J. Lightner (Ed.): AHFE 2018, AISC 779, pp. 196–203, 2019.
https://doi.org/10.1007/978-3-319-94373-2_22

**Tasks Performed in Dialysis.** In order to provide patients with safe and highly satisfactory treatments, guidelines are provided to govern tasks performed by MEs [3, 4]. These can be divided broadly into two types: (1) establishing treatment conditions (device settings and blood circulation assembly, needle insertion) for each patient, and (2) monitoring and responding to issues, such as device misconfiguration, bleeding caused by extracorporeal circulation of blood, and low blood pressure. Each of these is carried out both before and during treatment. An example of these tasks is shown in Table 1.

**Table 1.** Main tasks carried out by MEs

| |
| --- |
| • Patient identification |
| • Verification of type of dialyzer being used |
| • Verification of type of anticoagulant being used |
| • Determination of water removal volume/rate |
| • Verification of doctor's orders |
| • Blood pressure checks |
| • Needle insertion |
| • Health history interview |
| • Taping blood circuits |
| • Verification of blood removal conditions |

**RESILIENT BEHAVIORS in Dialysis.** Guidelines have been provided for the tasks noted in Table 1, but because such personal characteristics of each patient, as blood vessel shape and appropriate blood pressure values, are particular to the patient [5, 6], MEs must adjust such treatment conditions as the positions of "needle insertion" and "blood circuit taping," and "determination of water removal volume/rate" accordingly. Moreover, because the criteria for determining whether there is a defect differs for each patient, for confirmation of blood removal status, failure monitoring in accordance with this is required. Furthermore, items that affect patient satisfaction (the details of requests related to treatment conditions on the day of the procedure) are also individualized. In addition to this, the ME must adjust treatment conditions according to the physical condition of the patient on the day of the procedure. For example, "health history interview" requires that an inquiry be added to the prescribed history item in accordance with the patient's physical condition [7]. Moreover, the ME must also adjust the "determination of water removal volume/rate" of the patient each day of treatment. Because changes in the physical condition of the patient - such as the lowering of blood pressure - occur in real time, the ME must deal with these appropriately [3].

In this way, because conditions surrounding hemodialysis treatment are varied, MEs must fully understand these requirements, with resilient behavior required for each task's actions. It is worth noting that RESILIENT BEHAVIORS indicates the specific actions undertaken by ME for each task. For example, with "taping blood circuits," this corresponds to "performing taping according to the needle insertion position on the day of treatment, arrangement of blood circuits, and body motion during patient's procedure." In this way, all MEs involved in treatment perform appropriate RESILIENT BEHAVIORS, according to the situation, and thus it is felt that each patient can be provided with safe and highly satisfactory dialysis. It is therefore important to evaluate and strengthen the competence of new MEs with regards to such RESILIENT BEHAVIORS [8].

**RESILIENT BEHAVIORS Assessments.** Research on these types of competency assessments related to RESILIENT BEHAVIORS in medical treatment has been carried out. The NOTSS system [9] for evaluating a surgeon's nontechnical behavior is a well-known example of this. However, the chief subject of such research was acute medical treatment (surgery, anesthesiology) where responding to changes in real time was critical.

Meanwhile, in addition to responding to real-time situations in hemodialysis, it is also critically important to: (1) finely tune the setting of treatment conditions according to the physical characteristics of each patient; (2) reflect patient needs when it comes to safety issues; and (3) change the criteria for determining the presence or absence of malfunctions during treatment for each patient. Thus, it is important to carry out competency assessments that take into account the characteristics unique to such medical treatment for chronic diseases.

**The Goal of this Research.** Based on Miller's Pyramid, which is a representative model for evaluating clinical competence, in this study, we classified the ME competence that Maeda et al. [10] called for and examined the characteristics of dialysis competence assessments.

# 2   Methods

## 2.1   Competence for RESILIENT BEHAVIORS of Hemodialysis ME

Maeda et al. [10] clarified a total of 29 RESILIENT BEHAVIORS that present difficulties for new MEs and organized 100 items needed for competency in order to carry these RESILIENT BEHAVIORS out.

**Knowledge of Situations to be Understood (28 Items).** [This indicates] the grasping of the physical condition and characteristics – such as the characteristics of blood vessels - of the patient at the time of past procedures. Moreover, [this also indicates a] knowledge of historical information regarding the content of requests made by the patient during past procedures, such as "the ability to grasp how, and places where, tape is to be affixed."

**Criteria for Interpreting Situations (20 Items).** [This indicates] the grasping of criteria for judging whether or not there is a problem with the physical condition of the patient at the time of treatment. Examples include "grasping the criteria for judging whether or not the blood removal status of each patient is defective or not," as well as whether the issue in question is of an urgent nature.

**Knowledge of Future Situations to be Predicted (6 Items).** [This indicates] the ability to predict problems with the physical condition of the patient that can occur during procedures. Examples include "the ability to predict poor physical conditions when the patient's water removal rate is high."

**Knowledge Necessary for Decision Making (24 Items).** [This indicates the] understanding the knowledge necessary to determine how to carry out RESILIENT BEHAVIORS in accordance with the situation. Examples include "coming to an understanding of when it is easiest to discover any internal bleeding."

**Communication (11 Items).** [This indicates] a knowledge of specific methods for gathering information from each patient and communicating this information. Examples include "knowing how to ask simple questions of patients who are reluctant to communicate." Moreover, [this also indicates] the ability to disseminate information to other MEs and doctors, such as "the ability to determine the proper timing to consult a doctor," and understanding methods for consultation on treatment.

**Attitude (7 Items).** [This indicates] being prepared when referring to a doctor's instructions and trying to find the causes of a problem.

**Teamwork (4 Items).** [This indicates] properly grasping how to cooperate with other MEs in providing treatment.

## 2.2   Miller's Pyramid [11]

Miller [11] divided the evaluation targets of clinical competence in clinical practice into the four stages shown in Fig. 1, indicating the evaluation methods suitable for each stage.

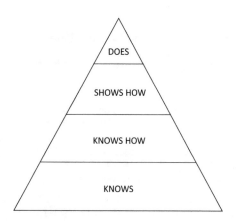

**Fig. 1.** Miller's pyramid [11]

In assessing exactly what is carried out with "Does", 360° evaluations and supervisor assessments are appropriate. OSCE (Objective Clinical Capability Assessment Test) and the like are suitable in evaluating how "Shows How" can indicate what to do. "Knows-How" indicates whether the individual know what to do; a case-based system is suitable in assessing this. "Knows" evaluates what one knows as knowledge, so multiple choice and verbal tests are appropriate.

### 2.3    Procedures Involved in the Present Study

We classified 100 items of competence [10] from Miller's viewpoint of which competency level a new ME should acquire.

## 3    Results and Discussions

Classification results are indicated in Fig. 2.

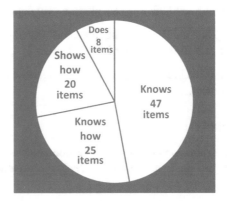

**Fig. 2.**  Competence classification results

### 3.1    Items Classified as "Knows" and "Knows-How"

Seventy-two out of 100 items were classified. Examples are shown in Table 2.

**Table 2.**  Major competencies classified as "Knows" and "Knows-how"

| Competence | Knows | Knows-how |
|---|---|---|
| • Understands the characteristics of each patient's blood vessels | ✓ | |
| • Knows the maximum amount of water removed so far for each patient | ✓ | |
| • Understands the minimum to be asked when inquiring about patient medical history | ✓ | |
| • Understands where tape should not be applied for each patient | ✓ | |
| • Understands where/how to attach tape as per each patient's wishes | | ✓ |
| • Understands how to measure blood pressure as per each patient's wishes | | ✓ |

As with "characteristics of blood vessels of each patient," these are related to an understanding of historical information, such as the physical condition and physical characteristics of the patient at the time of past treatments. Because 72 items are an extremely large number, the question of how much historical information to grasp is felt to greatly affect RESILIENT BEHAVIORS performance.

Put another way, if MEs possess historical information as knowledge, or even if they just know how to keep track of historical information, it is felt that it is relatively easy to carry out RESILIENT BEHAVIORS based on that. For example, in order to perform RESILIENT BEHAVIORS with the "taping of blood circuit" task, the ME must have knowledge of "where tape should not be applied for each patient" and "where/how to attach tape as per each patient's wishes." On the other hand, with this knowledge, acting based on this (i.e., taping) is made easy, with even new MEs able to complete this task without incident.

Moreover, it is felt that it is best to carry out assessments of these cognitive competencies by oral examination or investigations, using actual cases, as opposed to observations and practical tests. However, when conducting health history interviews, it is felt that [considering] what kind of historical information should be understood beforehand, when taping is more effective, then asking where the patient would like to have the tape attached. This is because in many cases the ME does not record information on all the patients, but rather refers to past dialysis records as needed. In other words, the ME that knows what historical information to obtain can gather this information appropriately from historical dialysis records and similar data and once this information is obtained, can easily carry out RESILIENT BEHAVIORS, meaning that they only have to ask for the information they need.

With medical care for acute conditions, techniques are needed for information collection itself, and even when collecting information, acting on this information is not easy. That is, these characteristics are considered to be specific to medical care for acute conditions.

### 3.2  Major Competencies Classified as "Show-How" and "Does"

Twenty-eight out of 100 items were classified. Examples are shown in Table 3.

**Table 3.** Major competencies classified as "Show-how" and "Does"

| Competence | Shows-how | Does |
|---|---|---|
| • Can also inquire in detail about problems that have come up since the last meeting | ✓ | |
| • Can ask patients, reluctant to answer, simple YES/NO questions | ✓ | |
| • Can advocate for his/her position when stating his/her opinion to the physician | ✓ | |
| • Does not accept physician's orders without question | | ✓ |
| • Appropriately estimates the degree to which he/she can make decisions by him/herself | | ✓ |

These consist mainly of competencies necessary for communication between the patient and the ME, such as "interviews," and between the doctor and the ME, such as "verifying doctor's orders." Unlike cognitive competencies classified as "Knows" or "Knows-how," these involve a level of competence that cannot be demonstrated simply by knowing procedures.

For example, in a patient interview for dialysis, which is a medical treatment for chronic illness, some patients may be reluctant to respond to ME questions because they "are always answering these types of questions." If the interview is not conducted properly in such situations, there is a possibility that patients, with infectious diseases, cannot be isolated or the medicine to be administered to the patient cannot be selected appropriately. Therefore, it is critical for medical safety reasons that MEs make full use of the competencies listed in Table 3, to properly "carry out" patient interviews. Communication between the doctor and the ME is also important in terms of accurate transmission of instructions.

Such competencies are observable, and are assumed to be effective in evaluation by clinical observation or practical test as well as with NOTSS performed in acute disease medical care.

## 4  Conclusion

With the present research, with regards to competence assessments for RESILIENT BEHAVIORS, we clarified the characteristics of dialysis, a medical treatment for chronic illness, by referring to Miller's Pyramid model. As a result, in many tasks, because grasping historical information, at the time of past procedures for each patient, greatly affects RESILIENT BEHAVIORS, most competencies consisted of the knowledge (Know, Know-how) for grasping historical information. Because these are cognitive competencies, it was thought that it would be best to carry out evaluations by oral examinations that ask knowledge-based questions. On the other hand, similar to competency assessments of medical care for acute illnesses, with tasks that require communication with patients and physicians, it is assumed that evaluations by clinical observation and practical testing were possible.

## References

1. Kadokawa, T.: Hemodialysis Patient Management for Resident. Igaku-syoin, Tokyo (2011). (in Japanese)
2. Toseki-ryoho-goudou-iinkai (ed.): Handbook of Hemodialysis. Kyodo-Isho-Shuppan, Tokyo (2015). (in Japanese)
3. Nihon-Toseki-Ikai (ed.): Standard Dialysis Operation Manual for Dialysis Medical Accident Prevention. Sansyusya, Tokyo (2015). (in Japanese)
4. Nihon-Toseki-Ikai (ed.): Rinsyo-Kougaku-goudou-Iinkai: Guidelines for Medical Engineers (2012). (in Japanese)
5. Simono, R., Tsuru, S., Iizuka, Y.: A model for describing work process at hospitals. J. Jpn. Soc. Qual. Control **41**(2), 213–224 (2011)

6. Tsuru, S.: Visualization, structuring and standardization for clinical knowledge. Manag. Syst. J. Jpn. Ind. Manag. Assoc. **24**(1), 15–20 (2014)
7. Ando, R.: Establish a relationship of trust between dialysis patients and medical staff. In: Akiba, T., Akizawa, T. (eds.) Dialysis Therapy NEXT XIII, pp. 110–120. Igaku-Tosho-Shuppan, Tokyo (2009). (in Japanese)
8. Ozaki, M., Arimoto, K.: Necessity of lifelong education and safe procedures for hospitals. Jpn. J. Clin. Dial. **21**(5), 571–576 (2005)
9. Yule, S., Flin, R., Paterson-Brown, S., Maran, N., Rowley, D.: Development of a rating system for surgeons' non-technical skills. Med. Educ. **40**(11), 1098–1104 (2006)
10. Maeda, Y., Suzuki, S., Komatsubara, A.: Competencies necessary for medical staff to deal with the situational changes during hemodialysis treatment. Jpn. J. Ergon. **51**(suppl), 232–233 (2015)
11. Miller, G.E.: The assessment of clinical skills/competence/performance. Acad. Med. **65**(9), 63–67 (1990)

# Patient Safety

# Reducing Medication Errors and Increasing Patient Safety: Utilizing the Fault Tree Analysis

Maryam Tabibzadeh[✉] and Anjana Muralidharan

Department of Manufacturing Systems Engineering and Management,
California State University, Northridge,
18111 Nordhoff Street, Northridge, CA 91330, USA
maryam.tabibzadeh@csun.edu,
anjana.muralidharan.749@my.csun.edu

**Abstract.** According to the 2000 Institute of Medicine Report on Building a Safer Health System, experts estimated that 8000 Americans die every year from preventable medication errors. It is believed that these errors annually affect more than 7 million patients with the cost of approximately $21 billion across all care settings. Despite some developed studies on analyzing the contributing causes of medication errors, there is a need for the development of more robust, systematic methodologies to identify their root causes and provide preventive measures to avoid their recurrence. This paper proposes a methodology, which is an integration of Failure Modes and Effects Analysis (FMEA) and Fault Tree Analysis (FTA), to first identify one of the top most important categories of medication error and then analyze its contributing and root causes. In this study, we develop FTA for administration errors, as they are highly occurring and very severe among other medication error categories.

**Keywords:** Medication errors · Medication administration errors
Patient safety · Fault tree analysis
Failure Modes and Effects Analysis (FMEA)

## 1 Introduction

According to the 2000 Institute of Medicine Report on Building a Safer Health System [1, p. 26], experts estimated that between 44,000 and 98,000 Americans die every year from preventable medical errors that occur in hospitals. Among these deaths, 8000 are attributable to medication errors [2]. Medication error is the third highest cause of deaths in the U.S. The causes for medication errors originate from various sources. Medication errors constitute between 5.3 to 20.6% of all errors occurring in healthcare settings [3]. They account for one out of 131 outpatient deaths and one out of 854 inpatient deaths [1, p. 27]. Moreover, in a review of the U.S. death certificates between 1983 and 1993, it was found that 7,391 individuals passed away due to medication errors in 1993 while this number was 2,876 in 1983, which indicates a large increase (2.57-times more) [1, p. 32]. In this 10-year period, outpatient deaths due to medication errors rose 8.48-times compared with a 2.37-times increase in inpatient deaths [1, p. 33].

© Springer International Publishing AG, part of Springer Nature 2019
N. J. Lightner (Ed.): AHFE 2018, AISC 779, pp. 207–218, 2019.
https://doi.org/10.1007/978-3-319-94373-2_23

According to a study by da Silva and Krishnamurthy [4] in 2016, preventable medication errors affect more than 7 million patients and cost almost $21 billion annually across all care settings. Medication errors occur due to different factors such as wrong drug selection; prescription writing; drug administration; lack of knowledge; slips and memory lapses; equipment failure and inexperienced staff including pharmacists, nurses, physicians, supportive personnel and clerical staff [5, 6]. Medication errors are categorized as prescription, transcription, dispensing and administration errors. Prescription errors are characterized as wrong medication determination for a patient [7]. Transcription errors are those that occur due to data entry error that is commonly made by human operators [8]. Dispensing errors are those that occur between a pharmacist and a patient in a drug store [9]. Finally, administration errors occur due to discrepancies between the recommended medication for a patient and the medication treatment the patient receives from the prescriber or administer [10].

Despite some developed studies on analyzing the contributing causes of medication errors, there is a need for the development of more robust systemic methodologies to identify their root causes and provide preventive measures to avoid their recurrence. This will contribute to increasing patient safety in healthcare settings.

This paper proposes a methodology, which is an integration of a Failure Modes and Effects Analysis (FMEA) and a Fault Tree Analysis (FTA), to first identify one of the top most important categories of medication errors and then analyze its contributing and root causes. The described medication error category has been identified by reviewing previous studies that already performed an FMEA and also through the analysis of provided statistics on the most frequent and influential medication errors. Based on that, we have developed our FTA to identify the root causes of the above-mentioned identified medication error category. The study and the analysis of previous case studies have also been utilized in conducting our fault tree analysis and the identification of root causes.

In the context of medication errors, to our knowledge, there are very few studies that have utilized FTA to analyze these errors. Even those studies have mainly identified some of the failure modes or faults that led to medication errors, and they have not usually investigated the main root causes of those identified failure modes. In addition, we have attempted to work systematically and focus on top most important medication errors, by identifying them through an FMEA.

The structure of the remaining of the paper is as follows: Sect. 2 reviews some of the main already developed methodologies to analyze medication errors. Section 3 discusses our proposed methodology to analyze the main contributing causes of medication errors; Medication Administration Errors (MAE) to be specific, to detect and prevent these errors. Section 4 provides some discussions and recommendations in the context of medication errors prevention. Finally, Sect. 5 provides some concluding points.

## 2   Literature Review

There have been several studies in the context of medication errors and their adverse effects in the healthcare industry. Some of these studies have utilized methodologies such as Six Sigma Define, Measure, Analyze, Improve, and Control (DMAIC), Root

Cause Analysis (RCA), FMEA, Socio-Technical Probabilistic Risk Assessment (ST-PRA) and FTA to analyze some of the contributing causes of medication errors with the purpose of preventing them or reducing the risk of their occurrence.

The first category of utilized methods for the analysis of medication errors is the Six Sigma DMAIC methodology to reduce and/or prevent these errors and their adverse effects. Kumar and Steinebach [11] and Al-Kuwaiti [12] have used Six Sigma methodologies to find the root causes of medication errors and reduce them. Similar to these two studies, Buck [13], with the help of experts, has applied the Six Sigma methodology to reduce medication and laboratory errors in the Froedtert Hospital in Milwaukee, Wisconsin, and increase patient safety. In the case of medication errors, Froedtert Hospital's processes for medication delivery were evaluated to be able to design an approach to reduce the likelihood of errors [13].

As another category of utilized methods, Teixeira and Cassiani [14] have used root cause analysis to detect, reduce, and prevent medication errors. According to this study, 24.3% of medication errors were due to dosage errors and 22.9% were related to schedule errors [14]. The RCA was implemented to identify the root causes of these errors and necessary recommendations were provided to prevent the occurrence of the errors.

Chiozza and Ponzetti [15] and Montesi and Lechi [16] have applied failure modes and effects analysis to identify the most severe medication errors after ranking them accordingly. As a result of using the FMEA technique, *identification errors* were found to be the most commonly occurring error. Introduction of patient barcoding reduced the error rates [15].

Sociotechnical probabilistic risk assessment is another method that has been utilized by Comden et al. [17] for medication errors investigation through the identification and analysis of related failure modes. ST-PRA is a powerful tool to use in the healthcare industry to prevent medication errors.

Finally, Cherian [18] has used FTA to analyze the contributing causes of errors in medication delivery. In the first top-level fault tree, medication delivery has been divided into three major sub-systems of the physician, the nurse and the pharmacy [18]. In this study, medication errors can occur due to independent errors by either of these sub-systems, which are the type of errors committed by one link in the medication chain that cannot be detected and therefore prevented by the other links. In another case, medication errors can be the ones that as a result of interaction between the links, can be detected, but may not be, because of oversight failures. In the next step, a separate fault tree has been developed to analyze each of the cases of those independent and dependent errors. It is however noteworthy that the analysis of the contributing causes of those errors has not been further developed and extended to the level of identifying the root causes.

In this section, we provided a literature review on the utilized methodologies by different studies for the analysis of medication errors in the healthcare industry. Each of the described studies have been successful in some aspects and have had limitations in other aspects.

# 3  Methodology

In this paper, we have proposed a systematic methodology, which is an integration of an FMEA and a FTA. This contributes to the identification of the top most important categories of medication errors through FMEA and the analysis of the contributing and root causes of those identified errors through FTA. The reason for selecting the FTA is that based on the provided analysis in the literature review section, to our knowledge, there are very few studies that have applied this method for the analysis of medication errors. Even those specific studies have mainly identified various failure modes or faults that led to medication errors, and they have not usually investigated the main root causes of those identified failure modes. In addition, we have attempted to work systematically and focus on top most important medication errors, by identifying them through an FMEA.

For conducting an FMEA, there is a need to access necessary data regarding the likelihood of occurrence, severity and detectability of each failure mode; medication error in this context. Since we did not have access to real data from a healthcare setting, we have utilized the results and the provided data of other studies that already performed an FMEA. After identifying one of the top most critical medication errors, we have developed a series of fault trees, in each the undesirable event being placed on top of the tree, to identify the root causes of that error and the factors/errors that contributed to it.

Failure Modes and Effects Analysis is a step-by-step procedure for the identification of possible failure modes in the process of producing a product or providing a service. "Failures" are the errors or defects and "effect analysis" is the process of analyzing the effects and impacts of those failures. Failures are prioritized on how severe the errors are, how frequently they occur and how easily they are detected. Once prioritized, the top most identified errors are selected to develop necessary contingency and mitigation plans to eliminate their occurrence or reduce their negative consequences if they occur.

Fault tree analysis is a systematic method that examines the contributing causes of a basic event using a top-down approach. It is normally used to investigate potential faults, its failure modes and causes, and to quantify the contribution of each failure mode if data is available. Usually, there are two series of gates; AND and OR gates, used in a fault tree that illustrate how top-level events are connected to their lower-level contributing causes. If either one of the input events are responsible for the occurrence of the output event, then the input events are connected using an OR gate. Else if both input events are responsible for the occurrence of the output event, then they are connected using an AND gate. In the developed fault trees in this paper, we have only used OR gates based on the nature and the necessity of our analysis.

## 3.1  Medication Administration Errors (MAEs): The Selected Top Error

Medication errors are usually classified as prescription, transcription, dispensing and administration errors. Mansouri et al. [19] conducted an analysis to study the severity and occurrence of medication errors in Iran. The results indicated the following breakdown for each of the stated categories of medication errors: prescribing errors,

29.8%–47.8%; transcribing errors, 10.0%–51.8%; dispensing errors, 11.3%–33.6%; and administration errors, 14.3%–70%. In this study, administration errors have the highest average percentage of occurrence comparing to the other three categories.

In a study by Yang and Grissinger [20], from the Pennsylvania Patient Safety Authority, a total of 813 medication errors were reported that were categorized as wrong patient. 38.3% of errors mostly occurred during transcription, 43.4% occurred during administration, 12.1% during prescribing and 5.2% during dispensing. This also shows that in that context, administration errors had the highest percentage of occurrence among other errors.

In another study, Aronson [5] states that the percentage distribution of medications errors are as follows: 30% associated to prescription errors, 25% to dispensing errors and 40% to administration errors. This study also concludes that administration errors were the highest of all.

Lisby et al. [21], from the Aarhus University Hospital of Denmark, conducted a study to investigate the frequency of medication errors. The study reported that the frequencies were: (1) Transcription: 56%, (2) Administration: 41%, (3) Ordering: 39% and (4) Dispensing: 4%. In this study, administration errors were the second highest frequently occurring errors. The study also concluded that 50% of all errors occurred due to missing actions, which indirectly led to administration errors.

Finally, Allard et al. [22] discusses a study by the Harvard Medical Practice Study on adverse drug events occurring in hospitalized patients. Results showed that 49% of errors occurred in the prescribing stage, 26% in administration, 14% in dispensing and 11% in transcription. They also analyzed error recovery, in which errors were more likely to be recovered in the prescribing and the dispensing stage but not in the administration stage. This shows that even though the occurrence of errors in the administration stage was less than the prescribing stage, because these errors cannot be recovered easily, they seem more fatal than the ones in the prescribing stage.

Based on the analysis of the above-mentioned studies, we concluded that medication administration errors are highly occurring and one of the most severe among other medication errors. Therefore, our fault tree analysis has been specifically performed on MAEs to analyze and identify their contributing and root causes.

## 3.2   Development of Fault Trees for Medication Administration Errors

Before illustrating and describing any of our developed fault trees for the analysis of medication administration errors, we would like to state that these fault trees, the captured contributing factors in them and the root causes of those factors have been developed and determined through extensive research and the analysis of several studies and published sources.

In the first step, we have developed a fault tree to capture the top-level contributing causes of medication administration errors. As shown in Fig. 1, MAEs occur due to errors made by the physician or the nurse or sometimes both. A physician alone can cause an administration error or a nurse alone can cause such an error. Therefore, it is not necessary that both the physician and the nurse contribute to causing an administration error. Hence, the nodes physician and nurse are linked by an OR gate.

In one level lower in the fault tree in Fig. 1, no proper information about the medication, wrong medication dose, wrong medication, wrong time of administering the medication and wrong patient can each contribute to an administration error by the physician. From the nurse perspective, wrong medication dose, wrong medication, wrong time of administering the medication, wrong patient, error in the method of medication administration and rule violation can be the contributing causes of the nurse administration error.

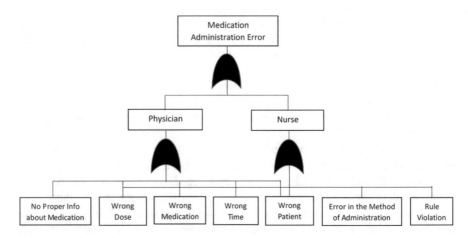

**Fig. 1.** Overall fault tree for the analysis of medication administration errors

In the next step, we have developed a separate fault tree to analyze each of the stated errors/faults in the bottom layer of our illustrated fault tree in Fig. 1. In this paper however, due to page limitation, we have only presented and described four of those fault trees that investigate the contributing and root causes of wrong medication dose by the physician, wrong medication dose by the nurse, wrong medication by the physician and wrong medication by the nurse. These four fault trees are illustrated in Figs. 2 through 5, respectively.

In Fig. 2, the fault tree for the analysis of a wrong medication dose by the physician has been developed. In this figure, the immediate causes of such an error are lack of knowledge about drugs and human errors. They are both linked with an OR gate because occurrence of either one can lead to the wrong dose by the physician. In one step further, lack of knowledge about drugs has its own causes: no proper education and lack of sufficient training. These two factors are also linked with an OR gate since either of them can contribute to lack of knowledge about drugs.

Human errors, as another contributing factor for the wrong medication dose by the physician, can be caused due to lack of attention and responsibility, haste and negligence, and fatigue and stress. The last two stated factors can occur due to high workload, which itself can be caused by insufficient number of staff and/or ineffective scheduling.

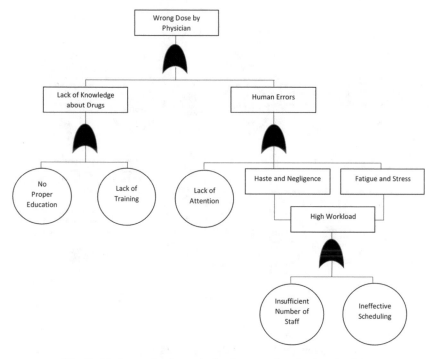

**Fig. 2.** Fault tree for the analysis of wrong dose by the physician

In Fig. 3, the fault tree for the analysis of a wrong medication dose by the nurse has been developed. In this figure, the immediate causes of such an error are incorrect dose specified by the physician, prescription error, patient's request to alter the dose, trusting senior colleagues, miscommunication between the nurse and the physician and human errors. The incorrect dose by the physician has been already described before in Fig. 2. Prescription error can occur due to the following causes: illegible handwriting by the physician, improper use of points, use of abbreviations and improper use of zeros. Two examples for an improper use of points and zeros are: (1) writing .5 mL instead of 0.5 mL and (2) writing 5.0 mL instead of 5 mL for a drug dose. It is instructed to always use a leading zero before a decimal expression of less than one; e.g., 0.5 mL, since the point might be missed, and conversely, never use a terminal zero; e.g. 5.0 mL, since failure to see the decimal can result in a 10-fold overdose.

Human errors, as another contributing factor for the wrong medication dose by the nurse (Fig. 3), have been further broken down into the causes of lack of attention and responsibility, haste and negligence, and fatigue and stress. The last two stated factors can occur due to high workload, which itself can be caused by insufficient number of staff and/or ineffective scheduling.

Figure 4 illustrates the developed fault tree to analyze the contributing causes of a wrong medication by the physician. In this figure, the immediate causes of such an error are lack of knowledge about drugs, inaccurate information in the patient's records, different diagnosis by another physician and human errors. Lack of knowledge

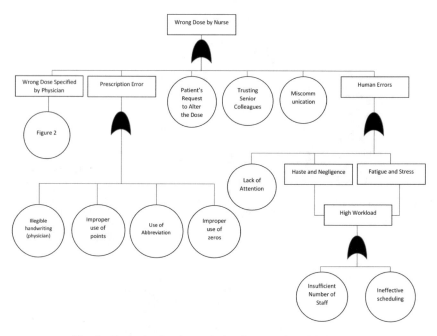

**Fig. 3.** Fault tree for the analysis of wrong dose by the nurse

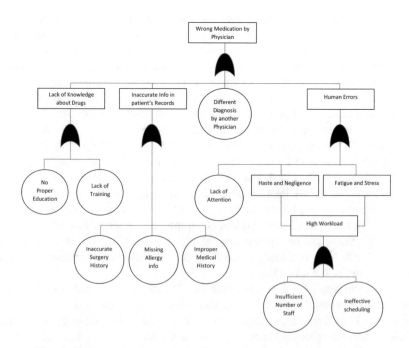

**Fig. 4.** Fault tree for the analysis of wrong medication by the physician

about drugs can be due to no proper education or lack of sufficient training. Inaccurate information in the patient's records can be because of missing allergy information, inaccurate medical history about the patient and missing surgery history of the patient. Finally, human errors, as another contributing factor for a wrong medication by the physician, have been broken down the same way as it was explained in Figs. 2 and 3.

Figure 5 illustrates the developed fault tree for the analysis of the contributing causes of a wrong medication by the nurse. In this figure, the immediate causes of such an error are interruptions during drug administration, inadequate written communication with the physician, lack of training and experience, inaccurate information in the patient's records, trusting senior colleagues, problems with medicine supply and storage and human errors. Inadequate written communication can be usually caused by illegible handwriting and use of abbreviations by the physician. Inaccurate information in patient's records can be due to missing allergy information, inaccurate surgery history and improper medical history. Finally, human errors, as another contributing factor for a wrong medication by the nurse, have been broken down the same way as it was explained in Figs. 2 through 4.

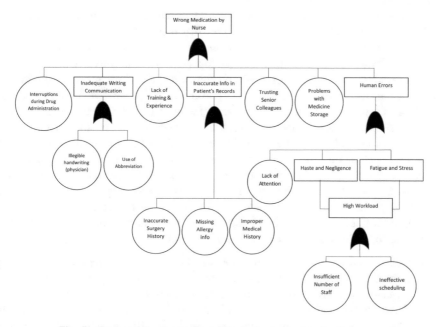

**Fig. 5.** Fault tree for the analysis of wrong medication by the nurse

# 4   Discussions and Some Recommendations

In the previous section, some of the developed fault trees for the analysis of different categories of medication administration errors were illustrated and described. Our analysis of those fault trees indicates that several contributing factors and root causes play a critical role in the occurrence of MAEs. The mostly occurring critical factors in our developed fault trees; the ones illustrated in this paper and the other ones that we could not present in the paper due to page limitation, are as follows: no proper education for the physician; lack of training and experience for both the physician and the nurse; insufficient number of staff and ineffective scheduling. The last two stated factors contribute to high workload, which itself can cause haste, negligence, fatigue and stress.

The next most commonly occurring contributing factors and root causes in our fault trees were illegible handwriting, improper use of zeros and points and inaccurate information in patient's records such as missing allergy information, no proper medical and surgical history, as well as the complications that the patient is suffering from.

Ineffective communication plays a critical role in causing medication administration errors as well. Different categories of communication and interaction exist in this case. First of all, miscommunication between the physician and the nurse; e.g. the physician does not provide the nurse with details on the method of administering the prescribed medication or the nurse does not contact the physician when in doubt, can contribute to issues such as administering a wrong medication or a wrong dose for the correct medication. Ineffective communication of the physician with the patient and not providing him with proper instructions on the prescribed medication and its side effects is another category that can lead to MAEs.

In a broader perspective, when reviewing the stated captured contributing causes of MAEs in our developed fault trees, we infer that many of these causes have organizational factors-related roots. Organizational factors such as personnel management issues, ineffective communication and interoperability among involved key players, lack of standard and well-documented procedures and economic pressure (production and productivity versus safety) play a major role in causing what we have captured in our analyzed models. In fact, organizational factors have been identified as the root causes of accumulated errors and questionable decisions made by personnel and management not only in different healthcare settings, but also in many safety-critical industries, such as offshore drilling, transportation sector and nuclear power plants.

It is also noteworthy that although we utilized our developed methodology for the analysis of medication administration errors, this methodology can be applied to analyze any other category of medication errors as well as any other errors in general.

Based on this analysis, the following are some specific recommendations that can contribute to preventing the stated commonly occurring errors:

1. Physicians have to be properly educated and hired based on their knowledge. They also need to be properly trained before treating patients. Only highly experienced and well-trained physicians should be allowed to treat patients.
2. High workload should be avoided for both physicians and nurses. High workload can be avoided by hiring more staff and scheduling shifts effectively. This in turn will reduce human errors due to fatigue, stress, haste, negligence, and lack of attention and responsibility.
3. Prescription error can be avoided by using computerized prescriptions in hospitals. This will avoid illegible handwriting, improper use of zeros and points and ambiguous writing by physicians.
4. If proving a hand-written prescription, proper use of points and zeros are essential. In addition to what was described before on always using a leading zero before a

decimal expression of less than one; e.g., 0.5 mL and conversely, never using a terminal zero; e.g. 5.0 mL, it is recommended to, when possible, avoid the use of decimals. For instance, prescribe 500 mg instead of 0.5 g.

5. Accurate patient records like allergy information of patients, and medical and surgery history of patients should be maintained by hospital administration to avoid wrong patient errors.
6. Physicians should provide proper information about the medication and its side effects to patients while prescribing. They also need to provide proper instructions regarding the method of administrating the medication to the nurse.
7. Nurses should contact the physician in case of any doubts in the method of administrating the medication and not take their own decisions. In addition, they should not act upon patient's request. They should also not take decisions based on senior colleagues' opinions.

# 5  Conclusion

In this paper, we proposed a system-oriented methodology to investigate some of the contributing and root causes of medication administration errors, as a major category of medication errors in healthcare settings. Our methodology was an integration of failure modes and effects analysis and fault tree analysis to first identify one of the top most critical categories of medication errors (using FMEA) and then analyze its main contributing factors and root causes (using FTA).

Our analysis using the stated methodology indicated that lack of proper education for physicians; lack of training and experience for both the physician and the nurse; insufficient number of staff and ineffective scheduling were the mostly observed contributing causes of MAEs. Illegible handwriting, improper use of zeros and points and inaccurate information in patient's records were also observed in several of our developed fault trees for the analysis of MAEs. Finally, ineffective communication between the physician and the nurse and also between the physician and the patient have a major role in causing these types of errors. We also recognized that many of these identified factors have roots in organizational factors. After this analysis, we provided some specific recommendations to prevent the identified root causes from occurring, which in turn will reduce the occurrence of medication administration errors.

# References

1. Kohn, L.T., Corrigan, J.M., Donaldson, M.S., McKay, T., Pike, K.C.: To Err is Human: Building a Safer Health System. Committee on Quality of Health Care in America. Institute of Medicine. National Academy Press, Washington, D.C. (2000)
2. Phillips, D.P., Christenfeld, N., Glynn, L.M.: Increase in US medication-error deaths between 1983 and 1993. Lancet **351**, 643–644 (1998)
3. Bindler, R., Baynd, T.: Medication calculation ability of registered nurses. J. Nurs. Scholarsh. **23**(4), 221–224 (1991)

218    M. Tabibzadeh and A. Muralidharan

4. da Silva, B.A., Krishnamurthy, M.: The alarming reality of medication error: a patient case and review of Pennsylvania and National data. J. Community Hosp. Intern. Med. Perspect. **6** (4) (2016). https://doi.org/10.3402/jchimp.v6.31758
5. Aronson, J.: Medication errors: what they are, how they happen, and how to avoid them. QJM: Int. J. Med. **102**, 513–521 (2009). https://doi.org/10.1093/qjmed/hcp052
6. Manasse, H.R.: Medication use in an imperfect world: drug misadventuring as an issue of public policy, part 1. Am. J. Hosp. Pharm. **46**, 929–944 (1989)
7. Barber, N., Rawlins, M., Franklin, B.D.: Reducing prescribing error: competence, control and culture. Qual. Saf. Health Care **12**, 129–132 (2003)
8. Fahimi, F., Ariapanah, P., Faizi, M., Shafaghi, B., Namdar, R., Ardakani, M.: Errors in preparation and administration of intravenous medications in the intensive care unit of a teaching hospital: an observational study. Aust. Crit. Care **21**, 110–116 (2008)
9. Bohand, X., Simon, L., Perrier, E., Mullot, H., Lefeuvre, L., Plotton, C.: Frequency, types, and potential clinical significance of medication-dispensing errors. Clinics **64**(1), 11–16 (2009)
10. Gladstone, J.: Drug administration errors: a study into the factors underlying the occurrence and reporting of drug errors in a district general hospital. J. Adv. Nurs. **22**, 628–637 (1995)
11. Kumar, S., Steinebach, M.: Eliminating US hospital medical errors. Int. J. Health Care Qual. Assur. **21**(5), 444–471 (2008)
12. Al-Kuwaiti, A.: Application of Six Sigma methodology to reduce medication errors in the outpatient pharmacy unit: a case study from the King Fahd University Hospital, Saudi Arabia. Int. J. Qual. Res. **10**(2), 267–278 (2016)
13. Buck, C.: Application of Six Sigma to reduce medical errors. In: ASQ World Conference on Quality and Improvement Proceedings, p. 739. American Society for Quality, January 2001
14. Teixeira, T.C., de Cassiani, S.H.: Root cause analysis: evaluation of medication errors at a university hospital. Rev. Esc. Enferm. USP **44**, 139–146 (2010). https://doi.org/10.1590/s0080-62342010000100020
15. Chiozza, M.L., Ponzetti, C.: FMEA: a model for reducing medical errors. Clin. Chim. Acta **404**, 75–78 (2009)
16. Montesi, G., Lechi, A.: Prevention of medication errors: detection and audit. Br. J. Clin. Pharmacol. **67**, 651–655 (2009)
17. Comden, S.C., Marx, D., Murphy-Carley, M., Hale, M.: Using probabilistic risk assessment to model medication system failures in long-term care facilities. In: Henriksen, K., Battles, J. B., Marks, E.S., Lewin, D.I. (eds.) Advances in Patient Safety: From Research to Implementation. Concepts and Methodology (AHRQ Publication No. 05–0021–2. Section: Cognition, Systems, and Risk), vol. 2, pp. 395–408. Agency for Healthcare Research and Quality, Rockville (2005)
18. Cherian, S.M.: Fault tree analysis of commonly occurring medication errors and methods to reduce them. Texas A&M University (1994)
19. Mansouri, A., Ahmadvand, A., Hadjibabaie, M., Kargar, M., Javadi, M., Gholami, K.: Types and severity of medication errors in Iran; a review of the current literature. DARU **21**, 49 (2013)
20. Yang, A., Grissinger, M.: Wrong-patient medication errors: an analysis of event reports in Pennsylvania and strategies for prevention. PA Patient Saf. Rep. Syst. (PA-PSRS) **10**, 41–49 (2013)
21. Lisby, M., Nielsen, L.P., Mainz, J.: Errors in the medication process: frequency, type, and potential clinical consequences. Int. J. Qual. Health Care **17**, 15–22 (2005)
22. Allard, J., Carthey, J., Cope, J., Pitt, M., Wood-ward, S.: Medication errors: causes, prevention and reduction. Br. J. Haematol. **116**, 255–265 (2002)

# Emory Healthcare's Safe Patient Handling Program

Kathy Norris$^{(\boxtimes)}$

Emory Healthcare, 1364 Clifton Rd. NE, Atlanta, GA 30341, USA
kathy.forde@emoryhealthcare.org

**Abstract.** Nursing staff are ranked sixth for highest at-risk for musculoskeletal injuries. Nurses may manually lift up to 2.7 tons in 12 h. Patients are admitted to the hospital sicker and heavier creating a physical challenge for nursing staff. Emory Healthcare launched a Safe Patient Handling Study in 2007 with an ergonomic analysis. 24% of the hospital injuries and 41% of skilled care nursing facility injuries were due to repositioning and transporting patients. The workers' compensation costs were up to $4 million yearly. Lift equipment trials were set up. Emory's Safe Patient Handling Program was implemented in November 2009. A dedicated safe patient handling nurse oversaw training and lift equipment installation. Challenges included maintaining lift sheets and consistent equipment utilization. With nursing education and administrative support, there was a 12.5% cumulative reduction in injuries in 2014. Emory Healthcare is dedicated to keeping nursing staff safe and injury free.

**Keywords:** Safe patient handling · Emory's Occupational Injury Management
Nursing lift assists · Nursing injury prevention programs

## 1 Healthcare in the Future

Quality healthcare is of the utmost importance in the future for longevity. People are living longer healthier lives up into their 90's. Having dedicated, healthy and qualified staff is important for the delivery of proper healthcare. Employment of licensed practical and vocational nurses is projected to grow 12%, registered nurses 15% and nurse practitioners up to 31% from 2016 to 2026. This is faster than the average for all occupations. As the baby-boom population ages, the overall need for healthcare services is expected to increase primarily because of an increased emphasis on preventive care and demand for healthcare services from an aging population [1].

## 2 Physical Demands of Patient Care

The Bureau of Labor Statistics lists nursing staff in sixth place for highest at-risk occupations, for strains and sprains including nurse technicians, orderlies and attendants [2]. Nursing personnel are among the highest at risk for musculoskeletal disorders. The leading cause of these healthcare employees' injuries is patient lifting, transferring, and repositioning injuries, which constitute a significant risk to the health

© Springer International Publishing AG, part of Springer Nature 2019
N. J. Lightner (Ed.): AHFE 2018, AISC 779, pp. 219–225, 2019.
https://doi.org/10.1007/978-3-319-94373-2_24

and welfare of those employees under the Occupational Safety and Health Act of 1970 [3]. It is estimated a nurse may manually lift up to 1.8 tons in an eight-hour shift that equates to 2.7 tons in a twelve-hour shift. For private industry and local government hospitals, which are predominantly medical and surgical hospitals, the most common event leading to injuries in 2015 was overexertion and bodily reaction, which includes injuries from lifting or moving patients [4].

People are living longer quality lives so it is important to protect the health and the welfare of nursing personnel. There is national recognition of the physical stress endured by nursing staff caring for patients at the bedside. Congress proposed bill H.R.4266 Nurse and Health Care Worker Protection Act in 2015. This bill requires the Department of Labor to establish a standard on safe patient handling, mobility, and injury prevention to prevent musculoskeletal disorders for health care workers. The standard must require the use of engineering and safety controls to handle patients [3]. The standard must require health care employers to: 1. develop and implement a safe patient handling, mobility, and injury prevention program; 2. train their workers on safe patient handling, mobility, and injury prevention; and 3. post a notice that explains the standard, procedures to report patient handling-related injuries, and workers' rights under this Act. The Department of Labor must conduct unscheduled inspections to ensure compliance with the standard. This bill amends title XVIII (Medicare) of the Social Security Act to apply the standard to hospitals receiving Medicare funds [3].

Patients are being admitted to the hospital sicker and heavier at Emory Healthcare. It is not uncommon to have a 600 lb. patient. In 2016, the State OF Obesity Report in Georgia reported 31.4% of Georgia adults were overweight. They are ranked 20th highest in the United States [5]. This presents a physical challenge for new resident nurses as well as experienced nurses. These days nurses are working bedside at times into their 60's.

# 3   Evolution of the Emory Safe Patient Handling Program

Emory Healthcare has always been on the forefront of promoting safety for our nursing staff. The Employee Occupational Injury Management Department launched a Safe Patient Handling and Movement Study in 2007 to develop a standardized process to reduce back and shoulder injuries in the nursing staff. Two ergonomists from Hill-Rom conducted an onsite evaluation. It was estimated 24% of the total injuries (229 employees), in our two primary hospitals, were due to patient handling. In the Emory skilled care facility, it accounted for 41% of the total injuries (62 employees). Injuries primarily occurred with repositioning patients in bed and transporting the patients in beds and stretchers. With onsite physical therapy, 39% of over 300 injuries treated were from the nursing staff. The estimated total direct and indirect workers' compensation costs were between $1.9 million to $4 million per year.

Based on the Safe Patient Handling and Movement Study, the Emory team set up lift equipment trials. The Emory Healthcare Safe Patient Handling Team evaluated many lifting and transfer devices on designated nursing units. The staff recommended purchasing the Liko Overhead Lifts and lift sheets.

The Safe Patient Handling Program was implemented in November 2009. A safe patient handling nurse coordinator was designated to oversee the staff training and installation of the patient lifts. The staff utilized the Liko Lift System, which could hold up to 440 lbs. with a lift sheet. Some patient rooms were set up with two lifts to accommodate an 880 lbs. patient. The Viking Lift and Sara Steady were mobile lifts utilized. Transfers sheets have been utilized to include the Angel Slider, plastic slide transfer boards and the Tortoise patient slider.

## 4   The Emory Safe Patient Handling Program

The Safe Patient Handling (SPH) Coordinator is employed under the Emory Occupational Injury Management Department. The SPH Coordinator constantly monitors the injuries that occur due to moving patients. Training programs are provided on a regular basis. The training programs have expanded to New Resident Nursing Training and a Smooth Moves New Employee Orientation Program. The Radiology Department transporters and radiology technologists were provided training for the mechanical lifts and motorized stretchers. Mitigation programs include a one on one interview with the injured staff member to assess if the lift system could have been utilized. Unit specific analysis is used to determine the lifting equipment needs. Entity specific data, i.e. type of injury such as lumbar or shoulder strain and the location of incidence, is provided to nursing management. The patient handling injuries are included in the Nursing Quality Index. Pilot programs are set up as designated by the staff.

The Safe Patient Handling (SPH) Coordinator provides multiple avenues for training. Emory Healthcare has an Intranet Site with Department Specific information for the Nursing Department. There is a dedicated Safe Patient Handling Site. It includes the contact for the SPH Coordinator, training videos, and a checklist for training. There is information on how to purchase the lift sheets and accessories. The SPH coordinator is always communicating with the staff to assess ways to avoid musculoskeletal injuries.

Challenges in the beginning included maintaining the lift sheets on inpatient units and having the staff consistently utilize the lift equipment. The lift sheets were embroidered and separated out from the hospital linen. Some of the lift sheets were accidently thrown into the regular laundry and never returned. The electrical mobile lifts were not always plugged in on the inpatient floor. If this occurred, the equipment was not functional at the time of the staff needed to utilize the electrical mobile lift. Lift champions were recognized on the inpatient units to promote the utilization of the lift assists. With significant continual nursing staff education and administrative support, there was a 12.5% cumulative reduction in injuries in 2014. A policy was set up and established which now requires that the staff have to utilize the lift equipment for patient handling to avoid musculoskeletal injures.

# 5    Safe Patient Handling Statistics

Overall, cumulative reported injuries reduced for 230 employees in 2015 to 201 employees in 2017. Of these injuries, cumulative yearly recordable patient handling injuries (those that required medical care) reduced from 153 in 2014 to 125 in 2017. Our reported injuries have reduced even with increasing our nursing staff. Emory Healthcare has added over 125 nursing staff positions between 2014 and 2017 with the addition of a new Emory Hospital Tower on our Emory University Campus (Figs. 1 and 2).

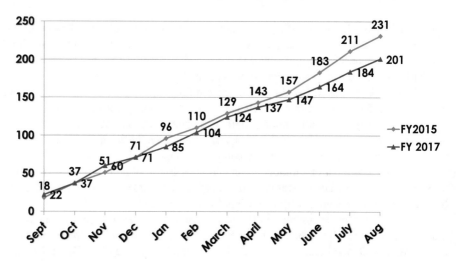

**Fig. 1.** Cumulative patient handling reported injuries from September 2014 to August 2017

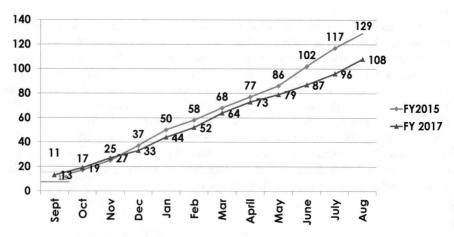

**Fig. 2.** Cumulative reportable patient handling injuries from September 2014 to August 2017

In 2016, one Cardiothoracic ICU unit averaged eight injuries per year. They did have patients weighing over 600 lbs. They piloted a study where each ICU bed was prepped with a lift sheet positioned on the bed prior to the patient occupying the bed. Backup lift sheets were readily available. The staff attended the Liko Lift training. From May 2016 to February 2017, there were only two patient handling injuries (Fig. 3).

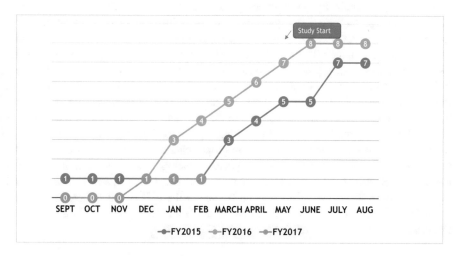

**Fig. 3.** Emory University Hospital Cardiothoracic ICU pilot study results

# 6  Injury Prevention with Lift and Transfer Devices

Emory Healthcare Hospital encourages each nursing department to evaluate the best lifting/transfer device and method for their inpatient unit. One nursing unit has a Lift Turn Team schedule. On each shift, the staff will pair up to turn and reposition each patient on the floor every two hours. With this system, the nursing staff member should only have to turn and reposition patients one time per twelve-hour shift. Some inpatient units utilize the Angel Sliders and another unit utilizes the Tortoise Patient Slider. Some inpatient units have ordered smaller Liko lift slings that can support a patient's leg or arm to assist with positioning the patient's arm or leg for dressing changes or cleaning the patient. Patient transfer boards are standardly used to move a patient from a bed to a stretcher.

The Emory Occupational Injury Management Physical Therapy Department teams up the Safe Patient Handling Coordinator to provide an injury prevention program. From physical therapy statistics of discharged patients, it was determined the primary injuries occurred to the back, shoulders and wrists. The injury prevention program is designed to review proper posture and body mechanics to help the employee position themselves for success. The goal is to work efficiently and reduce physical stress to the employee's low back, shoulders and wrists. The staff in instructed to use a neutral power grip position to move patients in bed to reduce wrist strains. Moving a patient up in bed abducting the arm from the side can lead to a rotator cuff strain. The staff is trained to move patients up in bed by rotating the shoulders with their arms at their side when moving a patient up in bed. There are joint in-services given by the SPH Coordinator and the physical therapist as needed to train the staff with the injury prevention techniques and to become efficient utilizing the lift devices.

Other aspects of safe patient handling involve moving patents in beds and stretchers. Emory Healthcare opened a new Hospital Tower in September 2017. It is connected to the main Emory University Hospital via a two level bridge. There is a dedicated bridge to transport inpatients from their hospital beds to other areas for testing and for surgery. The bridge has a slight elevation between the two hospital areas. Three StaminaLift TS5000 Bed and Stretcher Movers were purchased to assist the staff with moving the patients. The Radiology Department also purchased electronic stretchers. Some of the new patient beds are motorized. This allows ease of the staff in transporting the patient safely on the inclined bridge way. A transporter is also stationed on the bridge to move the patients in the bed with the StaminaLift TS5000. This allows the nursing staff to dedicate their time and energy to care for the patients.

It is also important for the staff to have proper clearance in the inpatient rooms, the Operating Room, Radiology and other specialty testing areas. It is important to clear the area of electrical cords and equipment. Emory Healthcare has added larger sized inpatient rooms. They also utilize special Booms in the ICU rooms to help easily open the ICU room up and tuck away the electrical cords and tubing off the floor for patient transfers from the bed to stretchers.

## 7 Conclusion

Emory Healthcare employs over 3000 nurses and 850 nurse technicians in our three primary hospitals alone. With Emory Healthcare and Emory University personnel combined, our staff has increased from 20,000 to 40,000 in the past ten years. Between 2005 to 2015, Emory Healthcare reduced the worker's compensation costs by 1.34 million dollars with twice the staff. Emory Healthcare's Safe Patient Handling Program has made a significant impact on reducing the work related injuries and overall costs. With our expanding hospital system, it is important to keep our nursing staff healthy, safe and free to concentrate on providing quality patient care. At Emory Healthcare, we know that together we can achieve great things. Our motto at Emory Healthcare is that we are all in this together to provide quality and safe patient care.

## References

1. Bureau of Labor Statistics: U.S. Department of Labor, Occupational Outlook Handbook, Licensed Practical and Licensed Vocational Nurses. https://wwwbls.gov/ooh/healthcare/licensed-practical-and-licensed-vocational-nurses.htm. Accessed 30 Jan 2018
2. Bureau of Labor Statistics Incidence rates are compared across private hospitals, private construction industries, and private manufacturing industries

3. H.R.4266-Nurse and Health Care Worker Protection Act of 2015. Sponsor Rep. Conyers, John, Jr. [D-MI-13], Introduced 16 December 2015
4. Dressner, M.A.: Hospital workers: an assessment of occupational injuries and illnesses. Monthly Labor Rev. (2017). https://doi.org/10.21916/mlr.2017.17
5. The State of Obesity: Better Policies for a Healthier America released August 2017

# The Impacts on Patient Safety of Changes in the Design of Medical Products and Devices Used in Patient Care Settings

Helen J. A. Fuller[1(✉)], Timothy Arnold[1,2], Nancy Lightner[3], and Tandi Bagian[1]

[1] National Center for Patient Safety, Ann Arbor, USA
{Helen.Fuller,Timothy.Arnold4,Tandi.Bagian}@VA.gov
[2] University of Michigan College of Pharmacy, Ann Arbor, USA
[3] Veterans Engineering Resource Center, Indianapolis, USA
Nancy.Lightner@VA.gov

**Abstract.** Changes in medical product or device design can have important implications in patient safety. An altered device interface may change the ability of a clinician to use the device properly, even if the underlying functionality of the device is the same. When a new device is brought into a health care setting, issues may occur at various stages, including acquisition, deployment, and continuing education. This paper examines reported patient safety events related to the introduction of new or changed devices into the health care environment. Communication was found to be a root cause of some events. In particular, lack of communication to the end user of product differences can result in misuse in the patient care setting. Recommendations include increased clinician input at the product selection and deployment stage and documentation of changes in product interface or use instructions to improve end user training and point-of-use aids.

**Keywords:** Human factors · Health care · Usability · Patient safety

## 1 Introduction

There is a great body of literature regarding inadvertent harm in health care. The famous Institute of Medicine report *To Err is Human* provided a wake-up call on the magnitude of the problem and helped to engage experts in disparate domains to address the topic of errors in health care [1]. Since then, there has been increased interest in examining how systems engineering and human factors can help to explain how harm occurs and suggest possible solutions, e.g., [2–5]. The United States Food and Drug Administration (FDA) offers recommendations for manufacturers for applying human factors to the design of medical devices and describes national and international consensus standards related to human factors and medical devices [6].

The field of human factors addresses the capabilities and limitations of people and how these influence the physical and cognitive interactions between humans and systems [7]. Health care human factors focuses on interactions with systems in the health care environment, including electronic health records, medical devices, and clinical products.

© Springer International Publishing AG, part of Springer Nature (outside the USA) 2019
N. J. Lightner (Ed.): AHFE 2018, AISC 779, pp. 226–233, 2019.
https://doi.org/10.1007/978-3-319-94373-2_25

Some examples of inadvertent patient harm are tied to the use of health care products and devices. Clinicians and human factors practitioners are increasingly describing the occurrence in health care settings of product or device use errors, which occur because of how a product or device is used rather than from a malfunction.

Human factors literature tells us that design changes may have impacts on usability and error tolerance [7]. Some changes may improve usability if, for example, they provide a better fit with the user's physical or cognitive capabilities, allow use in a way that better fits the user's workflow, fits better with the user's mental model, or are more error-tolerant [4]. For example, a manufacturer changed the design of a thermal fuse intended to stop the flow of oxygen from an oxygen tank to a patient in the event of a fire. Previously, the fuse was unidirectional and would not work if inserted backwards; the new design is bidirectional and works when inserted in either orientation.

Other design changes may decrease usability. This may occur due to design changes that make the product harder to use, but also because the new product design may fail to provide clear indications of its current state or to match the user's expectations of how the product should work based on the user's experience with similar products. For example, a transport monitor indicated it was in demonstration mode with a small, inconspicuous "D" on the screen [8]. If users missed that signal, they would operate under an incorrect understanding of the patient's condition.

In the best case, the user will realize that she or he does not know how to use the product; in the worst case, the user is accustomed to the product working one way and does not realize there is a change that impacts correct product use. In addition, a user may realize the product is different but forgets during high-pressure situations.

Manufacturers may sometimes be faced with systems goals that conflict with safety goals, leading to required constraints in design. For example, having a demonstration mode for the transport monitor described above meets an important training need, and making it look very similar to the screen during actual use improves the fidelity of training.

New items are routinely introduced into health care settings. There may be new products developed, or the design of currently available products may change with updates. A new contract may mean different products are brought into the health care facility. In addition, shortages or recalls can result in a rapid change from one product to another.

## 2 Methods

To identify cases of design changes impacting patient safety, we reviewed incident reports, including close calls, from multiple facilities in a large health care system in the United States. From these, we identified a subset of reports that were related to product or device usability. We then performed an in-depth review of the reports, including contacting reporters for additional information, in order to extract aspects related to human factors. The result is several case studies of how design changes can impact patient safety in the health care setting.

# 3   Case Studies

**Case 1: Oxygen Tank.** Several facilities reported concerns about the design of a new portable oxygen E tank. With the old tank, the user could start the flow of oxygen using only a valve on the top of the tank's regulator to set the desired rate. The new tank required the user to turn a separate valve, on the side of the regulator, prior to setting the flow rate with the valve on the top.

At one facility, a nurse first encountered the new tank during a night shift when she needed oxygen for a patient. At first, she was unsure of how to operate the tank, but she was able to obtain oxygen flow after some trial and error. She reported her concern at morning rounds, and the clinicians determined that due to a communication failure, they had not received training on the new design.

After learning about the new design, clinicians reported that they were concerned that users would think oxygen was flowing to the patient based on the setting on the top valve and not realize that the tank was not on. If the clinician is focused on the top valve, it is easy to miss seeing that there is an additional valve on the side of the regulator. A diagram of the how to operate each oxygen tank is shown in Fig. 1.

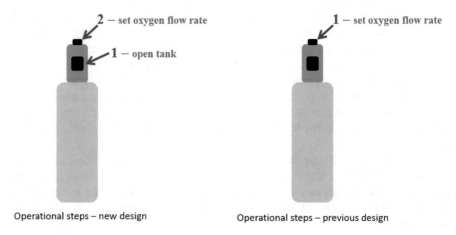

Operational steps – new design          Operational steps – previous design

**Fig. 1.**   Diagram of oxygen tanks showing steps to operate. The new design requires that the user must open the tank using Valve 1 and then set the desired flow of oxygen using Valve 2. The previous design only had one valve.

Upon further review, the presence of the new oxygen tanks was due to a contracting change that resulted in a different manufacturer providing portable oxygen tanks for in-hospital use. In at least one facility, the contracting process did not include consultation with patient safety or clinicians prior to creating the contract and accepting the new tank. Increased collaboration may have allowed the facility to identify and avoid or mitigate the hazard at an earlier stage.

In addition, there was a communications failure that resulted in clinicians not receiving the intended training on the new tanks prior to their introduction into the facility.

After interviewing contracting and patient safety staff at three facilities, we learned that one key aspect of the contract change was the ability of the supplier to provide the tanks on the schedule the facility needed. The tank design met basic requirements, and the design of the new tank was actually considered superior by the manufacturer, because they claimed it makes it safer to store and transport pressurized gas.

**Case 2: Scalpel Strength.** A second case involved a scalpel that was used for outpatient procedures in a health care facility. During use, the blade snapped. The surgeon reported that the scalpel felt less sturdy than the scalpel he was accustomed to using during this procedure. It is possible that the scalpel may have struck an anatomic structure or a surgical clip during the procedure, but the surgeon had never experienced this problem with previous designs and felt that the failure was due to the design of the new product.

The facility had switched scalpel suppliers twice in order to purchase on contract. In addition, the facility wanted to avoid known safety issues with a different design that consisted of a disposable blade and a reusable handle that needed to be reprocessed between uses. The facility had found that staff sometimes forgot to remove the blade for disposal in the sharps container, which could result in staff injury and potential exposure to blood borne pathogens. In solving one problem, they may have introduced a different one, demonstrating what can happen when there are necessary tradeoffs in two systems goals, both emphasizing safety.

**Case 3: IV Bag Text Color.** Users at a facility identified a potential hazard caused by a labeling change. One manufacturer changed their design of an IV bag containing heparin by replacing red text with black text. This design change may have been intended to improve readability, because red text on a bag of clear fluid has low contrast. However, the unintended consequence was that the change made the IV bag look similar to a different product. Figure 2 contains an illustration of (A) the previous design, (B) the new design, and (C) a standard IV bag of normal saline.

The concern regarding the changed IV bag design was identified by a pharmacy technician during inpatient pharmacy distribution tasks. The heparin bag was stored next to normal saline in the storage area. The large block of red text, though difficult to read, was a salient characteristic of the bag for individuals with normal color vision, and it is possible that clinicians, perhaps subconsciously, used it as a cue to identify the IV bag as containing a potentially hazardous substance. By removing this cue, the manufacturer increased the design similarity between the two products and may have increased the risk of selecting an unintended product, possibly resulting in patient harm.

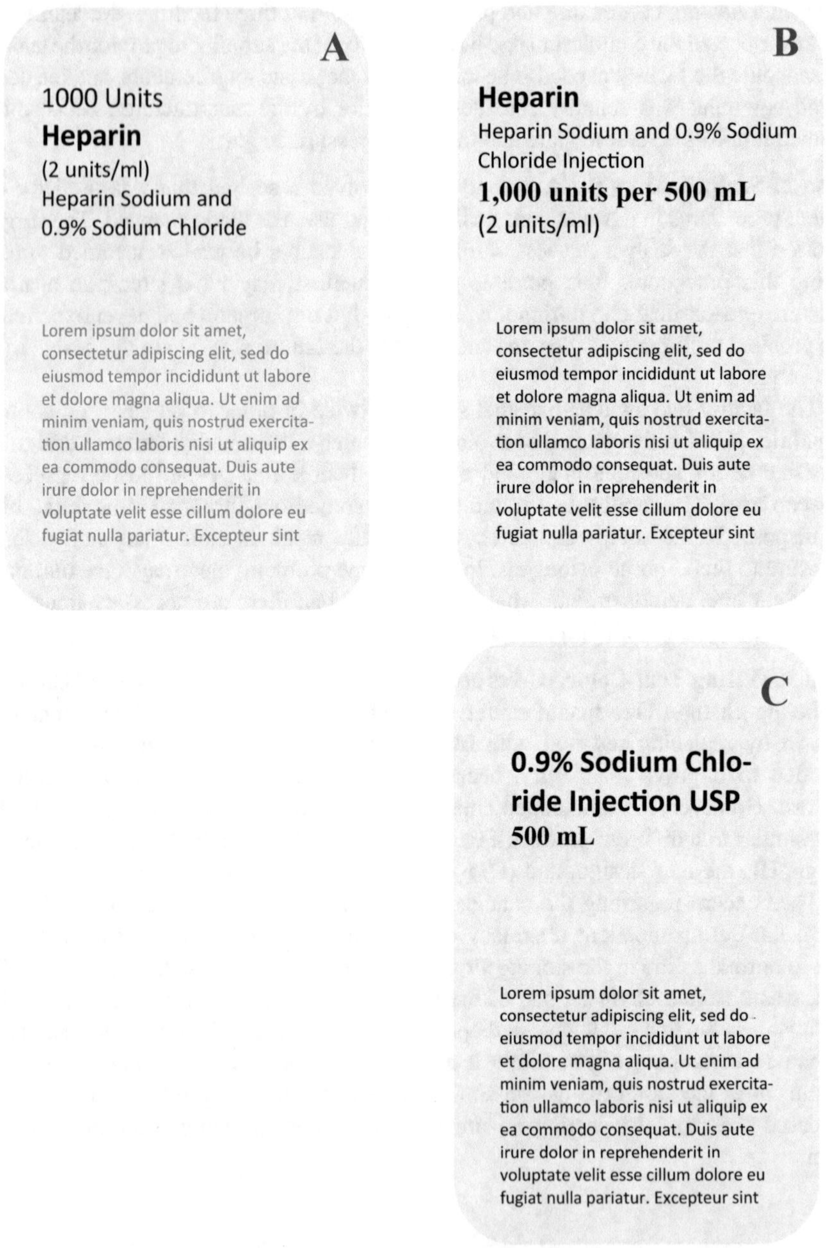

**A**

1000 Units

**Heparin**

(2 units/ml)
Heparin Sodium and
0.9% Sodium Chloride

Lorem ipsum dolor sit amet,
consectetur adipiscing elit, sed do
eiusmod tempor incididunt ut labore
et dolore magna aliqua. Ut enim ad
minim veniam, quis nostrud exercita-
tion ullamco laboris nisi ut aliquip ex
ea commodo consequat. Duis aute
irure dolor in reprehenderit in
voluptate velit esse cillum dolore eu
fugiat nulla pariatur. Excepteur sint

**B**

**Heparin**

Heparin Sodium and 0.9% Sodium
Chloride Injection

**1,000 units per 500 mL**

(2 units/ml)

Lorem ipsum dolor sit amet,
consectetur adipiscing elit, sed do
eiusmod tempor incididunt ut labore
et dolore magna aliqua. Ut enim ad
minim veniam, quis nostrud exercita-
tion ullamco laboris nisi ut aliquip ex
ea commodo consequat. Duis aute
irure dolor in reprehenderit in
voluptate velit esse cillum dolore eu
fugiat nulla pariatur. Excepteur sint

**C**

**0.9% Sodium Chlo-
ride Injection USP**

**500 mL**

Lorem ipsum dolor sit amet,
consectetur adipiscing elit, sed do
eiusmod tempor incididunt ut labore
et dolore magna aliqua. Ut enim ad
minim veniam, quis nostrud exercita-
tion ullamco laboris nisi ut aliquip ex
ea commodo consequat. Duis aute
irure dolor in reprehenderit in
voluptate velit esse cillum dolore eu
fugiat nulla pariatur. Excepteur sint

**Fig. 2.** This is an illustration of the design change of an IV bag of heparin. The original design is (A), and the new design is (B). Compare each to a bag of normal saline (C). For a user selecting a bag quickly without reading the text, it may be more likely for him or her to confuse Bag B with Bag C than to confuse Bag A with Bag C.

# 4   Discussion

While new designs may be beneficial, there is also the potential for harm from product or device changes. Failure to use a product or device correctly to deliver the desired treatment, error by omission, may mean the patient does not receive the intended treatment. Using a product or device incorrectly may introduce new hazards, which may be made more dangerous because they are unexpected or go unrecognized. Finally, the change may result in a failure of users to differentiate between two products or devices, contributing to them using the wrong one.

This paper examined a sample of reported patient safety events related to the introduction of new or changed products and devices into the health care environment. It discussed the stages at which changes could be made to reduce the probability of patient harm. Communication was found to be a root cause of some events. In particular, lack of communication to the end user of the differences in the product or device can result in misuse in the patient care setting. Recommendations include a consistent process for obtaining clinician input at the product or device selection and deployment stage and documentation of changes in product or device interface or use instructions to improve end user training and point-of-use aids.

Users may encounter interface changes due to new products or devices entering a facility that are different than those used previously or due to a change in the product or device design for an otherwise familiar product (Fig. 3). The introduction of a new or changed products and devices into a health care system should trigger actions on the part of the facility.

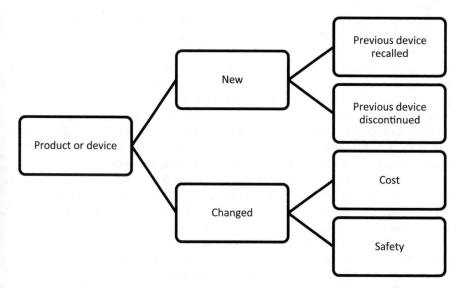

**Fig. 3.** Users may encounter new product or device interfaces due to new products or devices entering a facility or design changes in currently used products or devices.

Facilities should utilize human factors techniques to consider designs in the context of expected and possible uses. They should consider relevant characteristics of users, tasks, and environments [14]. It is particularly important to identify what users are accustomed to using and whether there are significant changes in the user interface or design. Human factors practitioners have described the importance of a multifaceted, team-based approach that utilizes the knowledge and experience of clinicians when addressing human factors in health care environments [9].

Similarly, manufacturers should incorporate human factors and usability experts and perform a full risk analysis, including considering unintended consequences, when making a design change [10, 11]. It is not sufficient to make a change that is supported by human factors principles or to conduct a limited usability evaluation that focuses only on a component of the use; manufacturers must take into account the full impact of the change given the users and the context of use. The FDA also addresses the need for manufacturers to perform a risk assessment, consider unintended consequences, and conduct testing to determine whether a change significantly affects safety [12]. It is challenging, perhaps impossible, to predict the introduction of every risk. Therefore, a rigorous post-implementation monitoring process should be implemented to examine usability.

Patient harm may be avoided if users are trained to identify unintended or unexpected use and encouraged to report concerns to patient safety professionals in their organizations. Aggregating user concerns could help to identify products with usability issues. In addition, it is very important to involve end users, patient safety professionals, and human factors professionals in the product acquisition process. Each of these roles can bring to the discussion important and distinct information based on specialized training.

There are multiple possible facility responses to identified usability issues. Research has identified a tendency in health care to blame the user, but this is seldom a useful or fair response [13]. Often, a more effective but also more difficult solution is replacing a problematic product or device. The facility could also increase point-of-use aids such as instructions and signs. These should be available and obvious to the user at the time of use. It is important to develop these with input from human factors engineers and to include end-user testing. Another possible solution is training, but this is generally considered a weak fix for multiple reasons [5, 7]. Staff turnover and scheduling difficulties make it difficult to train all users. In addition, users tend to fall back on what they are most familiar with in times of urgent action.

Changes in medical product or device design can have important implications in patient safety. Changing the user-facing parts of a product or device may change the ability of a clinician to use the item properly, even if the underlying functionality is the same. When a new product or device is brought into a health care setting, failures in successful adoption of the item into the clinical care environment may be introduced at many different stages, including acquisition, deployment, and continuing education. The omission of clinician input at the product selection stage is common, and clinicians may not realize the product or device has changed until patient harm occurs. A robust solution involves a team-based approach that includes the necessary technical knowledge, familiarity with the environment of use, and experience with human factors, usability, and systems-based thinking to evaluate the product or device, prior to purchase, while accounting for the full context of use.

**Acknowledgments.** We would like to thank everyone at the National Center for Patient Safety for their commitment to patient safety. There were no relevant financial relationships or any source of support in the forms of grants, equipment, or drugs. The authors declare no conflicts of interest. The opinions expressed in this article are those of the authors and do not necessarily represent those of the Veterans Administration.

# References

1. Kohn, L.T., Corrigan, J.M., Donaldson, M.S. (eds.): To Err is Human: Building a Safer Health System. National Academy Press, Washington, DC (1999). Institute of Medicine
2. Zhang, J., Johnson, T.R., Patel, V.L., Paige, D.L., Kubose, T.: Using usability heuristics to evaluate patient safety of medical devices. J. Biomed. Inform. 36(1–2), 23–30 (2003)
3. Fairbanks, R.J., Wears, R.L.: Hazards with medical devices: the role of design. Ann. Emerg. Med. 52(5), 519–521 (2008)
4. Weinger, M.B., Wiklund, M.E., Gardner-Bonneau, D.J. (eds.): Handbook of Human Factors in Medical Device Design. CRC Press, Boca Raton (2010)
5. Russ, A.L., Fairbanks, R.J., Karsh, B.T., Militello, L.G., Saleem, J.J., Wears, R.L.: The science of human factors: separating fact from fiction. BMJ Qual. Saf. 22(10), 802–808 (2013)
6. FDA: Applying Human Factors and Usability Engineering to Medical Devices (2011)
7. Wickens, C.D., Lee, J., Liu, Y., Becker, S.G.: An introduction to human factors engineering (2004)
8. Gosbee, J.: Human factors engineering and patient safety. Qual. Saf. Health Care 11(4), 352–354 (2002)
9. Catchpole, K.: Spreading human factors expertise in healthcare: untangling the knots in people and systems (2013)
10. Dekker, S.: The Field Guide to Understanding Human Error. Ashgate Publishing Ltd. (2014)
11. Pritchett, A.R., Strong, A.C.: Integrating cognitive engineering into industry design teams. J. Cogn. Eng. Decis. Mak. 10(2), 134–137 (2016)
12. FDA: Deciding When to Submit a 510(k) for a Change to an Existing Device (2017)
13. Johnson, T.R., Tang, X., Graham, M.J., Brixey, J., Turley, J.P., Zhang, J., Patel, V.L.: Attitudes toward medical device use errors and the prevention of adverse events. Joint Comm. J. Qual. Patient Saf. 33(11), 689–694 (2007)
14. Fuller, H.J., Bagian, T.M.: Task excursion analysis: matching the tool to the user, environment, and task. In: Proceedings of the International Symposium on Human Factors and Ergonomics in Health Care, vol. 3, no. 1, pp. 203–206. SAGE Publications, New Delhi, June 2014

# Patient Perceptions of the Use of a Technology-Augmented Healthcare System for the Self-care of Type 2 Diabetes Mellitus and/or Hypertension

Mian Yan[✉]

Institute of Physical Internet, School of Electrical and Information Engineering,
Jinan University (Zhuhai Campus), Zhuhai 519070, China
yanmian@jnu.edu.cn

**Abstract.** The use of consumer health information technologies (ITs) has been escalating among chronically ill patients to enhance the quality of disease self-care. Yet, studies examining the feasibility of such technologies among populations of in-home self-care patients are rare. This study provides the research community with a preliminary assessment of the feasibility of consumer health IT. A total of 38 patients with type 2 diabetes and/or hypertension were enrolled in the study. A tablet-based chronic disease self-monitoring system was set up in patient homes to facilitate disease self-monitoring for a duration of 12 weeks. Patient perceptions about seven variables indicating the feasibility of the system were collected at 2 weeks and 12 weeks post-implementation. Results showed that the healthcare system tested in this study was feasible from patients' perspectives. Further research is needed to verify the findings in larger samples with longer durations, and assess its feasibility from other aspects.

**Keywords:** Consumer health information technology · Disease self-care
Feasibility study

## 1 Background and Objectives

The prevalence of type 2 diabetes and hypertension has been growing among populations through past decades, increasing the chances of developing life-threatening complications such as stroke, heart failure, and other cardiovascular diseases; Continuous glycemic and hypertensive control is required to prevent evolving such complications [1]. Self-monitoring of blood glucose (BG) and blood pressure (BP), which allows patients acquire prompt information about their vital signs and help get better control of disease conditions, is suggested as one good practice among these patients [2, 3].

It has been progressively common for patients to conduct self-monitoring at home owing to the broad availability and low cost of the conventional BG/BP measurement devices in the market. However, patients' adherence to BG/BP self-monitoring is suboptimal [4, 5]. To facilitate disease self-monitoring and provide better healthcare quality, consumer health information technologies (ITs), incorporating with innovative ways of information sharing, communicating, and decision making, are becoming

© Springer International Publishing AG, part of Springer Nature 2019
N. J. Lightner (Ed.): AHFE 2018, AISC 779, pp. 234–239, 2019.
https://doi.org/10.1007/978-3-319-94373-2_26

popular. Benefits of implementing consumer health ITs have been well documented in the literature [6, 7]. Yet, research studies examining the feasibility of such technologies among populations of in-home self-care patients were less studied.

To this end, this study aimed to assess the feasibility of consumer health IT for the self-care of type 2 diabetes mellitus and/or hypertension in a home care setting.

## 2 Materials and Methods

### 2.1 Chronic Disease Self-monitoring System

The consumer health IT used in this study was a technology-augmented chronic disease self-monitoring system that comprised of a 10-inch touchscreen tablet computer and a two-in-one BG/BP meter. The interactive system was developed on the basis of human factors approaches and feedback from patients with chronic diseases. The primary application of this system was to help patients measure, record, and track their BG and BP. The measurement records can be saved and retrieved for review. Structured graphs and tables were used to present the vital sign records, where abnormal measurement values were displayed with red color, and values within the normal range were displayed with black color. Educational videos were incorporated into the system to provide patients with pertinent health information, such as how to conduct self-care, collocate diet, and take exercise.

### 2.2 Outcome Measurement

Variables indicating the feasibility of the consumer health IT were selected in a review of previous literature of technology acceptance and adoption. Two variables drawn from the Technology Acceptance Model [8] and its extensions [9, 10], perceived usefulness and perceived ease of use, were used to measure the degree to which patients believe that using the chronic disease self-monitoring system would be useful and free of effort; Perceived behavioral control [11] and application-specific self-efficacy [12] were employed to examine patient perceptions of the internal ability and external constraints to perform disease self-monitoring; Subjective norm [13, 14] was measured to understand how patients were influenced by others' opinions regarding the acceptance or non-acceptance of the disease self-monitoring system; Attitude [15] and behavioral intention [16] were examined to understand patient feelings and intentions toward using the system to perform disease self-monitoring.

The measurement scales were adapted from previous mentioned validated research works and were rated on a seven-point Likert-type scale, whereby 1 indicates "very strongly disagree", 2 indicates "strongly disagree", 3 indicates "disagree", 4 indicates "neutral", 5 indicates "agree", 6 indicates "strongly agree", and 7 indicates "very strongly agree".

## 2.3 Participants

Participants of the study were recruited from three health service centers of a non-profit health service network that provided healthcare and services to the community. The site managers of the health service centers first contacted potential patients and invited them to attend the recruitment talk, where the purpose of the study and applications of the disease self-monitoring system were introduced. On-site screenings were conducted for potential participants who were interested in the study to confirm their eligibilities. Inclusion criteria for enrollment were: (1) age of 18 years or above with a diagnosis of type 2 diabetes and/or hypertension for at least 3 months' duration, (2) taking oral hypoglycemic and/or antihypertensive medications, (3) normal (or corrected-to-normal) vision, (4) no cognitive or physical impairment, (5) the ability to learn and perform tablet computer-based disease self-monitoring, and (6) the ability to understand written and spoken Chinese. Patients with unstable or life-threatening conditions were excluded.

## 2.4 Study Procedures

This study received institutional review board approval of the author's institution. After getting the informed consents, sociodemographic information of the participants was obtained including age, gender, education level, living status, and self-reported computer experience. A brief training session was carried out to teach participants to use the disease self-monitoring system. Patients were provided with the system at no cost and were encouraged to use the devices to measure their vital signs and perform other disease self-management activities as recommended by their healthcare providers. Technical support was provided upon the requirement of the participants throughout the study. A questionnaire comprised of the seven variables was administered to participants at 2 weeks (T1) and 12 weeks (T2) post-implementation.

## 2.5 Data Analysis

Data collected at T1 and T2 were used to examine patient perceptions about the feasibility of the health IT to perform disease self-monitoring. At each time point, arithmetical means with standard deviations and 95% confidence intervals of the average rating scores for each variable were calculated. Two-tailed paired samples t-test was conducted to detect the changes in rating scores over time. Prior to conducting the analysis, the assumption of distribution normality for all variables was tested. IBM SPSS statistics package for Window was used for data analysis.

# 3   Results

## 3.1   Sample Characteristics

A total of 38 patients were enrolled in this study and returned 38 valid responses at both T1 and T2. Sociodemographic characteristics were calculated and presented in Table 1.

**Table 1.** Sample characteristics.

|  | Participants ($n = 38$) |
|---|---|
| Males/females | 15/23 |
| Mean age (*Standard deviation*) | 69.2 (9.4) years |
| Education |  |
| Primary school or below | 22 (57.9%) |
| Secondary school | 12 (31.6%) |
| College or above | 4 (10.5%) |
| Living status |  |
| Live alone | 11 (28.9%) |
| Live with family | 27 (70.1%) |
| Self-reported computer experience |  |
| None | 23 (60.5%) |
| Beginner | 10 (26.3%) |
| Competent | 5 (13.2%) |

## 3.2  Variables Indicating Feasibility

Results from descriptive statistics showed the disease self-monitoring system had a considerable level of feasibility among in-home self-care patients (see Table 2). The lower bounds of the average rating score for all variables at both time points surpassed five at the 95% confidence level, indicating that patients were substantially "agree": (1) using the disease self-monitoring system was useful and free of effort, (2) they had the sense of control and efficacy to use the system, (3) patients' important others would support their use of the system, and (4) they had positive attitudes and intentions toward using the system to perform disease self-monitoring.

**Table 2.** Descriptive statistics of the variables ($n = 38$).

| Variable |  | Mean (*SD*) | 95% CI |
|---|---|---|---|
| Perceived usefulness | T1 | 5.59 (0.70) | [5.35, 5.82] |
|  | T2 | 5.62 (0.74) | [5.37, 5.86] |
| Perceived ease of use | T1 | 5.47 (0.82) | [5.20, 5.74] |
|  | T2 | 5.59 (0.67) | [5.36, 5.81] |
| Perceived behavioral control | T1 | 5.46 (0.69) | [5.23, 5.68] |
|  | T2 | 5.54 (0.71) | [5.31, 5.77] |
| Application-specific self-efficacy | T1 | 5.55 (0.80) | [5.29, 5.81] |
|  | T2 | 5.57 (0.63) | [5.36, 5.78] |
| Subjective norm | T1 | 5.32 (0.72) | [5.08, 5.55] |
|  | T2 | 5.39 (0.78) | [5.14, 5.65] |
| Attitude | T1 | 5.57 (0.71) | [5.34, 5.81] |
|  | T2 | 5.57 (0.72) | [5.33, 5.81] |
| Behavioral intention | T1 | 5.50 (0.83) | [5.23, 5.77] |
|  | T2 | 5.42 (0.90) | [5.13, 5.72] |

*Note: SD* indicates standard deviation; CI = confidence interval; T1 and T2 indicate 2 weeks and 12 weeks post-implementation, respectively.

### 3.3 Paired Samples Statistics

The normality assumption was considered satisfied, as the absolute values of skewness and kurtosis of the variables at both time points were less than 1 [17, 18]. Results from the paired samples t-test revealed none significant differences between T1 and T2. The effect size indicated by Cohen's d also suggests little differences between the mean values of the variables at both time points [19]. Table 3 presents the results of the paired samples t-test.

**Table 3.** Paired samples *t*-test results for each of the variables.

| Variable | $t(37)$ | $p$ | 95% CI | Cohen's $d$ |
|---|---|---|---|---|
| Perceived usefulness | −0.27 | 0.79 | [−0.28, 0.21] | −0.05 |
| Perceived ease of use | −1.22 | 0.23 | [−0.32, 0.08] | −0.16 |
| Perceived behavioral control | −0.85 | 0.40 | [−0.28, 0.12] | −0.12 |
| Application-specific self-efficacy | −0.17 | 0.87 | [−0.23, 0.19] | −0.02 |
| Subjective norm | −0.63 | 0.53 | [−0.33, 0.18] | −0.10 |
| Attitude | 0.00 | 1.00 | [−0.21, 0.21] | 0.00 |
| Behavioral intention | 0.53 | 0.60 | [−0.22, 0.38] | 0.09 |

*Note: $p$ = two-tailed $p$-value; CI = confidence interval; Cohen's $d$ indicates the standardized difference between mean values of the variable at T1 and T2.*

## 4    Conclusions

This study assessed the feasibility of a technology-augmented disease self-monitoring system among patients with type 2 diabetes and/or hypertension. The healthcare system tested in this study was shown to be feasible from patients' perspectives. Further research is needed to verify the findings in larger samples with longer durations, and assess its feasibility from other aspects.

**Acknowledgments.** The study was conducted with the support of the Fundamental Research Funds for the Central Universities (grant no. 21618317).

## References

1. American Diabetes Association: Standards of medical care in diabetes-2014. Diabetes Care **37**(Supplement 1), S14–S80 (2014)
2. Cappuccio, F.P., et al.: Blood pressure control by home monitoring: meta-analysis of randomised trials. BMJ **329**(145) (2004)
3. Karter, A.J., et al.: Self-monitoring of blood glucose levels and glycemic control: the northern california kaiser permanente diabetes registry∗. Am. J. Med. **111**(1), 1–9 (2001)
4. Patton, S.R.: Adherence to glycemic monitoring in diabetes. J. Diab. Sci. Technol. **9**(3), 668–675 (2015)
5. Baral-Grant, S., et al.: Self-monitoring of blood pressure in hypertension: a UK primary care survey. Int. J. Hypertens. **2012**, 1–4 (2011). (Article ID 582068)

6. Barlow, J., et al.: A systematic review of the benefits of home telecare for frail elderly people and those with long-term conditions. J. Telemed. Telecare **13**(4), 172–179 (2007)
7. Hailey, D., Roine, R., Ohinmaa, A.: Systematic review of evidence for the benefits of telemedicine. J. Telemed. Telecare **8**(Suppl. 1), 1–7 (2002)
8. Davis, F.D.: Perceived usefulness, perceived ease of use, and user acceptance of information technology. MIS Q. **13**(3), 319–340 (1989)
9. Venkatesh, V., Davis, F.D.: A theoretical extension of the technology acceptance model: four longitudinal field studies. Manage. Sci. **46**(2), 186–204 (2000)
10. Venkatesh, V., Bala, H.: Technology acceptance model 3 and a research agenda on interventions. Decis. Sci. **39**(2), 273–315 (2008)
11. Taylor, S., Todd, P.A.: Understanding information technology usage: a test of competing models. Inf. Syst. Res. **6**(2), 144–176 (1995)
12. Agarwal, R., Sambamurthy, V., Stair, R.M.: Research report: the evolving relationship between general and specific computer self-efficacy—an empirical assessment. Inf. Syst. Res. **11**(4), 418–430 (2000)
13. Finlay, K.A., Trafimow, D., Moroi, E.: The importance of subjective norms on intentions to perform health behaviors. J. Appl. Soc. Psychol. **29**(11), 2381–2393 (1999)
14. Finlay, K.A., Trafimow, D., Jones, D.: Predicting health behaviors from attitudes and subjective norms: between-subjects and within-subjects analyses. J. Appl. Soc. Psychol. **27**(22), 2015–2031 (1997)
15. Ajzen, I.: The theory of planned behavior. Organ. Behav. Hum. Decis. Process. **50**(2), 179–211 (1991)
16. Venkatesh, V., et al.: User acceptance of information technology: Toward a unified view. MIS Q. **27**(3), 425–478 (2003)
17. Bulmer, M.G.: Principles of Statistics. Dover Books on Mathematics, vol. 252. Dover Publications, New York (1979)
18. Posten, H.O., Robustness of the two-sample t-test. In: Rasch, D., Tiku, M.L., (eds.) Robustness of Statistical Methods and Nonparametric Statistics, pp. 92–99. D. Reidel Publishing Company, Dordrecht (1984)
19. Cohen, J.: Statistical Power Analysis for the Behavioral Sciences, 2nd edn. Lawrence Erlbaum, Hillsdale (1988)

# The WireSafe™ for Preventing Retained Central Venous Catheter Guidewires: Clinical Usability

Maryanne Mariyaselvam[1(✉)], Darcy Pearson[2], Robin Heij[2], Emad Fawzy[3], and Peter Young[2]

[1] Lucy Cavendish College, The University of Cambridge,
Lady Margaret Road, Cambridge, UK
mm2100@cam.ac.uk

[2] The Queen Elizabeth Hospital NHS Foundation Trust,
Gayton Road, Kings Lynn, Norfolk, UK
darcymichaelpearson@hotmail.com,
robin.heij@virgin.net, peteryoung101@gmail.com

[3] Sheikh Khalifa Medical City,
Al Karamah Street, Abu Dhabi, United Arab Emirates
emadffawzy@yahoo.com

**Abstract.** Retained objects are the most frequent harmful error in US hospitals. Central venous catheter insertion requires the use of a guidewire, which the clinician can forget to remove during the procedure. The guidewire can move into the circulation and to the heart and must be retrieved by an invasive surgical procedure, causing upto 20% mortality. Checklists alone depend upon a robust safety culture at all times, with all individuals, in all circumstances and so are only moderately robust and have been shown to fail in complex and disparate healthcare systems. An engineered solution (WireSafe™), forces the clinician to remove a guidewire before they are able to access the equipment required to complete the procedure, this makes this error all but impossible. The WireSafe™ also has design features which facilitates the speed and safety of the routine task which is important when dealing with rare but catastrophic events.

**Keywords:** Human factors · Engineering · Patient safety · Medical
Hospital · Never event · Sentinel event · Anesthesiology · Critical care

## 1 Background

Medical errors cause 400,000 patient deaths a year in the USA [1]. Retained foreign objects (including guidewires) are the most frequent harmful error, or Sentinel event, identified annually by the Joint Commission. It is estimated that more than 5 million central venous catheters (CVC) are inserted every year in the United States (US) [2]. CVCs are used in healthcare for administering medications which cannot be given through peripheral venous lines and for monitoring venous pressures. The most standard CVC insertion technique utilizes the Seldinger method, whereby a needle is inserted into the patient's vein, a guidewire is then inserted through the needle and

© Springer International Publishing AG, part of Springer Nature 2019
N. J. Lightner (Ed.): AHFE 2018, AISC 779, pp. 240–247, 2019.
https://doi.org/10.1007/978-3-319-94373-2_27

positioned inside the vein (needle then removed), a catheter is threaded over the guidewire and inserted into the vein. The guidewire is then removed and discarded and the catheter is secured in place using sutures. However, this technique is associated with the error of guidewire retention. A retained CVC guidewire can travel to the heart, causing complications such as thrombosis, arrhythmias and cardiac perforation, with a reported mortality of up to 20% mortality [3]. Retained guidewires have a reported incidence of 1:3,291 procedures in the literature [4] and are classified as a never events. Never events are rare errors that should not occur and are preventable provided the correct safety measures have been implemented [5]. Due to the preventable nature of these errors, and to ensure that hospitals introduce preventative measures, in the USA insurers do not pay for the additional costs associated with a never event [6]. Whilst undertaking work to determine the nature of the error after a retained guidewire never event occurred in our hospital, we analyzed the clinical procedure, observing clinicians undertake the task of CVC insertion to determine the point at which a retained guidewire would be likely to occur. We conducted a literature search to understand the nature of the error reported in case studies and were given access to the last 10 years of UK National Reporting and Learning System (NRLS) database of retained guidewire never events. On analysis of the data we determined that a retained guidewire occurs at a single critical point in the clinical procedure: this is the moment when the catheter is placed over the guidewire and before it is secured in place. At this point, if the clinician is distracted, they can forget that they have not removed the guidewire and push the catheter and guidewire together into the vein, causing the guidewire retention. Through these observational studies understanding of how the error occurs, we a preventative safety solution: the WireSafe™.

## 2    Guidewire Retention: Incidence in the National Health Service

The incidence of retained guidewires are reported to be 1:3221 [7] and 1:3291 in the literature [4]. In the UK national health service (NHS), hospitals are required to report their never event errors to the National Reporting and Learning System. We applied for and were given confidential and anonymised data on retained guidewires between 2004 and 2015 for analysis. We sought to determine the reported incidence, location and timing of recognition of guidewire retention. The data was analysed by two independent investigators and queries were adjudicated by a 3rd investigator. There were 239 cases of retained guidewires identified in the NRLS database. We found the incidence of retained guidewires was increasing annually in the NHS (Fig. 1) and occurs about twice a month in the NHS [8]. It is likely that this rising incidence is due to an increase in the reporting and a move towards an open and learning culture in the healthcare system. However, it does show that the incidence of retained guidewires is not decreasing and still indicates the need to develop safety mechanisms to prevent the error. We determined the time of recognition of guidewire retention and found that only 25% of retained guidewires were recognized during the procedure, 23% were recognized on the check radiograph and 52% were recognized after the 1st check radiographs, on subsequent interventions such as further radiological investigations, manipulation of the catheter or catheter removal. This data highlighted that most guidewires were forgotten and only identified after the conclusion of the procedure. In terms of forgotten guidewires, it is unsurprising that less than a third were identified on the check x-ray. Interpretation of the x-ray for retained guidewires has poor sensitivity and other confounders such as the rarity of the error or the presence of other catheters, which make recognition of guidewire retention poor. This data highlights that efforts to prevent retained guidewires should be concentrated on prevention and recognition prior to completion when guidewire retrieval is possible and immediately achievable.

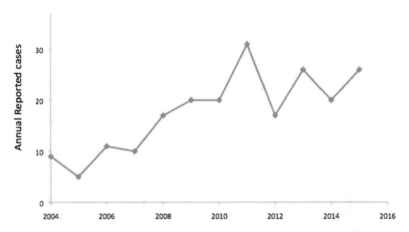

**Fig. 1.** The annual reported incidence of CVC retained guidewires to the National Reporting and Learning System, National Health Service, England, 2004–2016.

## 3   Veterans Health Administration Study (2018)

The VHA, the largest integrated healthcare system in the USA, analyzed their patient safety reporting system (2000–2016) to determine the demographics and contributing factors of retained guidewires [1]. Of a total of 391 cases, 101 were evaluable. The error occurred in all grades (trainee residents accounted for 36%) and the majority occurred in non-emergent (elective) situations (79%). The guidewire was discovered during the procedure in 38% of cases. After the check x-ray, within 24 h a further 31% were discovered and months or years later in some cases. This indicates that the normal error is simply forgetting to remove the guidewire rather than a technical error or the patient's circulation sucking the guidewire in or the guidewire fracturing (91% of cases were whole guidewires). Indeed, common root causes included inexperience (perhaps with a heightened cognitive load experienced by the operator), poor standardization (increasing complexity and resultant cognitive load), distractions and only 23% lacked a checklist. The latter implies that up to 77% of guidewires may be retained despite the use of checklists, indicating the fallibility of checklists for rare events due to creeping complacency and alert fatigue. The process of CVC insertion requires continuation of a complex procedure and multitasking of both operator and assistants, at and after the time of guidewire removal, and the operator is gowned, scrubbed, gloved and in a sterile field and may well defer the checklist until a more manageable time after completion so as not to disrupt the process. The authors conclude that guidewire loss is mostly an omission error, caused by missed steps in a process which requires memory and attention for each step with the error only becoming apparent after completion of the process. Checklists properly performed can be beneficial but require a robust culture at all times with all individuals and so are only moderately robust. The authors recommend that equipment design using a forcing function that do not allow clinicians to complete the insertion process, such as the WireSafe™, should be recommended.

## 4    The WireSafe™: An Engineered Forcing Function to Prevent a Never Event

The WireSafe™ (Venner Medical, Singapore) is an engineered safety solution being implemented by the NHS, the largest semi-integrated health system in the world, through the NHS innovation Accelerator programme and supported by the publically funded Academic Health Science Networks. The WireSafe™ is a novel locked procedure pack, designed to prevent the never event of retained guidewires. The WireSafe™ contains the equipment required to complete a CVC insertion after the guidewire is normally removed from the patient: the suture, suture holder, countertraction forceps and dressings. In order to gain access to the equipment and finish the procedure, the guide wire is used as a key to open the locked pack. Thereby when inserting a CVC, the clinician must remove the guidewire from the patient in order to complete the procedure (Fig. 2). The efficacy and use of a prototype WireSafe™ was demonstrated in a simulation study and reported at the Applied Human Factors and Ergonomics conference 2017 [9]. We presented a simulation study and described a clinical scenario which replicated a CVC insertion. The CVC catheter was inserted into the right internal jugular vein of a mannequin model, and it had the guidewire clearly visible within the lumen and easily retrievable with artery forceps if the participant recognized the error. The trolley placed by the beside of the mannequin had either the WireSafe™ or the standard equipment needed to complete the procedure, and participants were randomized using envelope randomization. An ECG machine displayed ectopic beats and was used as an indicator for the participants. The scenario which was based on a real life incidents, as detailed in the NRLS database, described that the clinician was called away part way through CVC insertion. Participants were randomized to standard or WireSafe™, were asked to assess the situation, complete the CVC insertion and undertake any safety checks prior to authorizing the CVC for use. We found in the standard group 80% of participants failed to recognize the guidewire in the catheter lumen. The WireSafe™ was 100% effective in preventing guidewire retention at completion of CVC insertion (20% standard v 100% PP, n = 20, $p < 0.001$) [10]. Following the development and regulatory approval the WireSafe™ is now used in clinical practice.

# WireSafe™

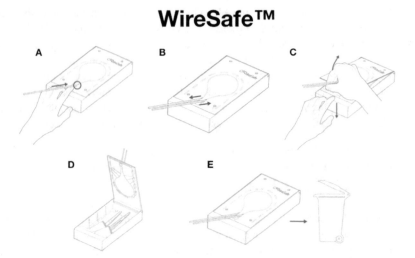

**Fig. 2.** How to use the Venner WireSafe™, (A) the guidewire is inserted into the channel in the lid of the device, (B) the guidewire is pushed through the channel until both ends protrude out of the device, (C) the ends of the guidewire are used as a handle to open the box (lifting up and counter traction on the ledge), (D) the WireSafe™ is opened and the contents (suture, suture holder, counter-traction forceps, dressings) are used to secure the CVC in place and complete the procedure, (E) the contents can be easily disposed into the bin. Images used with permissions from Venner Medical Technologies.

## 5   WireSafe™: Clinical Usability

We implemented the WireSafe™ into our intensive care units (ICUs) and operating rooms (OR) for CVC insertion. A phased introduction involved teaching the residents, attending physicians and assistants who would normally undertake these procedures how to use the WireSafe™ during CVC insertions, (instructions on how to use the WireSafe™ are also available on the bottom of the box). After clinical introduction, we conducted a retrospective usability study to determine whether the device was suitable for preventing the retained guidewires and for ease of use during clinical practice. We surveyed 10 ICU physicians and 10 anesthetists who had used the WireSafe™ whilst inserting CVCs. Physicians were asked standardized questions on their clinical experience of inserting CVCs, whether they had used the WireSafe™, in which clinical scenarios and to remark on any problems when using the device. Physicians were also asked their opinion on the ease of use of the WireSafe™ during CVC insertion, and any general likes or dislikes to the change in the CVC procedure when using the WireSafe™. There was a broad range of experience in inserting CVCs (3 and 1000 CVCs in their careers). All stated that they had used the WireSafe™ in their clinical practice and 225 WireSafe™'s had been used in total. Of those surveyed, 20/20 had used the WireSafe™ to insert a CVC in unconscious patients, 7/20 had used it in awake patients and 4/20 had used it in agitated patients. All clinicians stated that there were no problems in using the WireSafe™ for CVC insertions in these patients. Participants stated that they found the CVC insertion process easier (10/20) with the WireSafe™ and the remaining (10/20) found no difference to previous practice, whilst preventing retained guidewires. Most participants (16/20) stated using the WireSafe™ was more convenient for clearing up sharps at the end of the procedure and the remaining 4/20 found no difference compared to previous practice. All 20 participants stated they approved of the WireSafe™ for CVC insertions and would continue to support its use for the safety benefits.

# 6  Using the WireSafe™ to Improve Sharps Disposal

Sharps injuries have a recorded incidence as high as 99% in surgical trainees and have a human and economic burden on healthcare systems estimated in excess of $500,000 per hospital/year [11]. Safety devices, safer needle types and disposal methods may reduce the incidence of sharps injuries. Although the WireSafe™ is primarily designed to prevent the never event of guidewire retention, we found that after implementation, clinicians have found the WireSafe™ convenient for point of care sharps and wire disposal. Sharps are placed in the WireSafe™ and the guidewire left in the channel used to open the device. During an observational study of Anesthesiologists [12] disposing of sharps following cvc insertion, before (Control) and after the implementation of a safety solution (WireSafe™), sequential procedures were observed. Investigators informed the staff only that they were observing the whole procedure for quality improvement purposes. Safe technique was defined as following hospital policy, with a sharps bin brought to the clinician or the procedure trolley wheeled to the sharp's bin. Unsafe technique involved throwing sharps, hand carriage to sharps disposal or leaving sharps for others to clear up. Safe disposal of sharps was increased from 60% to 100%. The total average CVC placement time was similar in both groups (standard 16 min v WireSafe™ 14.5 min, p = ns) and the sharps clear up time was less in the WireSafe™ group (standard 11.6 min v WireSafe™ 9.5 min, p < 0.05). There was one sharps injury in the control group period requiring extended occupational health surveillance. Despite clear guidance, sharps disposal practice is poor and the WireSafe™ encouraged better decision making at the bedside.

# 7  Technique to Remove a Retained Guidewire: Salvage Technique

The NHS England National Reporting and Learning System (NRLS) database 2004–2015 reported 239 guidewire retentions of which on only one occasion was suction reportedly applied to the distal lumen prior to removal. If recognized early (38% of cases in the VHA database and 25% of cases in the NHS database), the guidewire is more likely to be still in the catheter lumen. A common technique for guidewire removal is to clamp the catheter at the skin and pull the assembly back, however, if the guidewire has passed beyond the skin level, this is likely to be ineffective as the guidewire will be left in the patient's body. We tested a rapid suctioning technique prior to clamping to improve the chances of success, using a bench model with a guidewire placed 2 cm into the distal tip of a CVC catheter simulating a wire about to embolise [13]. The CVC was positioned in a quarter circle conformation and the tip and guidewire was submerged in a water bath simulating the circulation. A 20 ml syringe was attached to the distal lumen and strong suction was continuously applied for 5 s by vigorously retracting the plunger and guidewire retraction measured. We tested 3 CVCs, 2 vascaths and 2 wide-bore introducers 10 times each. Success was determined by the wire moving back into the catheter thereby improving the chances of clamping and removal. The rapid suck technique successfully retracted the wire in all cases and for all catheters. We concluded that the intraluminal position of a retained guidewire may be unknown, may be difficult to see on x-ray, and delays or patient manipulation may cause further migration. If there has been a decision to remove the catheter then suction should be applied first to retract the wire.

# 8   Chest Drain Guidewire Retention

A common procedure to place chest drains uses a wire guided technique and is associated with a complication of wire retention in the patients chest if the clinician forgets to remove it. We have adapted the WireSafe™ by changing the contents for use in wired chest drain insertion, and conducted a simulation study to test the efficacy of the safety solution in this setting. Randomizing 20 chest drain competent doctors, but with no knowledge of the WireSafe™, to standard or WireSafe™ groups, they were presented with a scenario to complete, where a colleague who had been urgently called away midway during a chest drain insertion. A simulation manikin had a 12G drain in-situ with a visible guidewire 'accidentally' left in the lumen. If asked, the assistant stated only that the WireSafe™ was a new procedure pack containing the sutures and dressings which could be used as a sharps repository after placement. The WireSafe™ prevented guidewire retention (100% WireSafe™ v 10% Standard, n = 20, p < 0.001, Fisher's Exact test). In the WireSafe™ group participants underwent searches of trolley, floor and/or sharps bin before the realization of the intra-luminal location of the wire and all were safely removed. In this scenario, we used a systems approach to align the latent failures in the system and all but force the error to occur and our participants were given a false pretext for the experiment, to distract focus, so that would be unable to unintentionally alter the results. With this approach, in the standard group, the participants reliably fell into the error trap, and did not recognize the guidewire in situ. In the WireSafe™ group, the participants did not initially recognize the guidewire retention, however when attempting to complete the procedure, the device forced participants to search for the guidewire. The WireSafe™ was 100% successful in preventing the never event of chest drain guidewire retention alongside facilitating fixation and sharps disposal.

# 9  Summary

The WireSafe™ is a fail safe engineered solution which prevents a clinician from forgetting to remove a guidewire during central venous catheter and chest drain insertion by only allowing access to the equipment needed to complete the procedure by using the guidewire as a key. This provides a simple, elegant solution to the second commonest never event in emergency medicine, preventing patient harm, whilst facilitating normal practice.

# References

1. Cherara, L., Sculli, G.L., Paull, D.E., Mazzia, L., Neily, J., Mills, P.D.: Retained guidewires in the veterans health administration: getting to the root of the problem. J. Patient Saf. E pub ahead of print (2018)
2. McGee, D.C., Gould, M.K.: Preventing complications of central venous catheterization. N. Engl. J. Med. **348**, 1123–1133 (2003)
3. Williams, T.L., Bowdle, A.T., Winters, B.D., Pavkovic, S.D., Szekendi, M.K.: Guidewires unintentionally retained during central venous catheterization. J. Assoc. Vasc. Access. **19**, 29–34 (2014)
4. Vannucci, A., Jeffcoat, A., Ifune, C., Salinas, C., Duncan, J.R., Wall, M.: Retained guidewires after intraoperative placement of central venous catheters. Anaesth Analg. **117**, 102–108 (2013)
5. The never events policy framework. An update to the never events policy. Department of Health, NHS (2012). https://improvement.nhs.uk/resources/never-events-policy-and-framework/
6. Milstein, A.: Ending extra payment for "never events" — stronger incentives for patients' safety. N. Engl. J. Med. **360**, 2388–2390 (2009)
7. Omar, H.R., Sprenker, C., Karlnoski, R., Mangar, D., Miller, J., Camporesi, E.M.: The incidence of retained guidewires after central venous catheterization in a tertiary care centre. Am. J. Emerg. Med. **31**, 1528–1530 (2013)
8. Mariyaselvam, M., Walters, H., Callan, C., Matthew, K., Jackman, S., Young, P.: Guidewire retention: reported incidence, location and timing of error. Eur. J. Anaesthesiol. **34** (2017). 16AP02–12
9. Mariyaselvam, M., Young, P.: Disaster scenario simulation for testing solutions to never events. In: Proceedings of the Conference 8th International Conference of Applied Human Factors and Ergonomics, Advances in Human Factors and Ergonomics in Healthcare and Medical Devices (2017)
10. Mariyaselvam, M.Z., Catchpole, K., Menon, D., Gupta, A., Young, P.: Preventing retained guidewires: a randomised controlled simulation study using a human factors approach. Anaesthesiology **127**, 658–665 (2017)
11. Makary, M.A., Al-Attar, A., Holzmueller, C.G., Sexton, B., Syin, D., Gilson, M.M., Sulkowski, M.S., Pronovost, P.J.: Needlestick injuries among surgeons in training. N. Engl. J. Med. **28**, 2693–2699 (2007)
12. Hodges, E., Gooch, E., Swan, T., Keable, S., Mariyaselvam, M., Young, P.: Sharp's disposal using the WireSafe during central venous catheter placement. In: Conference Proceedings of the British Association of Critical Care Nursing Conference BACCN. P06 (2017)
13. Mariyaselvam, M., Richardson, J., Sawyer A., Young, P.: Central venous catheter guidewire salvage technique to prevent a never event. Eur. J. Anaesthesiol. **34** (2017). 16AP04–8

# Designing for Social Support in a Mobile Health Application for Children and Adolescents

Jette Selent and Michael Minge[✉]

Cognitive Psychology and Cognitive Ergonomics, Technische Universität Berlin,
Marchstraße 23, 10587 Berlin, Germany
jette.selent@gmail.com, michael.minge@tu-berlin.de

**Abstract.** The experience of relatedness to others is a key intrinsic motivator for human behavior. Therefore, social support can be seen as a promising factor for enhancing intrinsic motivation, thus, leading to an improvement in health-promoting behavior. That is why in this study, an effort towards the development and user-centered evaluation of different design concepts for realizing social support in a mobile health application was made. The goal of this application is to improve treatment adherence in children and adolescents diagnosed with scoliosis that have to wear a back brace as their prescribed orthotic treatment. The application, in its current form, helps patients to track their brace wear time and provides them with knowledge about scoliosis. Additional features have been created in the form of storyboards, offering the possibility to provide and receive different types of social support as defined in the social support theory by House, i.e., appraisal, informational and emotional support. To test the effects of these support types on intrinsic motivation, the storyboards were evaluated in an online study, with 33 children and adolescents diagnosed with scoliosis. Results show that for informational and appraisal support, significant main effects could be observed, while emotional support did not substantially improve intrinsic motivation. The study was helpful in prioritizing the next implementation steps for the application and to justify the decisions empirically with data from a user's point of view.

**Keywords:** Social support · mHealth · eHealth · User-centered design
Evaluation · Scoliosis · Treatment adherence · Motivational design
Persuasion · Intrinsic motivation · Self-determination theory

## 1 Introduction

The ever-increasing importance of smartphones for peoples everyday lives is creating more and more opportunities to deeply influence formerly non-digitalized areas. Health related behavior and medical care, for example, seem to have a great potential for benefiting from mobile applications (apps) [1, 2].

Pursuing that goal, a multifaceted treatment system is being developed as a sub-project under the umbrella of the regional innovation cluster *BeMobil*, funded by the German Federal Ministry of Education and Research. The system is aiming to support

© Springer International Publishing AG, part of Springer Nature 2019
N. J. Lightner (Ed.): AHFE 2018, AISC 779, pp. 248–258, 2019.
https://doi.org/10.1007/978-3-319-94373-2_28

the treatment of children and adolescents that have been diagnosed with scoliosis, a physical deformity of the spine that occurs with a high prevalence of 6.2 up to 11.1% in German youth, depending on the specific age group regarded [3].

Supporting their treatment is necessary, since one of the main obstacles for successful treatment is the lack of adherence to the prescribed regimen. In a lot of cases, the most promising treatment method includes wearing an orthesis, a rigid orthopedic back brace that supports and lengthens the spine by utilizing the process of natural growth to straighten the back. Depending on the severity of the diagnosis, the brace needs to be worn for a considerable amount of time each day, as well as during therapeutic physical workouts. Since wearing the brace is oftentimes accompanied by discomfort, may result in unwanted attention from peers and does not result in immediate noticeable improvements of the deformity, the average wear time tends to be too short [4]. For that reason, measures need to be taken to assist and motivate patients in adhering to their prescribed regimen. *BeMobil* aims to achieve this by providing a combination of sensory-based braces that improve feedback and monitoring options for both the patients and their doctors, and a smartphone app [5]. The so-called *Scoliosis App* assists the young patients in monitoring their wear time, in scheduling and planning of doctors and physical therapy appointments, educates them playfully trough a quiz, and offers general information on the topic of scoliosis on an administrated news feed.

One of the most requested features, according to initial research done within the scope of the project, however, could not be implemented in the app so far: Social interaction or social support. Dannehl et al. [5] emphasize, that providing a stage for social support within the peer group, that is connected through similar life circumstances, obstacles and needs, holds a great potential for increasing the willingness and motivation to overcome reservations and drawbacks regarding the treatment. Reasons to expect these positive motivational outcomes can also be found in the research of Gardner and colleagues [6] as well as Pickett, Gardner and Knowles [7]. They were able to show that people report more positive attitudes towards situations inherenting a high potential for social support, as opposed to ones that don't provide such potential. Additionally, they found a heightened sensitivity for cues indicating the potential for social support in given situations. Especially in children and adolescents, stable and consistent social support is also connected to heightened general interest, more precise goal setting behavior as well as general well-being and positive emotional states [8].

Providing features facilitating social support between the patients using the app might therefore increase the motivation to use the app. And a more frequent utilization of the *Scoliosis App* would increase the chances of it having the aspired positive effect on the patient's treatment adherence.

## 1.1 Social Support

To study the effects of social support on motivation, app features were conceptually visualized that provided prototypical versions of three different social support types defined by House [9]: emotional support, informational support and appraisal support. Emotional support refers to the provision of love, trust, care and empathy, as well as respect [10] through members of a closely-nit social network. Informational support on the other hand is directed towards an improvement of the supported persons coping strategies for dealing with personal or environmental problems [11]. It follows the systemic approach of helping people help themselves [12, 13] by providing useful information, assisting in information selection and the validation of gained insights. Appraisal support is another form of support involving the transmission of information. The supporting person provides information relevant for the receiving persons self-evaluation and social comparison. That includes, mostly positive, feedback [14], affirmation [10] or cues for behaviors that will be positively evaluated by a desired social group [15]. The fourth type of social support after House [9], instrumental support, was not applied, since it's nature is rather non-fitting to the topic of social support provided within an app.

## 1.2    Intrinsic Motivation

Ryan and Deci [16] as well as Vallerand [17] describe, that intrinsic motivation leads to a heightened probability of showing a specific behavior that has a high potential of being stable over a long time period. Aspects like playfulness, learning experiences and the perceived development of competence are important factors for the acceptance of software products in particular [18–20] and can be seen as sources for intrinsic motivation [21]. Moreover, Cox, Miller and Mull [22], as well as Pelletier and Dion [23] were able to show that intrinsic motivation is especially valuable for health-related behaviors.

That is why the focus of this study was to evaluate the effect of social support on intrinsic motivation. The self-determination theory [24] is a well-established meta theory of intrinsic motivation taking relatedness into account as an important source of motivation. It is also connecting intrinsic motivation through the satisfaction of three basic needs - competence, autonomy and relatedness - to positive effects on wellbeing and the tendency to engage in health-benefiting behaviors [25–28].

For that reason, it was hypothesized that the integration of features facilitating social support through the *Scoliosis App* would lead to increased levels of intrinsic motivation.

## 2    Method

The goal of the present study was to determine the effect of three different types of social support on various facets of intrinsic motivation. Therefore, app features were prototypically developed to represent the three social support types described above. They were presented as individual sketches, each containing one app feature. Those features were developed in two different versions – providing the facilitation of social support vs. not providing it. Emotional support was realized through the feature for generating a personalized avatar either including emotional cues for friends to react to, or not. Informational support was facilitated through a news feed that was either filled by members of one's own social network (i.e., support) vs. through an automated online search for articles relating to scoliosis and its treatment (i.e., no support). Lastly, appraisal support could be provided through the feature assisting in the evaluation of the weekly brace wear time and the percentage achievement of the self-set weekly wear time goal. In the supported version connected users were able to react to each others wear time through "likes" or supportive and encouraging private messages. The combination of the three features either including or not including the option to offer and receive social support resulted in a storyboard, each consisting of three sketches. Those storyboards visualized the possible set of interactions with one's own network within the app (see Fig. 1).

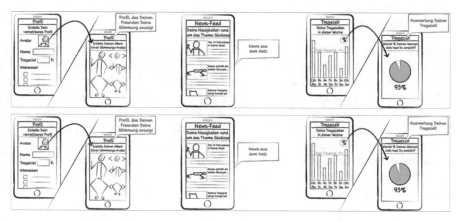

**Fig. 1.** Two of the eight storyboards that were evaluated in the online study. Top row: No emotional support, informational support, appraisal support; bottom row: Emotional support, no informational support, no appraisal support. The two versions of all three social support types were provided in every possible combination, resulting in eight different storyboards as stimuli.

## 2.1 Dependent Variables

The eight storyboards were rated on a 10-item semantic differential scale measuring the satisfaction of the three basic needs stated in the self-determination theory (i.e., competence, autonomy, relatedness), as well as two general factors related to intrinsic motivation (i.e., stimulation, acceptance) with two items each. The measurement scale was developed in advance of the study, following a multi-stepped procedure. The final German version of the questionnaire, as used in the present study, consisted of 10 word pairs measuring the above-mentioned five different components of intrinsic motivation. The factorial validity of the questionnaire was examined through a principle component analysis. The five components explain 79.57% of the items' total variance. Three scales (i.e., competence, stimulation, and acceptance) show an acceptable internal consistency with Cronbach's Alpha values between $\alpha = .741$ and $.767$. The results for relatedness ($\alpha = .653$) and autonomy ($\alpha = .506$) indicate that the internal consistency could still be improved for these scales.

Aside from rating the stimuli with the help of the semantic differential scale, participants were asked to rank the eight storyboards reviewed and give a brief explanation to their choice of preference. In the end, participants were given the chance to give further qualitative information on things they liked, disliked or were missing in the app as shown.

## 2.2    Study Design

The independent variable social support was manipulated through three factors (i.e., emotional support, informational support, appraisal support). All factors were realized in two manifestations (i.e., support provided vs. not provided). The fully-crossed $2 \times 2 \times 2$ study design resulted in a set of eight stimuli, representing the distinct sets of feature combinations. In repeated measures, all participants rated the full set of stimuli in counterbalanced order.

## 2.3    Participants

Participants were contacted through various social media groups, scoliosis related online forums, in medical treatment facilities specializing in the treatment of scoliosis as well as through a contact data set gathered in a previous *BeMobil* study. Thirty-four scoliosis patients participated in the online study. One 39 year old participant was excluded from the data set due to their age not conforming to the targeted user group. The remaining participants were 15.73 years old on average, spanning from 9 to 20 years. A greater number of participants was female (f:m = 29:4), which is not problematic due to the higher prevalence of scoliosis in girls as opposed to boys [29–31]. The participants reported wearing a back brace for a mean of 2.27 years (0–7 years) and a daily prescribed wearing time of 17.36 h (0–24 h).

# 3    Results

For data analysis, a $2 \times 2 \times 2$ multivariate analysis of variance with repeated measurements (MANOVA) was conducted. The multivariate test revealed significant main effects of appraisal support ($F(5,28) = 3.211, p < .05, \eta^2_{part.} = 0.364$) and informational support ($F(5,28) = 2.833, p < .05, \eta^2_{part.} = 0.336$), while emotional support did not significantly affect the subjective ratings ($F(5,28) = 0.566, p = .726, \eta^2_{part.} = 0.092$). An overview of the particular effects of the factor appraisal support on all dependent variables can be found in Table 1. It shows significant influences with regard to competence, relatedness and stimulation.

**Table 1.** Main effects of "appraisal support" on all dependent variables.

| Dependent variable | df1 | df2 | F | P | $\eta^2_{part.}$ |
|---|---|---|---|---|---|
| Autonomy | 5 | 28 | 2.187 | .149 | 0.064 |
| **Competence** | 5 | 28 | 4.492 | .042* | **0.123** |
| **Relatedness** | 5 | 28 | 17.662 | <.001** | **0.356** |
| **Stimulation** | 5 | 28 | 5.502 | .025* | **0.147** |
| Acceptance | 5 | 28 | 3.718 | .063(*) | 0.104 |

Figure 2 displays the descriptive statistics, indicating that participants reported higher values on all motivational facets for stimuli that included the facilitation of appraisal support.

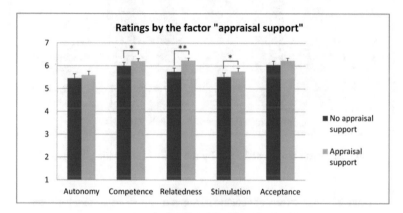

**Fig. 2.** Mean ratings and standard errors of the means (SEM) by the factor "appraisal support".

When looking at informational support, only the dependent variable relatedness was substantially influenced by this factor (see Table 2).

**Table 2.** Main effects of "informational support" on all dependent variables.

| Dependent variable | $df1$ | $df2$ | $F$ | $P$ | $\eta^2_{part.}$ |
|---|---|---|---|---|---|
| Autonomy | 5 | 28 | 0.196 | .661 | 0.006 |
| Competence | 5 | 28 | 0.044 | .835 | 0.001 |
| **Relatedness** | **5** | **28** | **6.878** | **<.013\*** | **0.177** |
| Stimulation | 5 | 28 | 5.502 | .627 | 0.007 |
| Acceptance | 5 | 28 | 0.002 | .966 | <0.001 |

Mean ratings indicate that relatedness was rated higher in case of provided informational support (see Fig. 3).

As for emotional support, no significant effects were obtained (see Table 3).

At the end of the survey, participants were asked to rank the storyboards according to their preference. Median ranking positions of the storyboards were compared for each of the factors appraisal, informational, and emotional support. Results show that differences in the expected direction were empirically found for appraisal support, only. Design solutions that facilitated appraisal support were highly preferred over those that did not offer features for appraisal support (see Fig. 4). No differences were obtained with respect to the factor informational support. Against the preliminary expectations, design solutions that facilitated emotional support were slightly less preferred as opposed to solutions without emotional support.

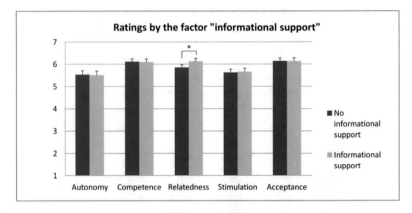

**Fig. 3.** Mean ratings and SEM by the factor "informational support".

**Table 3.** Main effects of "emotional support" on all dependent variables.

| Dependent variable | df1 | df2 | F | P | $\eta^2_{part.}$ |
|---|---|---|---|---|---|
| Autonomy | 5 | 28 | 1.188 | .284 | 0.036 |
| Competence | 5 | 28 | 0.002 | .969 | <0.001 |
| Relatedness | 5 | 28 | 0.358 | .554 | 0.011 |
| Stimulation | 5 | 28 | 0.295 | .591 | 0.009 |
| Acceptance | 5 | 28 | 0.042 | .838 | 0.001 |

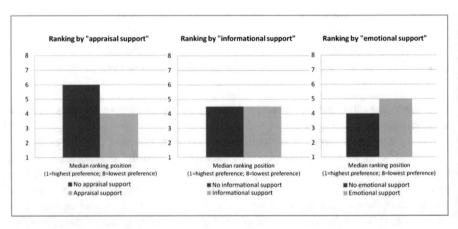

**Fig. 4.** Median ranking positions of the storyboards including the factors appraisal support (left), informational support (middle) and emotional support (right).

# 4 Discussion

The results of the analysis of variance have indicated that the additional features representing a facilitation of appraisal support have the highest impact on intrinsic motivation. This result corresponds with the finding that the possibility to provide and receive appraisal support leads to a higher preference of the apps feature set, expressed through the ranking position. In this study, features enabling the exchange of appraisal support between users were the possibility to share individual wear times of the back brace with ones network, and to define and communicate personal treatment goals with others. Connected app users were given the opportunity to react to others accomplishments, wear times and goals through private messages or "likes", an appreciative interaction form that is widely known due to social networks like *facebook*. Based on the findings, the integration of such features that correspond to the facilitation of appraisal support should have the highest priority in the further development of the *Scoliosis App*. Part of this effort should be the identification of additional features including the chance to provide and receive appraisal support. Possible ways to do so might be found in the extension of some features that are already integrated in the app. The option to share and react to results of the knowledge quiz for example, or group based physiological therapeutic exercises instructed through the app might be good starting points.

Informational support, more precisely the option to share personalized information and individually relevant knowledge regarding topics related to scoliosis, can be seen as the second most important feature when designing for social support. Even though informational support did not directly improve the subjective rating of neither competence nor stimulation, it had a substantial impact on the feeling of relatedness to others. However, looking at the ranking positions depending on the presence of the related feature, the facilitation of informational support did not affect the preference of the feature set for better or for worse.

The results with regard to the facilitation of emotional support were somewhat unexpected. When analyzing the effect on the components of intrinsic motivation, no significant influences on the subjective ratings were obtained. Surprisingly, the ranking positions even showed a slight tendency towards a higher preference if no feature for emotional support was provided. However, qualitative statements of the participants helped to uncover possible explanations for this finding. A surprisingly high number of respondents indicated that sharing emotions through an avatar might be complicated and a continuous update might be stressful. Furthermore, participants expressed concerns about privacy issues. Some were also worried about negative ramifications of unintended or even absent reactions, i.e., "what happens, if I feel sad and get no reply". Consequently, it was decided to postpone the implementation of emotional support in the further development of the application.

Regardless of the specific features decided on, every implementation of the facilitation of social support needs to take the cost of administration into account. As a software supporting a medical treatment, the app deals with a highly sensitive topic. Measures need to be taken to make sure that the communication between the users is safe and secure, publicly available information (e.g., comments, news recommendations) is free of harm- and hurtful content, and there is no way of exploitation of the young user group [32]. Additionally, privacy settings must be easily accessible and understandable [33].

### 4.1 Limitations

When interpreting the results of this study, some limitations need to be considered. First and foremost, children and adolescents with scoliosis are a very heterogeneous group. Especially due to the large age range that needs to be catered to, problems to find the right interactions and features may arise. The reason is, that children and adolescents undergo various psychological, social and physical developmental stages during the age period in question [34, 35]. Therefore, a sample size of 33 participants might not adequately represent the full range of individual needs and preferences with regard to the intended support system. Since the age associated developmental changes could play a particularly important role when designing for social support, age differences should be considered in a more systematic way than it was possible to realize in the present online study.

Second, in the present study the different types of social support have been implemented by specific features (or a characteristic set of features). In order to generalize the results, a greater variety of features representing the support types would be necessary.

Third, the design solutions were presented as storyboards, i.e., low-fidelity prototypes. Therefore, the material did not allow for the experience of real interactions with the software. In a next step, interactive prototypes could be used to validate the findings [36].

Finally, in order to investigate the validity of the results the additional features offering the chance to receive or provide social support need to be reevaluated in a real-life use case and over a longer period of usage. The real user experience over time might not be adequately captured by a one-time measurement.

## 5   Conclusion

In this contribution, possible solutions for the facilitation of social support in a mobile health application for children and adolescents with scoliosis were presented. The design solutions have been evaluated in a very early phase of the development process following a user-centered design approach. While features that improve appraisal and informational support were identified as particularly important to enhance intrinsic motivation, emotional support led to inconsistent and unexpected results. Therefore, the implementation of features representing emotional support were postponed. The results were helpful in prioritizing the next implementation steps of the application and to justify the decisions empirically with data from a user's point of view.

**Acknowledgments.** This research has been supported by the German Federal Ministry of Education and Research (BMBF) as part of the innovation cluster *BeMobil*. We would like to thank all participants and project members.

# References

1. Boulos, M.N.K., Wheeler, S., Tavares, C., Jones, R.: How smartphones are changing the face of mobile and participatory healthcare: an overview, with example from ecaalyx. BioMed. Eng. OnLine **10**(1) (2011). 24, http://www.biomedical-engineering-online.com/content/10/1/24, https://doi.org/10.1186/1475-925x-10-24
2. Luxton, D.D., McCann, R.A., Bush, N.E., Mishkind, M.C., Reger, G.M.: mHealth for mental health: integrating smartphone technology in behavioral healthcare. Prof. Psychol. Res. Pract. **42**(6), 505–512 (2011)
3. Kamtsiuris, P., Atzpodien, K., Ellert, U., Schlack, R., Schlaud, M.: Prävalenz von somatischen Erkrankungen bei Kindern und Jugendlichen in Deutschland. Bundesgesundheitsblatt-Gesundheitsforschung-Gesundheitsschutz **50**(5), 686–700 (2007)
4. Weinstein, S.L., Dolan, L.A., Wright, J.G., Dobbs, M.B.: Effects of bracing in adolescents with idiopathic scoliosis. N. Engl. J. Med. **369**(16), 1512–1521 (2013)
5. Dannehl, S., Doria, L., Kraft, M.: Verbesserung der Therapiemitarbeit durch interaktive Rückmeldungen in einem sensorbasierten Unterstützungssystem. In: Weisbecker, A., Burmester, M., Schmidt, A. (eds.) Mensch und Computer 2015 Workshopband, pp. 93–99 (2015)
6. Gardner, W.L., Pickett, C.L., Brewer, M.B.: Social exclusion and selective memory: how the need to belong influences memory for social events. Pers. Soc. Psychol. Bull. **26**(4), 486–496 (2000)
7. Pickett, C.L., Gardner, W.L., Knowles, M.: Getting a cue: the need to belong and enhanced sensitivity to social cues. Pers. Soc. Psychol. Bull. **30**(9), 1095–1107 (2004)
8. Wentzel, K.R.: Social relationships and motivation in middle school: the role of parents, teachers, and peers. J. Educ. Psychol. **90**(2), 202–209 (1998)
9. House, J.S.: Work Stress and Social Support. Addison-Wesley, Reading (1981)
10. Kahn, R.L., Antonucci, T.C.: Convoys over the life course: attachment, roles, and social support. In: Baltes, P.B., Brim, O.G. (eds.) Life-Span Development and Behavior, pp. 254–283. Academic Press, New York (1980)
11. Krause, N.: Social support, stress, and well-being among older adults. J. Gerontol. **41**(4), 512–519 (1986)
12. Kanfer, F.H., Reinecker, H., Schmelzer, D.: Selbstmanagement-Therapie. Springer, Heidelberg (2006)
13. Schmelzer, D.: Hilfe zur Selbsthilfe: Der Selbstmanagement-Ansatz als Rahmenkonzept für Beratung und Therapie. Beratung aktuell **1**(4), 1–20 (2000)
14. Malecki, C.K., Demaray, M.K.: What type of support do they need? Investigating student adjustment as related to emotional, informational, appraisal, and instrumental support. Sch. Psychol. Q. **18**(3), 231–252 (2003)
15. Langford, C.P.H., Bowsher, J., Maloney, J.P., Lillis, P.P.: Social support: a conceptual analysis. J. Adv. Nurs. **25**(1), 95–100 (1997)
16. Ryan, R.M., Deci, E.L.: Intrinsic and extrinsic motivations: classic definitions and new directions. Contemp. Educ. Psychol. **25**(1), 54–67 (2000)
17. Vallerand, R.J.: Toward a hierarchical model of intrinsic and extrinsic motivation. Adv. Exp. Soc. Psychol. **29**, 271–360 (1997)
18. Venkatesh, V.: Determinants of perceived ease of use: Integrating control, intrinsic motivation, and emotion into the technology acceptance model. Inf. Syst. Res. **11**(4), 342–365 (2000)
19. Hwang, Y., Yi, M.: Predicting the use of web-based information systems: intrinsic motivation and self-efficacy. In: Proceedings of the 2002 - Eighth Americas Conference on Information Systems, pp. 1076–1081 (2002)

20. Lee, M.K., Cheung, C.M., Chen, Z.: Acceptance of internet-based learning medium: the role of extrinsic and intrinsic motivation. Inf. Manag. **42**(8), 1095–1104 (2005)
21. Deci, E.L.: Conceptualizations of intrinsic motivation. In: Deci, E.L. (ed.) Intrinsic Motivation, pp. 23–63. Springer, Boston (1975)
22. Cox, C.L., Miller, E.H., Mull, C.S.: Motivation in health behavior: measurement, antecedents, and correlates. Adv. Nurs. Sci. **9**(4), 1–15 (1987)
23. Pelletier, L.G., Dion, S.C.: An examination of general and specific motivational mechanisms for the relations between body dissatisfaction and eating behaviors. J. Soc. Clin. Psychol. **26**(3), 303–333 (2007)
24. Ryan, R.M., Deci, E.L.: Self-determination theory and the facilitation of intrinsic motivation, social development, and well-being. Am. Psychol. **55**(1), 68–78 (2000)
25. Deci, E.L., Ryan, R.M.: Handbook of self-determination research. University Rochester Press, Rochester (2002)
26. Hagger, M.S., Chatzisarantis, N.L.: Integrating the theory of planned behaviour and self-determination theory in health behaviour: a meta-analysis. Br. J. Health. Psychol. **14**(2), 275–302 (2009)
27. Ng, J.Y., Ntoumanis, N., Thøgersen-Ntoumani, C., Deci, E.L., Ryan, R.M., Duda, J.L., Williams, G.C.: Self-determination theory applied to health contexts: a meta-analysis. Perspect. Psychol. Sci. **7**(4), 325–340 (2012)
28. Deci, E.L., Ryan, R.M.: Self-determination theory: a macrotheory of human motivation, development, and health. Can. Psychol. **49**(3), 182–185 (2008)
29. Deutsches skoliose netzwerk: was ist skoliose? (2017). http://www.deutsches-skoliose-netzwerk.de/index.php/ueber-skoliose-de-de/. Accessed 23 Aug 2017
30. Stücker, R.: Die idiopathische Skoliose. Orthopädie und Unfallchirurgie up2date **5**(01), 39–56 (2010)
31. Trobisch, P., Suess, O., Schwab, F.: Die idiopathische Skoliose. Deutsches Ärzteblatt **107**(49), 875–884 (2010)
32. Butler, B., Sproull, L., Kiesler, S., Kraut, R.: Community effort in online groups: who does the work and why. In: Leadership at a Distance: Research in Technologically Supported Work, pp. 171–194 (2002)
33. Taddicken, M.: The 'privacy paradox' in the social web: The impact of privacyconcerns, individual characteristics, and the perceived social relevance on different forms of self-disclosure. J. Comput. Mediat. Commun. **19**(2), 248–273 (2014)
34. Rutter, M.: Pathways from childhood to adult life. J. Child Psychol. Psychiatry **30**(1), 23–51 (1989)
35. Steinberg, L.: Cognitive and affective development in adolescence. Trends Cogn. Sci. **9**(2), 69–74 (2005)
36. Buchenau, M., Suri, J.F.: Experience prototyping. In: Proceedings of the 3rd Conference on Designing Interactive Systems: Processes, Practices, Methods, and Techniques, pp. 424–433 (2000)

# Developing Culturally Sensitive Care in Japan: Comparison of Competence in Healthcare and Education

Miyoko Okamoto[1]([✉]), Norihito Taniguchi[2], Manami Nozaki[1],
Yui Matsuda[3], and Naoko Saito[1]

[1] Juntendo University, Tokyo, Chiba, Japan
{myokamo,ma-nozaki,naosaito}@juntendo.ac.jp
[2] Nagoya University, Nagoya, Japan
taniguchi.norihito@i.mbox.nagoya-u.ac.jp
[3] University of Miami, Coral Gables, FL, USA
ymatsuda@miami.edu

**Abstract.** Competence in culturally sensitive care in healthcare has been included into the Japanese medical school curriculum since 2001 and will be integrated into the Japanese nursing school curriculum in 2018. Since the concept of competence in culturally sensitive care is new to the Japanese healthcare education, we need to gain knowledge about the concept from other forward-thinking countries. However, when introducing the concept of competence in culturally sensitive care from foreign countries to Japan, the knowledge and experiences of those countries should be considered.

**Keywords:** Cultural competence · Intercultural competence
Healthcare education · Multicultural society

## 1 Introduction

The number of foreign residents in Japan in 2016 was tallied at approximately 2,400,000 people and 1.9% of the overall population [1]. As for their nationalities, the non-English speaking segment, such as China, South Korea, the Philippines, and Vietnam, accounted for about seventy percent of the total number of foreign residents.

Consequently, the Ministry of Health, Labour and Welfare in Japan introduced "the accreditation system for medical institutions accepting international patients" since 2012, and started "the environmental management project for admitting foreign patients into medical institutions" since 2013 [2]. They have recently led to a long-needed improvement in the healthcare system in Japan. Thus, caring for patients from diverse cultural backgrounds and competence in culturally sensitive care in healthcare are required.

Competence in culturally sensitive care in healthcare has been included into the Japanese medical school curriculum since 2001 and will be integrated into the Japanese nursing school curriculum in 2018. Since the concept of competence in culturally sensitive care is new to Japanese healthcare education, we need to gain knowledge

© Springer International Publishing AG, part of Springer Nature 2019
N. J. Lightner (Ed.): AHFE 2018, AISC 779, pp. 259–266, 2019.
https://doi.org/10.1007/978-3-319-94373-2_29

about the concept from other forward-thinking countries. However, when introducing the concept of competence in culturally sensitive care from foreign countries to Japan, the arguments and experiences of those countries are considered to be discussed.

## 2   Purpose of This Study

The purpose of this study is to understand how the concept of competence in culturally sensitive care has been developed by the study of related articles in English through comparing the fields of healthcare and education. Then, we will examine perspectives required to introduce the concept of competence in culturally sensitive care from foreign countries to Japanese healthcare education.

## 3   Methodology

The target articles in English in the fields of healthcare and education were extracted through the Web of Science spanning the last two decades, from January 1998 to December 2017. The keywords in the title, "culture" related words, such as cultural, intercultural, cross-cultural, multicultural and transcultural, and also "competence" but not "biology" related in the topic were used as common keywords. Additionally, we searched by dividing into two targeted disciplines, namely healthcare and education. Representative terms of the healthcare fields, such as, "health care sciences service" and "nursing", etc., were selected. Representative terms of the education fields, "education/educational research" and "education scientific discipline", etc., were used. Moreover, this study analyzed only open access articles written in English. Those articles were chronologically analyzed by discipline and by terms and definitions.

## 4   Results

The total of one-hundred seventy-seven articles were extracted. Among them, one-hundred ten articles from healthcare and sixty-seven articles from education fields were extracted. Yearly trends of published articles and the variety of terms are described below:

1. *Yearly trends of published articles*

In the healthcare field, the upward tendency was asymptotically from 2001, and the number was highest in 2017. In the education field, although a small scattered number of articles was seen from 2001, a gradually increase was seen each year since 2014 (See Fig. 1).

2. *Variety of terms*

As for culture related terms, a total of five categories: culture/cultural, cross-cultural, transcultural, multicultural and intercultural were used in the extracted articles. In both fields, the term "culture/cultural" was the most often used. In the healthcare field, the

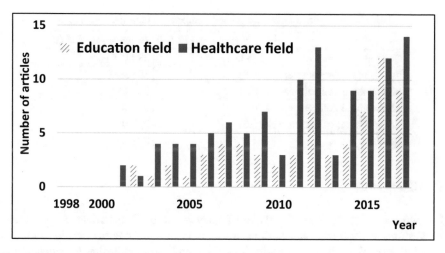

**Fig. 1.** Yearly trends of published articles about the competence in culturally sensitive care in the period 1998–2017.

terms "cross-cultural" and "transcultural" were followed by "culture/cultural". Moreover, there was a tendency to use the term "transcultural" for research in the nursing or psychiatric domain in the healthcare field. The term "intercultural" was used most specifically in the education field (See Table 1).

**Table 1.** Categories of culture related terms used in articles.

| Categories | *Healthcare* n = 110 (%) | *Education* n = 67 (%) |
|---|---|---|
| Culture/Cultural | 96 (87.3) | 36 (53.7) |
| Cross-cultural | 6 (5.5) | 7 (10.4) |
| Transcultural | 3 (2.7) | 1 (1.5) |
| Multicultural | 2 (1.8) | 3 (4.5) |
| Intercultural | 2 (1.8) | 20 (29.9) |

As for the term "competence", it was expressed along with culture related terms, a total of five categories were noted: cultural competence, intercultural competence, multicultural competence, transcultural competence and cross-cultural competence were seen (See Table 2). In the healthcare field, "cultural competence" was mainly used, and it was used in ninety-two articles of one hundred-ten articles. Moreover, the number of articles using "intercultural competence" in the healthcare field was only two.

On the other hand, in the articles from the education field, "cultural competence" was most widely used in thirty-eight articles of sixty-seven articles using the term. "Intercultural competence", however, was remarkably found in nineteen articles with it used in the title in the education field.

**Table 2.** Categories of culture related competence term used in articles.

| Categories | Healthcare n = 110 (%) | Education n = 67 (%) |
|---|---|---|
| Cultural competence | 92 (83.6) | 38 (56.7) |
| Intercultural competence | 2 (1.8) | 19 (28.4) |
| Multicultural competence | 1 (0.9) | 0 (0.0) |
| Transcultural competence | 1 (0.9) | 0 (0.0) |
| Cross-cultural competence | 0 (0.0) | 2 (3.0) |
| Others | 14 (12.7) | 8 (11.9) |

# 5 Discussion

The two major findings from the results of analysis will be discussed hereafter, namely implications of "culture" and various ways of expressing competence in culturally sensitive care. Then, finally, we will discuss its application in healthcare education in Japan.

*1. Implications of "culture"*

"Culture" means the customs and beliefs, art, way of life and social organization of a particular country or group, according to the Oxford dictionary (2014). In English, there are multiple interpretations as to what constitutes cultural difference and diversity. Culture has been cultivated from historically accepted or adapted diverse socio-political backgrounds.

"Bunka", which means culture in Japanese, is defined as collectively regarded physical and psychological accomplishments. It includes lifestyle and norms, such as technology, learning, art, morality, religion, and politics by the popular Kojien Japanese-Japanese dictionary (2008). In contrast to the English variety of terminology regarding culture, such as intercultural, cross-cultural and transcultural, Japan has only one term "i-bunka-kan", which literally translated as between cultures in Japanese. Therefore, it is considered that accurate interpretation of the concept of diversity from English to Japanese has a tendency to be limited in scope.

Japanese society, as a highly homogenous culture, may be influenced by its own stereotype. In addition, there is a tendency to interpret culture by stereotypical lifestyle and way of thinking of a racial group, and often automatically dividing members of a different cultural group into two poles, such as Japanese and non-Japanese. This kind of attitude can make the creation of multicultural society harder. Thus, "the multicultural coexistence promotion plan" led by the Ministry of Internal Affairs and Communications has been carried out since 2006 [3].

Among extracted articles in this study, the articles which targeted various cultural themes were included. For examples, there are culturally related articles concerning ethnic or racial issues which were published over the period of our research [4–9]. In addition, there were articles focusing on organizational culture [10, 11], and on specific professional culture [12–14]. Moreover, there were articles focusing on disability culture as a specific group [15–17], ethical culture [18, 19], gender identity [20], religious belief [21], health disparity issues [22, 23], and socio-economic status, [24], too.

The term "cross-cultural", was the most used culture related word between the two disciplines. In research, comparing a certain phenomenon among two or more nations, "cross-cultural" emerged as the common terminology across the two disciplines. The term "intercultural", however, was favored in the educational field, and "cultural" and "transcultural" were more likely to be used in the healthcare field.

"Intercultural" appeared to be used for the topic which has mainly developed in the education field between two disciplines, such as learning strategies in education [25, 26] and also educational programs for healthcare professionals in the healthcare field [27, 28]. This seems to be influenced by the intercultural education movement of Rachel D. Dubois originally initiated in the 1920s, and it has spread overall educational fields [29]. In fact, cultural factors were not formally integrated into healthcare curricula before the 1960s [30]. After that the concept of transcultural care was coined by Madeleine Leininger in 1978, with blended ideas of nursing and anthropology [31]. The concept of transcultural care has been developed only in specific fields such as nursing and psychiatry.

As described above, a bird's-eye view of "culture" shows that there are various perspectives. In an international society, however, the terminology is complicated. Therefore, it is necessary to understand that a targeted topic of cultural matters would be only one part of vast "culture", so we should carefully search the references. Since this broad view perspective has not yet fully permeated the Japanese society, we needs to illuminate this issue. In the lecture halls of Japanese healthcare education, it is very important to wipe away the narrow view of "culture", since there is a tendency of healthcare professionals to stereotype others into categories by labeling them [19].

## 2. Various ways of expressing competence in culturally sensitive care

The notation of "culture" as an adjective of competence had differences in the characteristics in the healthcare and education fields. Currently, "cultural competence" is a term mostly used in the healthcare field, and the term is shared in the broader healthcare fields, such as medicine, nursing, dental health, mental health, social work, etc.

It is said that the term "cultural competence" was first used in a paper about the mental health service delivery to the children of the minority group by Cross et al. in 1989 [32]. Cultural competence was defined by Cross et al. as "a set of congruent behaviors, attitudes, and policies that come together in a system, agency, or among professionals and enable that system, agency, or those professionals to work effectively in a cross-cultural situation" [33]. Then, furthermore refined, 'cultural competence is an ability of healthcare professional to provide legitimate, effective, and respectful service to people based on the understanding of differences and similarities between or among diverse cultural groups' [32]. Additionally, cultural competence is recognized as a patient safety strategy to increase the healthcare professionals' quality of care [34].

Standing on a broad cultural viewpoint, transcultural care or transcultural nursing is promoted to respect individual values, such as belief and religion, gender identity, also health determinants of socio-economic status, geographic region, and occupation [31, 35, 36]. Therefore, to accomplish the overall goal of reducing health disparities in society, culturally sensitive care has been developing in the healthcare field in its own peculiar way [32].

On the other hand, the term "intercultural competence" has been mainly used in the education field. An anthropologist, Edward, T. Hall contributed to intercultural study before the 1960s. The intercultural communication competence study has been developed since 1980, and the term "intercultural competence" appeared around 1990. However, there was confusion due to the wide interest in the competence in diverse disciplines as already described regarding healthcare related disciplines [29]. The definition of intercultural competence is 'the appropriate and effective management of interaction between people who represent different or divergent affective, cognitive, and behavioral orientations to the world' [37]. Additionally, scholars generally agree that intercultural competence has cognitive, affective, and behavioral dimensions, and contains two components namely, "effectiveness" as the ability to achieve one's goals in a particular exchange, and "appropriateness" as the ability to do so in a manner that is acceptable to the other person [29].

3. *Application in healthcare education in Japan*

In the current condition of each discipline and domain, the definition and the terminology of competency of culturally sensitive care slightly differ from each other and have not yet been unified [32, 37]. Such variability in terms are factors which bar access to transdisciplinary development and creates one-sidedness in which collaboration of the knowledge and experiences of each field are made difficult.

It is necessary to apply the competence in culturally sensitive care to healthcare education in Japan by fully utilizing the rich knowledge and experiences of the healthcare and education fields and by recognizing the mobility of the concept. Moreover, empirical studies which contribute to an international vision are important for the advancement of the practices related to culturally sensitive care and can lead to vital discussions across international and interdisciplinary circles.

# 6   Limitation

We limited our study to analyze open accessed articles published in English through the Web of Science from the last two decades namely 1998 to 2017. Consequently, some valuable articles may not be included in our study.

# 7   Conclusion

In order to apply competence in culturally sensitive care to Japanese healthcare education, it is necessary to fully utilize the knowledge and experiences from other forward-thinking countries. It is important to consider recognizing the mobility of the concept. Moreover, empirical studies which contribute to an international society into a vision are also needed for advancement in this area of study.

# References

1. Ministry of Justice, Japan. http://www.moj.go.jp/housei/toukei/toukei_ichiran_touroku.html. Accessed 10 Dec 2017
2. Ministry of Health, Labour and Welfare, Japan. http://www.meti.go.jp/commitee/kenkyukai/shoujo/iryou_coordinate/pdf/001_05_00.pdf. Accessed 10 Dec 2017
3. Ministry of Internal Affairs and Communications, Japan: the multicultural coexistence promotion plan. http://www.soumu.go.jp/kokusai/pdf/sonota_b6.pdf. Accessed 10 Dec 2017
4. Betancourt, J.R., Green, A.R., Carrillo, J.E., Ananeh-Firempong, O.: Defining cultural competence: a practical framework for addressing racial/ethnic disparities in health and health care. Public Health Rep. **118**(4), 293–302 (2003)
5. Johnson, R.L., Saha, S., Arbelaez, J.J., Beach, M.C., Cooper, L.A.: Racial and ethnic differences in patient perceptions of bias and cultural competence in health care. J. Gen. Intern. Med. **19**(2), 101–110 (2004)
6. Liaw, S.T., Lau, P., Pyett, P., Furler, J., Burchill, M., Rowley, K., Kelaher, M.: Successful chronic disease care for Aboriginal Australians requires cultural competence. Aust. N. Z. J. Public Health **35**(3), 238–248 (2011)
7. Carle, A.C., Weech-Maldonado, R., Ngo-Metzger, Q., Hays, R.D.: Evaluating Measurement equivalence across race and ethnicity on the CAHPS cultural competence survey. Med. Care **50**(9), 32–36 (2012)
8. Saha, S., Korthuis, P.T., Cohn, J.A., Sharp, V.L., Moore, R.D., Beach, M.C.: Primary care provider cultural competence and racial disparities in HIV care and outcomes. J. Gen. Intern. Med. **28**(5), 622–629 (2013)
9. Walters, K.L., Simoni, J.M., Evans-Campbell, T., Udell, W., Johnson-Jennings, M., Pearson, C.R., MacDonald, M.M., Duran, B.: Mentoring the mentors of underrepresented racial/ethnic minorities who are conducting HIV research: beyond cultural competency. AIDS Behav. **20**, 288–293 (2016)
10. Fung, K., Lo, H.-T., Srivastava, R., Andermann, L.: Organizational cultural competence consultation to a mental health institution. Transcult. Psychiatry **49**(2), 165–184 (2012)
11. Barksdale, C.L., Ottley, P.G., Stephens, R., Gebreselassie, T., Fua, I., Azur, M., Walrath, G.: System-level change in cultural and linguistic competence (CLC): how changes in CLC are related to service experience outcomes in systems of care. Am. J. Community Psychol. **49**(3–4), 483–493 (2012)
12. Paez, K.A., Allen, J.K., Carson, K.A., Cooper, L.A.: Provider and clinic cultural competence in a primary care setting. Soc. Sci. Med. **66**(5), 1204–1216 (2008)
13. Ohana, S., Mash, R.: Physician and patient perceptions of cultural competency and medical compliance. Health Educ. Res. **30**(6), 923–934 (2015)
14. Doorenbos, A.Z., Morris, A.M., Haozous, E.A., Harris, H.R., Flum, D.R.: Assessing cultural competence among oncology surgeons. J. Oncol. Pract. **12**(1), 61 (2016)
15. Eddey, G.E., Robey, K.L.: Considering the culture of disability in cultural competence education. Acad. Med. **80**(7), 706–712 (2005)
16. Hoang, L., LaHousse, S.F., Nakaji, M.C., Sadler, G.R.: Assessing deaf cultural competency of physicians and medical students. J. Cancer Educ. **26**(1), 175–182 (2011)
17. Roscigno, C.I.: Challenging Nurses' Cultural Competence of Disability to Improve Interpersonal Interactions. J. Neurosci. Nurs. **45**(1), 21–37 (2013)
18. Paasche-Orlow, M.: The ethics of cultural competence. Acad. Med. **79**(4), 347–350 (2004)
19. Constance, L.M.: Ehics and defining cultural competence: an alternative view. Nurs. Sci. Q. **29**(1), 21–23 (2015)

20. Hughto, J.M.W., Clark, K.A., Altice, F.L., Reisner, S.L., Kershaw, T.S., Pachankis, J.E.: Improving correctional healthcare providers' ability to care for transgender patients: development and evaluation of a theory-driven cultural and clinical competence intervenetion. Soc. Sci. Med. **195**, 159–169 (2017)

21. Whitley, R.: Religious competence as cultural competence. Transcult. Psychiatry **49**(2), 245–260 (2012)

22. Siegel, C.E., Haugland, G., Laska, E.M., Reid-Rose, L.M., Tang, D.-I., Wanderling, J.A., Chambers, E.D., Case, B.G.: The nathan kline institute cultural competency assessment scale: psychometrics and implications for disparity reduction. Adm. Policy Ment. Health Ment. Health Serv. Res. **38**(2), 120–130 (2011)

23. Weech-Maldonado, R., Elliott, M., Pradhan, R., Schiller, C., Hall, A., Hays, R.D.: Can hospital cultural competency reduce disparities in patient experiences with care? Med. Care **50**(11), 48–55 (2012)

24. McClellan, F.M., White III, A.A., Jimenez, R.L., Fahmy, S.: Do poor people sue doctors more frequently? Confronting unconscious bias and the role of cultural competency. Clin. Orthop. Relat. Res. **470**(5), 1393–1397 (2012)

25. Liaw, M.-L.: E-learning and the development of intercultural competence. Lang. Learn. Technol. **10**(3), 49–64 (2006)

26. Marie, Z.-V.A., Humberto, M.-D.J.: Experiential learning with global virtual teams: developing intercultural and virtual competencies. Magis-Revista Internacional De Investigacion En Educacion. **9**(8), 129–146 (2016)

27. Kaplan-Marcusan, A., Toran-Monserrat, P., Moreno-Navarro, J., Fabregas, M.J.C., Munoz-Ortiz, L.: Perception of primary health professionals about Female Genital Mutilation: from healthcare to intercultural competence. BMC Health Serv. Res. **9** (2009)

28. Stone, T.E., Francis, L., van der Riet, P., Dedkhard, S., Junlapeeya, P., Orwat, E.: Awaken ing to the other: Reflections on developing intercultural competence through an undergraduate study tour. Nurs. Health Sci. **16**(4), 521–527 (2014)

29. Lily, A.A.: Intercultural competence in higher education. In: International Approaches, Assessment and Application, pp. 7–18. Routlege (2017)

30. Mimi, J., Moffitt, S.R.: Transcultural nursing principles. J. Hospice Palliat. Nurs. **8**(2), 172–181 (2006)

31. Giger, J.N., Davishizar, R.E.: Transcultural Nursing: Assessment and Intervention, 7th edn. Mosby, St Louis (2016)

32. Duan-Ying, C.: A concept analysis of cultural competence. Int. J. Nurcing Sci. **3**, 268–273 (2016)

33. Cross, T.L., Bazron, B.J., Dennis, K.W., Mareasa, R.I.: Toward a culturally competent system of care. A monograph on effective services for minority children who are severely emotionally disturbed. CASSP Technical Assistance Center, Georgetown University Child Development Center (1989)

34. Julian Grant, Y.P., Guerin, P.: An investigation of culturally competent terminology in healthcare policy finds ambiguity and lack of definition. Aust. N. Z. J. Public Health **37**(3), 250–257 (2013)

35. Leininger, M.M.: Transcultural Nursing: Concepts, Theories, and Practices. Wiley, New York (1978)

36. Purnell, L.: Transcultural Health Care a Culturally Competent Approach, 4th edn. FA Davice, Philadelphia (2012)

37. Spitzberg, B.H., Changnon, G.: Conceptualizing intercultural competence. In: Deardorff, D.K. (ed.) The Sage Handbook of International Competence, pp. 2–52. Sage, Thousand Oaks (2009)

# Thai Nutrition Beliefs and Eating Behaviors Associated with Non-Communicable Diseases (NCDs)

Chanonya Chaiwongroj[✉]

College of Social Communication Innovation, Srinakharinwirot University,
114 Sukhumvit 23, Bangkok 10110, Thailand
chaiwong_non@hotmail.com

**Abstract.** This research investigates the Thai's nutrition beliefs and food consumption behaviors, comparing healthy subjects with those that have non-communicable diseases (NCDs). Convenience sampling was used, and 430 Thai residents agreed to participate. They filled out a five-part questionnaire that included personal data, health status, food consumption behaviors, communication channels for nutrition information and nutrition beliefs. A majority of them worked in an office with a salary of at least 20,000 baht per month (35%). Over 58% were females and had at least an undergraduate degree (49%). Of the 23% of the participants that had NCDs, their nutritional beliefs and eating behaviors were not significantly different than those participants that had no NCDs. In a digital age that includes LINE, Facebook and YouTube, 43% of the participants still said most of the information about nutrition comes from local television programs. There was a significant negative correlation between nutrition beliefs and actual eating behaviors, but it was so small as to have no predictive effect.

**Keywords:** Thai nutrition beliefs · Non-communicable diseases
Eating behaviors

## 1 Introduction

Non-Communicable diseases (NCDs) have risen to be a top public health priority in high-, middle-, and low-income countries alike. Most of the risk factors and high-risk behaviors upstream of NCDs have no symptoms, and people do not associate today's behavior choices with subsequent diseases. The World Health Organization (WHO) Global status Report (GSR 2010) on Noncommunicable Diseases 2010 showed that NCDs are the biggest cause of death in worldwide. In 2008, more than 36 million people died from NCDs, there are 48% from cardiovascular diseases, 21% from cancer, 12% from chronic respiratory diseases, and 3% from diabetes [1]. Moreover, from the WHO report in 2014, over 14 million deaths from NCDs occur between the ages of 30 and 70, of which 85% are in developing countries. Therefore, premature deaths are largely preventable by governments sector like public health ministry [2]. In Thailand, the mortality rate and prevalence of NCDs have been increasing during 2010–2014, especially in diabetes, hypertension, stroke and ischemic heart disease. The highest

© Springer International Publishing AG, part of Springer Nature 2019
N. J. Lightner (Ed.): AHFE 2018, AISC 779, pp. 267–273, 2019.
https://doi.org/10.1007/978-3-319-94373-2_30

NCDs incidence rate was in premature population (aged 30–69 years old) with the rate 28% in male and 19% in female which also higher than NCDs-WHO-target rate [3].

Noncommunicable diseases (NCDs), also known as chronic diseases, tend to be of long duration and are the results of a combination of genetic, physiological, environmental and behaviors factors. The main types of NCDs are cardiovascular diseases, cancers, chronic respiratory diseases (such as chronic obstructive pulmonary disease and asthma) and diabetes. WHO said, "These diseases are driven by forces that include rapid unplanned urbanization, globalization of unhealthy lifestyles and population aging. Unhealthy diets and a lack of physical activity may show up in people as raised blood pressure, increased blood glucose, elevated blood lipids and obesity." [4, 5]. To lessen the impact of NCDs on individuals and society, a comprehensive approach is needed requiring all sectors, including health, finance, transport, education, agriculture, planning and others, to collaborate to reduce the risk factors associated with NCDs, and promote interventions to prevent and control them.

The answer lies in "Health Promotion" and "Health Prevention" which involve changing the behaviors at multiple levels. Therefore, firstly it needs to understand and then apply the models that have been widely used to empower people to change their behaviors [1, 6]. Health knowledge is a key that everyone should have before practicing. Different areas have different health or nutrition beliefs depending to cultures and traditional beliefs. Therefore, these might be one reason that people have their own nutrition beliefs and caused them have healthy or unhealthy eating behaviors.

Nutrition beliefs have continued to generation-to-generation by words of mouth, sometimes there have no reasons to explain or support, for example, in Thai culture, if you have big wound, you have not to eat egg or sticky rice that might cause your wound infection. The truth is protein in egg help healing the wound. Another one is eating microwave food every day might get cancer and so on. In fact, there are so many myths or nutrition beliefs that floating around us especially on the internet [7, 8] such as:

1. Trans fat and saturated fats are bad; the truth is saturated fats have no effect on heart health at all.
2. Choosing a low-fat diet options; low fat products may be less healthy because they are loaded with sugar and salt to improve the taste.
3. Eating a heart-healthy diet means avoiding salt; some studies indicate that salt has no effect on cardiovascular health. The body needs salt to regulate fluid levels, so getting too little salt can lead to blood pressure is too low.
4. Avoid eggs that might cause heart disease; eggs have been demonized because their yolks contain high levels of cholesterol, but it turns out eggs are not the enemy. It is not the eggs themselves that are the culprit, but it often the food that company them, like bacon and sausage. Therefore, it is safe to eat as many as six eggs per week, according to the heart foundation.
5. Coffee cause disease; many people believed that coffee is detrimental to health because of the caffeine. The truth is coffee has many incredible health benefits. Coffee also contains cancer-fighting antioxidants that are the primary source of these free radical fighters.

There are many myths or nutrition beliefs that people may apply into their eating behaviors that might cause them unhealthy or having NCDs in near future.

In Thailand, government has paid for care treatment of health problems caused from over-eating behaviors more than 100,000 million baht per year [9]. Moreover, the severity of the NCDs may cause disability. It would better to decrease the risk factors to NCDs. Health prevention and promotion should be the absolute answer with huge problems. Ministry of Public Health runs many health campaigns for NCDs, but it might not too much successful. Why? One factor is people may have wrong beliefs or lack of health knowledge. Therefore, this paper aims to investigate the nutrition beliefs and identify the association between food consumption behaviors and nutrition beliefs with incidence of NCDs in Thai people who live in Bangkok. By comparing in NCDs and healthy people and ask for the channels that people get the health information.

# 2 Methodology

The method used in this study is questionnaire survey. Based on convenience sampling, data were collected from 430 subjects who lived in Bangkok and this research protocol was approved by the Srinakharinwirot University Social Science Institutional Review Boards. All of subjects signed the consent form before participating in this research.

## 2.1 Instrument

The questionnaire consisted of five main sections to explore a relationship between the incidence of NCDs and these variables: demographic profiles, health status, food consumption behaviors, communication channels for nutrition information, and nutritional beliefs.

The first section described characteristics of the respondents in term of gender, age, married status, education level, and salary.

The second section asked for health status that could identify non-NCDs and NCDs. In this research, NCDs are including diabetes, hypertension, chronic kidney disease, cardiovascular disease, cancer and stroke.

The third section explored the food consumption behaviors of the subjects. The 20-scaled items were rated on five scales. This section asked the frequency of eating food that may cause the subjects having NCDs, for example, eating junk food, having salty food, having soft drink or intake alcohol or smoking etc. Only four items that good for healthy life, like eating vegetables, having unsweetened fruits, having exercise for 30 min and having activities in house; cooking, housework, gardening.

The scales were run from 1 to 5 which mean the frequency of eating in each items. Scale 1 = never or rare, scale 2 = once a week, scale 3 = 2–3 times a week, scale 4 = 4–5 times a week and 5 = eating almost every day.

The forth section identified communication channels for nutrition information by rating from 1 to 5, which 1 mean always get information from this channel and 5 mean sometimes. The channels were television show, poster, leaflet, radio, nurse, magazine, and so on.

The last section of the questionnaire asked about the Thai nutrition beliefs that could show health knowledge of the participants. There were 20-items of nutrition beliefs that have 3 answers; "agree", "not agree" and "not sure". A score of 2 was awarded to "agree" answer, an 1 was for "not agree" and a zero was allocated to "not sure" answer.

## 2.2   Participants

The 430 survey samples consisted of 252 females and 178 males. The most of participants had the age range between 21–30 years old (27%), including; 31–40 years old (23%), 41–50 years old (14%), 51–60 years old (12%), >60 years old (12%) and <20 years old (8%), respectively. The majority education was 49% of undergraduate, 17% high school, 16% primary school and 7% of master degree level. Most of samples were office employee and had salary more than 20,000 baht.

From the total participants were identified into two groups; 278 healthy subjects and 100 NCDs subjects; 54 hypertension, 27 diabetes, 12 cardiovascular disease, 2 kidney disease, 3 cancer and 2 stroke, respectively.

## 2.3   Data Analyses

Descriptive statistics were used to describe respondents in term of the demographics and variables of interest. SPSS, $t$-tests, was conducted to analyze the association of nutrition beliefs, food-eating behaviors of NCDs and non-NCDs subjects. Statistical significance was denoted by a $p$-value $< 0.05$.

# 3   Results

## 3.1   Food Consumption Behaviors

In term of 20-items of the food consumption behaviors in the questionnaire were categorized into two behavior types:

1. 16-items of eating behaviors were the common risk factors to NCDs, such as junk food, salty food, soft drink, smoking and excessive intake of alcohol.
2. 4-items of healthy food and exercise, such as; eating vegetables, unsweetened fruits and doing housework.

The result showed that all of subjects have healthy eating behaviors because they have eating risky food for one a week and be non-smoking and non-alcoholic. Moreover, they have exercise almost every day like cooking, housework and gardening. Researcher also found that eating behaviors were not significantly different between NCDs and non-NCDs subjects as show in Table 1. Both of them were healthy eating behaviors.

**Table 1.** Outcome of food consumption behaviors between NCDs and non-NCDs subjects.

|          | N   | Mean | SD   | $t$  | $p$   |
|----------|-----|------|------|------|-------|
| Non-NCDs | 314 | 2.44 | 0.42 | 1.84 | 0.067 |
| NCDs     | 115 | 2.34 | 0.52 |      |       |

## 3.2    Communication Channels for Nutrition Information

A total of 430 subjects rated five channels for receiving nutrition information from the most channel to the least channel. The result showed the first rank was television show, leaflets, poster, nurses, and the last rank was radio program, respectively. Only 51 subjects chose other channels for the first rank, there were internet, Face Book, Line and You tube.

## 3.3    Nutrition Beliefs

All subjects in this research showed that they have nutrition beliefs in the right way, except only three beliefs got "not sure" answer. There were the adequate quantity of sugar and salt per one day and eat white rice is the cause for diabetes. Therefore, nutrition beliefs in both NCDs and non-NCDs subjects were not different significantly with $p$-value 0.16 ($p > 0.05$) as shown in Table 2.

**Table 2.**    Outcome of nutrition beliefs between NCDs and non-NCDs subjects.

|          | Number | Mean  | SD   | $t$    | $p$  |
|----------|--------|-------|------|--------|------|
| Non-NCDs | 314    | 26.92 | 4.23 | $-1.41$ | 0.16 |
| NCDs     | 115    | 27.56 | 3.79 |        |      |

Moreover, checking the correlation between nutrition beliefs and eating behaviors in both groups, it came out with very low negative correlation ($r = -0.15$, $p = 0.002$) even though it was a significantly effect.

# 4    Discussion

This research was to exam the Thai nutrition beliefs and eating behaviors associated with Non-Communicable diseases (NCDs). There have more healthy subjects than NCDs subjects, and the mean scores of food consumption behaviors of both groups were about 2.34 and 2.44. This score "2" means "once a week", this could explain that both groups have unhealthy eating behaviors once a week or sometimes 2–3 times a week. Because of female subjects more than male, the result of smoking and intake alcohol came out in score "1" (1 = never). Both subject groups have not different in eating behaviors and the nutrition beliefs. Hence, it might be interpreted that NCDs subjects may adjust their eating behaviors after they got one of NCDs. This result was different from other researches that explored in patients than in normal subject [6, 10–15], therefore the results were come out totally different. Researcher is interested in normal or healthy subjects than patient subjects because it is easy to apply health prevention and health promotion.

In not only Thailand, Kearney and his co-workers [16] studies about the attitudes towards the beliefs about nutrition and health in Republic of Ireland and Northern Ireland. They reported that it is necessary to understand the attitudes towards and beliefs about nutrition of the public for effective healthy eating promotion. Moreover, their result showed there was female, a majority of subjects, that they make conscious efforts to eat a healthy diet either most of the time or quite often. Like this research, the nutrition beliefs came out pretty good; subjects have corrected nutrition knowledge 18-items from 20-items. Only 2-items were answer mostly in "not sure". This nutrition knowledge is not difficult, there is the quantity of sugar and salt should take in one day. It could imply that health promotion in Thailand was not work. Wongwatananakul *et al.* [17] reported that during 2002–2012, primary prevention shared the minority in overall resources for NCDs prevention. In addition, economic cost of NCDs treatment was 11 times higher than TEPP (total expenditure on prevention and promotion) for NCDs. Therefore, it is time for Thai government put the priority in NCDs prevention and control. The channels are so important to release the health information also, even though many nutrition and health information are floating around in the internet, social media, Line and Face Book. How to give credits that information, especially data from the social media? This research found television show was the first rank that they received nutrition knowledge. It may be TV programs (in Thailand) about health always have physicians or specialist doctors give the health information. In spite of internet and social media, tons of health and nutrition knowledge run around us with no reliability data sources. Finally, nutrition and health information would launch via television program for enhancing healthy eating behaviors for prevention of NCDs.

NCDs are the chronic diseases that caused mortality and disability for worldwide. It has been the magnitude problems for long time even though WHO cooperated with many countries to control the incidence of NCDs. The risk factors of NCDs were come from the unhealthy eating behaviors and lack of exercise or activities. People do understand about the causes and effects of NCDs, but the incidence of NCDs in Thai still high. We need to take it seriously for preventing and promoting the healthy behaviors and nutrition knowledge, therefore people would have eating behaviors in the right way.

# 5    Limitations

This study samples were not enough to identify the associated of nutrition beliefs and eating behaviors and the result cannot be generalized. In addition to the convenient sampling might not be suitable, it should apply with other sampling methods to get diversity of eating behaviors. Moreover, this research is cross-sectional design that might not get the practical behaviors of the subjects. Further research should apply other research design and sampling method.

**Acknowledgements.** This research was supported by the research fund of College of Social Communication Innovation, Srinakharinwirot University. Researcher greatly appreciated this support and all of participants who answered the questionnaire.

# References

1. Dobe, M.: Health promotion for prevention and control of non-communicable diseases: unfinihed agenda. Indian J. Public Health **56**(3), 180–186 (2012). https://doi.org/10.4103/0019-557X.104199
2. World Health Organization.: Noncommunication Diseases Country Profiles (2014). http://www.who.int/nmh/publications/ncd-profiles-2014/en
3. Srivanichakorn, S.: Morbidity and Mortality situation of non-communicable diseases. (Diabetes type 2 and Cardiovascular diseases) in Thailand during 2010–2014. Disease Control J. **43**(4), 370–390 (2017)
4. World Health Organization: Noncommunicable Diseases Fact Sheet; Update, June 2017. http://www.who.int/mediacentre/factsheets/fs355/en/
5. GBD 2015 Risk Factors Collaborators. Global, Regional, and National Comparative Risk Assessment of 79 Behavioral, Environmental and Occupational, and Metabolic Risks or Clusters of Risks, 1990–2015: A Systematic Analysis for The Global Burden of Disease Study 2015. Lancet **388**(10053), 1659–1724 (2016)
6. Brotons, C., Drenthen, A.J.M., Durrer, D., Moral, I.: Beliefs and attitudes to lifestyle, nutrition and physical activity: the views of patients in Europe. Fam. Pract. **29**, i49–i55 (2012). https://doi.org/10.1093/fampra/cmr091
7. Hilmantel, R.: 10 Healthy-Eating Myths (2014). https://www.womenshealthmag.com/food/healthy-eating-myths/slide/11
8. The 15 Biggest Nutritional Beliefs Busted by Science Customer Testimonials. https://www.dietspotlight.com/15-nutritional-beliefs-busted/
9. Intarakamhang, U.: Health Literacy: Measurement and Development. Behavioral Science Research Institute, Srinakharinwirot University, Bangkok, pp. 1–21 (2016)
10. Hankey, C.R., Eley, S., Leslie, W.S., Hunter, C.M., Lean, M.E.J.: Eating habits, beliefs, attitudes and knowledge among health professionals regarding the links between obesity. Nutr. Health Public Health Nutr. **7**(2), 337–343 (2003)
11. Acheampong, I., Haldeman, L.: Are nutrition knowledge, attitudes, and beliefs associated with obesity among low-income hispanic and african american woman caretakers? J. Obesity, 1–8 (2013). http://dx.doi.org/10.1155/2013/123901
12. Phoemphun, N., Thongbai, W., Numkham, L.: Effects of a behavior changing program on the health behavior and nutrition of overweight employees in the workplace. Rama Nurs. J. **22**(2), 177–191 (2016)
13. Jangwang, S., Pittayapinune, T., Chutipattana, N.: Factors related to self-care behavior for prevention of diabetes mellitus and hypertension among population groups at risk. South. Coll. Netw. J. Nurs. Public Health **3**(1), 110–128 (2016)
14. Wichitthonchai, C.: The factors associated with food consumption behaviors of cardiac and arterial diseases patients, queen sirikit heart center of the northeastern region. Khon Kaen Univ. Srinagarind Med J. **27**(4), 340–346 (2012)
15. Kinosian, B., Glick, H., Garland, G.: Cholesterol and Coronary Heart diseases: Predicting risks by levels and ratio. Ann. Internal Med. **121**, 641–647 (1994)
16. Kearney, J.M., Gibney, M.J., Livingstone, B.E., Robson, P.J., Kiely, M., Harrington, K.: Attitudes toward and beliefs about nutrition and health among a random sample of adults in the Republic of Ireland and Northern Ireland. Public Health Nutr. **4**(5A), 1117–1126 (2001)
17. Wongwatanakul, W., Viriyathron, S., Prakongsai, P.: Trend in financing for prevention and control of non-communicable diseases (NCDs) in Thailand, 2002–2012. J. Health Sci. **25**(4), 571–582 (2016)

# Improving Japanese Nursing Education by Understanding "Intercultural Competence"

Norihito Taniguchi[1]([⊠]), Miyoko Okamoto[2], Yui Mastuda[3], and Manami Nozaki[2]

[1] Nagoya University, Nagoya, Japan
taniguchi.norihito@i.mbox.nagoya-u.ac.jp
[2] Juntendo University, Tokyo, Chiba, Japan
myokamo@juntendo.ac.jp
[3] University of Miami, Coral Gables, FL, USA
ymatsuda@miami.edu

**Abstract.** There are approximately 2.4 million international residents in Japan in 2016. Seventy percent of these residents do not speak English. However, medical and nursing schools emphasize education in Medical English, rather than taking a broader approach that encompasses diverse cultures. This is why current healthcare professionals struggle in dealing with international patients, especially those from non-English speaking countries. Therefore, shifting the viewpoint from how we can technically support international patients to how we can improve the intercultural competence of healthcare professionals is critical. the aim of this literature review is to examine the similarities and differences between the intercultural competence in pedagogy and healthcare in Japan and the US by comparing literatures from both fields, and by clarifying how intercultural competence has been conceptualized as well as its significance. Results show that when comparing the concept of intercultural competence in pedagogy and healthcare, while the components are similar, the historical background of the concept and the social contexts in use are different (between the two disciplines). In order to understand the concept of intercultural competence, it is critically important to define Japan's own interdisciplinary concept of intercultural competence in both healthcare and pedagogy.

**Keywords:** Cultural competence · Intercultural competence
Nursing education

## 1 Introduction

There are approximately 2.4 million international residents in Japan as of 2016 (see, Japan's Ministry of Justice website). Seventy percent of these residents do not speak English. Despite this, the Japanese government implemented the Japan Medical Service Accreditation for International Patients policy in 2012, and the Foreign Patient Acceptance Environment Improvement project in 2014. However, as of today, for example, only two institutions in Aichi prefecture are accredited through the above system as of today. Providing subsidy to medical institutions is also application based and unlimited, which might cause a regional disparity among international residents in

© Springer International Publishing AG, part of Springer Nature 2019
N. J. Lightner (Ed.): AHFE 2018, AISC 779, pp. 274–282, 2019.
https://doi.org/10.1007/978-3-319-94373-2_31

terms of accessibility to healthcare throughout Japan. In addition, according to preliminary research, there is pushback against these Japanese government policies at healthcare sites. These policies make it necessary not only to arrange for medical interpreters in multiple languages, but also to understand diverse cultures, customs, religions, etc. This includes differences, such as healthcare system differences between the home country of international patients, and different views on health and healthcare decision-making [1]. Moreover, medical and nursing schools emphasize providing medical English education, not intercultural education to understand diverse cultures. There is a huge disparity between assumed medical "English" education and actual onsite practice [2, 3].

For these reasons, current healthcare professionals struggle in dealing with international patients, especially those from non-English speaking countries. Therefore, shifting the viewpoint from how we can technically support international patients to how we can improve the "intercultural competence" of healthcare professionals is critically important.

## 2    Aim of This Study

The term "intercultural competence" has been used in pedagogy and healthcare in Japan and the US for a long time. Therefore, the aim of this literature review is to examine the similarities and differences between the intercultural competence in pedagogy and healthcare in Japan and the US by comparing literature from both fields and by clarifying how intercultural competence has been conceptualized as well as its significance. The research questions that guide this study are as follows:

1. How is intercultural competence for healthcare professionals conceptualized in the healthcare field in Japan and the US?
2. What are the similarities and differences between the intercultural competence in pedagogy and healthcare in Japan and the US?

## 3    Methods

This study was carried out by conducting a systematic search through Google Scholar and Web of Science. We searched for articles in pedagogy and healthcare published from January 1987 to December 2017 by using the following keywords: cultural competence/transcultural competence/cross-cultural competence/intercultural competence/health/healthcare/medical/medicine/nursing

Firstly, more than 100 articles were systematically searched, but we selected several key articles that had an important influence (most cited) on the development of intercultural competence, explaining the discussion in Japan and US. Then, based on an analysis of literature, we compare the similarities and differences of intercultural competence between both fields in both countries, and finally synthesize the relevant literature rather than reporting the number of articles found per key word.

# 4  Results and Discussion

## 4.1  Development of Intercultural Competence in Pedagogy (or Other Fields Except Healthcare) in Japan

There is little discussion of intercultural competence in academics in Japan until the mid-1990s. During the 1960s, due to the expansion of Japanese trading companies and banks internationally, the number of children living overseas with their parents increased. We call these children "Kikyokushijo" in Japanese, and these children's unique educational issues, such as intercultural adaptation, intercultural contact, culture shock, intercultural experience, identity, intercultural understanding, and intercultural communication, were the main research topics in the field of intercultural education [4]. The closest concept at present of intercultural competence emerged from psychology during the 1990s. For example, according to Yamagishi [5], intercultural competence is defined as an integrated ability, a deeper level of ability to communicate, and an ability to deal with general culture different from one's own culture. (see Fig. 1.) Additionally, several authors mentioned similar concepts related to intercultural competence [e.g. 5, 6, etc.]. This literature is based on the scene of intercultural contact in psychology or the concept of intercultural ability has been studied with the development of the field of intercultural communication from 1980s to 1990s. Subsequently, with the exception of Yamagishi's book, there is hardly any literature on intercultural competence.

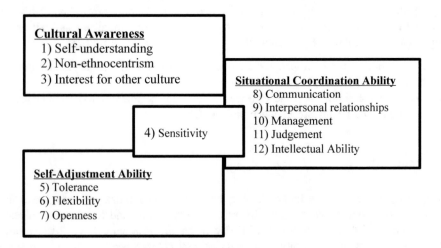

**Fig. 1.**  Factors of Intercultural Competence [5]

The Intercultural Education Society of Japan published a bulletin titled "Think about intercultural competence" in 2017 [7], but it was written from the perspective of a wide range of academic fields such as pedagogy, psychology and linguistics, and there was no discussion based on one common academic field on intercultural competence. While the term "intercultural competence" is used several times in the literature on pedagogy, it is cited from international literatures, and so there is currently very little literature where Japanese scholars independently defined "intercultural competence". Even if the term "intercultural competence" is not used, terms such as "cross-cultural adaptability", "international understanding ability", "cross-cultural communication ability", etc. are frequently used in the context of each academic field.

As described above, such confusion is seen presently in the development of the conceptualization of intercultural competence in Japan. Therefore, it is quite difficult to see the trajectory of intercultural competence in Japan's pedagogy, especially intercultural education.

### 4.2    Development of Intercultural Competence in Pedagogy in the US

According to Spitzberg [8], the idea of intercultural competence was first conceptualized after World War II. In the 1950s, the Cold War heightened the importance of business alliances, humanitarian problems, and political stability in other countries. The Peace Corps especially was a key organization in the stabilization of foreign countries with its foreign aid programs. The need to select and train individuals to serve in a culture effectively in the other countries were essential, which then stimulated a new movement and social scientific interest in the conceptualization of intercultural competence. In the 1970s, based on the experience of Peace Corp, 24 characteristics in Tonga were differentiated from highly successful to less successful volunteers [9]. Other literature discussed cross-cultural adjustment, effectiveness, etc. [e.g., 10]. In the 1980s, researchers focus more on communication, and developing and refining instruments to assess intercultural "communication" competence which were being studied multidimensionally. From the 1990s to 2000s, Spitzberg and Changnon conducted a comprehensive review of intercultural competence. Instead of defining intercultural competence itself, they modelized it into 5 categorize, which are Compositional Models, Co-orientational Models, Developmental Models, Adaptational Models, and Causal Path Models. Among five categories, the process model (including Causal Path Models) proposed by Deardorff [11] was most recent cited literature. In addition, the developmental model of intercultural sensitivity (included in the Development Models) proposed by Bennett [12] is still frequently used in the most recent literatures. Both are used to assess intercultural competence in the rubrics of Association of American College and Universities (cf. https://www.aacu.org/value/rubrics).

### 4.3    Comparison of Intercultural Competence in Pedagogy Between Japan and the US

Historically in Japan, in analyzing the development of intercultural competence, most of the discussion has been done in psychology or communication, not in intercultural education or higher education as in the US. In 1960s Japan, it was assumed that in the context of intercultural contact, communication issues in English would be the first priority, the second would be intercultural adaption in another country or culture, and the third might be acquisition of intercultural competence. In short, discussions on the mastery of intercultural competence in Japan first emerge as a debate in the 1990s, not since the 1950s as in like the U.S. And so, with this state of affairs in Japan as summarized by Spitzberg, we have not been able to reach the stage of modeling across a variety of academic disciplines, though this topic has been discussed in many independent fields. This is why the discussion of intercultural competence is more mature in the U.S. compared to Japan where there is still a question as to which position among the various models of intercultural competence is best. Consequently, the method of categorization used by Spitzberg makes possible a comparison of the idea of intercultural competence in both countries and will be used in this paper.

## 4.4    Development of Intercultural Competence in Healthcare in Japan

In Japan today, nursing school curricula does not incorporate intercultural competence in healthcare. Even in an upcoming school curriculum for nursing professionals (September 2017), as a study objective, it states that "Students can understand and support the life of people with diverse cultural background". It is not an exaggeration to say that detailed explanation and training method are not discussed.

Even though preliminary research in Japan considers the possibilities to introducing curricula that teach intercultural competence for domestic doctors [13] or of developing intercultural educational programs for perinatal caregivers [14], there is no paper discussing comprehensive educational methods aimed at improving intercultural competence. In other words, much of the literature related to intercultural competence in healthcare in Japan just explains or cites concepts of intercultural competence from US literatures or theories.

There is, however, one study which defines intercultural competence for nursing in Japan. That is Sugiura's thesis written in 2003 [15]. Sugiura compared the cultural competence between nurses who were Japan Oversees Corporation Volunteers and nurses working at municipal hospitals by quantitative analysis. Sugiura described the components of intercultural nursing as follows:

1. Knowledge of cultural specifics in intercultural competence nursing
2. Knowledge of general culture in intercultural competence nursing
3. Less of a tendency to avoid international patients
4. Recognition of own culture
5. Skills in intercultural nursing

Of note is that the intercultural competence that nurses acquired overseas and the intercultural competence of nurses that was acquired in Japan were slightly different. For example, the way of approaching international patients in the US medical system is not the same as that of the Japanese healthcare system. If the medical system, which is a premise of intercultural competence, is different from country to country, it is reasonable that the concept of intercultural competence within these systems would also be different. Therefore, introducing concept directly to healthcare facilities in Japan as-is might cause confusion. The ability to respond to international patients effectively and appropriately in the Japanese healthcare system would and must be intercultural competence carefully tailored to the context of Japanese healthcare delivery. It cannot be directly introduced from other countries without careful consideration. In short, what needs to be clarified are the differences between nurses who acquired intercultural competence inside of Japan versus those outside Japan. In that light, while Sugiura's paper might be critical in some ways, refining the concept of intercultural competence is much more essential than introducing it directly to the Japanese context.

## 4.5 Development of Intercultural Competence in Healthcare in the US

The term "intercultural competence" is conceptually similar to "cultural competence" in healthcare, and it is the most common term in the US to refer to optimal training outcomes for health professionals and trainees [16]. The conceptualization of cultural competence was started in the 1950 s' by Leininger [17]. Leininger did not mention the term "intercultural competence", but she conceptualized transurethral nursing and culturally congruent (competent) care. According to Leininger, first, transcultural nursing is defined as a legitimate and formal area of study, research, and practice, focused on culturally-based care beliefs, values, and practices to help cultures or subcultures maintain or regain their health (wellbeing) and face disabilities or death in culturally congruent and beneficial caring ways. Second, culturally congruent (competent) care means care that is meaningful and fits with cultural beliefs and lifeways [17]. Since Leininger, the definition of cultural competence in the US has been nearly equivalent to transcultural nursing or culturally congruent (competent) care.

In addition to Leininger's theory, Campinha-Bacote [18] developed the process model of cultural competence in 2002. According to Campinha-Bacote, "this model requires health care providers to see themselves as becoming culturally competent rather than already being culturally competent. This process involves the integration of cultural awareness, cultural knowledge, cultural skill, cultural encounters, and cultural desire." [18]. The assumptions of this theory are as follows (Fig. 2):

---

1) Cultural competence is a process, not an event.
2) Cultural competence consists of five constructs: cultural awareness, cultural knowledge, cultural skill, cultural encounters, and cultural desire.
3) There is more variation within ethnic groups than across ethnic groups (intra-ethnic variation).
4) There is a direct relationship between the level of competence of healthcare providers and their ability to provide culturally responsive health care services.
5) Cultural competence is an essential component in rendering effective and culturally responsive services to culturally and ethnically diverse clients.

---

**Fig. 2.** Assumptions of the Model by Campinha-Bacote

The most distinguished feature of Compinha-Bacote's view, compared to Leininger's views, is that cultural competence is a process, not an event, and one "in which the healthcare provider continuously strives to achieve the ability to effectively work within the cultural context of the client". Also, "the works of Leininger (1978) in the area of transcultural nursing and Pedersen (1988) in the area of multicultural development were combined to develop the constructs used in the model".

In the end, after these developments in intercultural competence, school curricula for cultural competence were created in the US, although the content of nursing school curricula vary according to state as of 2010s' [19, 20].

## 4.6    Comparison of Intercultural Competence in Healthcare Between Japan and the US

As discussed before, while Sugiura's paper deserves consideration for its treatment of intercultural competence, further research is necessary in order to formulate a concept of Japan's own intercultural competence in healthcare.

In contrast to Japan, in the US, Leinigher and Campinha-Bacotes theories have developed since the 1950's and are well-known all over the world. Yet, the applications of these concepts are not discussed in depth in Japan. Before that can happen, these needs to be a base provided of general education on culture. First identifying the concept of Japan's own intercultural competence in healthcare and then mixing that concept with American nursing education theory will lead to the formation of new hybrid theories suitable for the Japanese medical environment.

## 4.7    Comparison of Intercultural Competence in Pedagogy and Healthcare

While preliminary research in the US was advanced in comparison to Japan in both fields, we will examine the similarities and differences between pedagogy and healthcare, and then explain several conceptual challenges.

In terms of similarities Lilly [21] mentioned two points: first, effectiveness (the ability to achieve one's goals in a particular exchange) and appropriateness (the ability to do so in a manner that is acceptable to the other person) are two components of intercultural competence prevalent in literature. Second, there is a consensus among scholars that intercultural competence has cognitive, affective, and behavioral dimensions. In reviewing the selected literature [5, 8, 15, 17, 18], regardless of country and academic field, it is consistent that these two criteria are standards to define the intercultural competence in an interdisciplinary way.

Conversely, in terms of differences, unlike earlier literature, the concept of intercultural competence in healthcare has evolved under the influence of the "care" concept, separate from the evolvement of pedagogy. The influence of Leininger's theory is profound, and, as she used the term "culturally congruent care" rather than "intercultural competence" starting in 1950's, it is hypothesized that the concept of "care" has become a key term to separate the evolvement between both fields. For the same reason, the concept of culture in healthcare is strongly influenced by cultural anthropology, whereas in pedagogy it is influenced by a broader range of fields. The concept of culture in healthcare is more likely to include specific cultural nuances, while the concept of cultural in pedagogy encompasses general cultural nuances. Eventually, the concept of "cultural humility" emerged as a separate concept from the term "cultural competence" in the late 1990s. As with the concept of care, this was due to the fact that the concept of competence has an established meaning in healthcare [16]. Jann emphasizes that "to alert medical educators to the potential pitfalls and pitfalls inherent in the term "competence" when involved in cross-cultural interactions, the term "cultural humility" was proposed as an alternative to cultural competence (Tervalon & Murray-Garcia 1998)." From the concept of care and the concept of cultural humility, the concept of competence may have been intentionally avoided due to its established meaning. In this respect as well, we can follow the trajectory of independent development for the different concepts of intercultural competence in healthcare.

As stated, there are similarities and differences between the two disciplines of healthcare and pedagogy and, several challenges and limitations in comparing them should be noted. First, the definition of intercultural competence differs according to the academic field whether pedagogy or healthcare, and their definitions are currently still vague [8]. Second, measuring intercultural competence requires both theory and conceptual models to form a basis for measurement. Also, necessary is research into the validity and reliability of those measurement [22]. There is an established measurement for intercultural competence in pedagogy, but not in healthcare [23]. Third, Japan's healthcare situation (in political and social terms) is different from that of the US [21], and thus, when introducing intercultural competence to Japan, its own cultural background should be considered after a through discussion with overseas' researchers.

## 5 Conclusion

The number of international patients in the Japanese healthcare environment has rapidly increased in recent years, and it is urgent that healthcare professionals understand intercultural competence. As discussed in this paper, in order to understand the concept of intercultural competence, it is first necessary to define, measure and understand the intercultural competence. As medical environments may differ from country to country, another country's concept of intercultural competence should not be introduced directly into Japan. It is critically important to define Japan's own interdisciplinary concept of intercultural competence in both healthcare and pedagogy.

## References

1. Nakamura, Y.: Support for international residents in Japan, health and healthcare issues for international residents, Community Health **34**(11), 5–12 (2003)
2. Matsuo, H.: Present situation and issues of foreign maternal and child health medicine in Japan - Questionnaire survey of obstetric medical professional in Kobe-city. Perinatal Med. **34**(2), 261–264 (2004)
3. Adachi, Y., et al.: Problems in caring patients with different cultural background-a postal survey of public hospitals in Japan. Nursing J. Osaka Univ. **15**(1), 19–31 (2009)
4. Intercultural Education Society of Japan (2016): Education for 'people' to learn from different cultures, Akashi-shoten (2016)
5. Yamagishi, M.: Intercultural competence and training. In: Watanabe, F. (ed.) Psychology of Intercultural Contact, Kawashima-Shoten, pp. 209–219 (1995)
6. Mizuta, S.: Intercultural training. In: Nishida, et al. International Human Relations Theory, Seibunsha, pp. 234–259 (1989)

7. Intercultural Education Society of Japan: Think about intercultural competence, Intercultural Education, Kokusaibunkensha (2017)

8. Spitzberg, B.H., Changnon, G.: Conceptualizing Intercultural Competence. In: Deardorff, D. (ed.) The Sage Handbook of Intercultural Competence, pp. 1–52. Sage, Thousand Oaks (2009)

9. Harris Jr., J.G.: Identification of cross-cultural talent: the empirical approach of the Peace Corps. In: Brislin, R.W. (ed.) Culture Learning: Concepts, Applications, and Research, pp. 182–194. University of Hawaii, Honolulu (1977)

10. Benson, P.G.: Measuring cross-cultural adjustment: the problem of criteria. Int. J. Intercultural Relat. **2**, 21–37 (1978)

11. Deardorff, D.K.: The identification and assessment of intercultural competence as a student outcome of internationalization at institutions of higher education in the United States. J. Stud. Int. Educ. **10**, 241–266 (2006)

12. Bennett, M.J.: Towards a developmental model of intercultural sensitivity. In: Michael Paige, R. (ed.) Education for the Intercultural Experience. Intercultural Press, Yarmouth (1993)

13. Yokoyama, S., et al.: Building an empathetic medical communication model centered on intercultural competence, Ministry of Education, Culture, Science and Technology Grant-in-Aid for Scientific Research, Challenging Exploration Research, Research Result Report) (2014, 2015)

14. Igarashi, Y., et al.: Implementation and evaluation of perinatal care nurse development program to nurture susceptibility of multicultural coexistence, Ministry of Education, Culture, Sports, Science and Technology Grant-in-Aid for Scientific Research, Basic Research (C), Research Result Report) (2013–2016) (2016)

15. Sugiura, K.: Survey-based analysis of cultural competence in nursing an its predictors: comparison between nurses who were japan overseas cooperation volunteers and nurses working at municipal hospitals. J. Japanese Acad. Nurs. Sci. **23**(3), 22–36 (2003)

16. Murray-García, J., et al.: Rethinking intercultural competence, cultural humility in internationalizing higher education. In Deardorff, D. (ed.) Intercultural Competence in Higher Education, pp. 44–56. Routledge (2017)

17. Leininger, M.M.: What is transcultural nursing and culturally competent care? J. Transcult. Nurs. **10**, 9 (1999)

18. Campinha-Bacote, J.: The process of cultural competence in the delivery of healthcare service: A model of care. J. Transcult. Nurs. **13**, 181–184 (2002)

19. Calvillo, E., et al.: Cultural Competence in Baccalaureate Nursing Education. J. Transcult. Nurs. **20**(2), 137–145 (2009)

20. Axtel, S., Avery, M., Westra, B.: Incorporating cultural competence content into graduate nursing curricula through community-university collaboration. J. Transcult. Nurs. **21**(2), 183–191 (2010)

21. Arasaratnam-Smith, L.A.: Intercultural competence: an overview. In: Deardorff, D. (ed.) Intercultural Competence in Higher Education, pp. 7–18. Routledge (2017)

22. Paige, R.M.: Instrumentation in Intercultural Training. In: Landis, D. (ed.) Hand Book of Intercultural Training, pp. 85–128. Sage, Thousand Oaks (2004)

23. Hammer, M.R., Bennet, M.J., Wiseman, R.L.: Measuring intercultural sensitivity: the intercultural development inventory. Int. J. Intercult. Relat. **27**, 421–433 (2003)

# The Related Factors for Self-efficacy of Condom Use Among Adolescent Girls - Taking HPV Acquisition Preventing as an Example

Cheng-Chieh Tsai[1], Jing-Shia Tang[1], Tung-I Tsai[2], and Yu-Ching Tu[1(✉)]

[1] Department of Nursing,
Chung Hwa University of Medical Technology, Tainan, Taiwan
s58961353@gmail.com, pochacco2293@yahoo.com.tw
[2] Collaborative Innovation Center of China Pilot Reform Exploration
and Assessment-Hubei Sub-Center,
Hubei University of Economics, Wuhan, China

**Abstract.** Human papillomavirus (HPV) acquisition is caused by skin to skin contact, and the use of condoms reduces the risk of HPV acquisition. This study employed a cross-sectional design to investigate condom use self-efficacy and the expected results of adolescent girls using condoms to prevent HPV acquisition. The results showed that the standard index score of adolescent girls using condoms to prevent HPV acquisition was 68.5. The perceived condom use control, health locus of control, and expected result of condom use were significant predictors of condom use self-efficacy, which explained 30.00% of the total amount of variance in condom use self-efficacy. Furthermore, two regression models showed the statistic variation of condom use self-efficacy for those who have had sexual experience and those have not, which was 78.49% and 29.22% of the total amount of variance in condom use self-efficacy, respectively.

**Keywords:** Human papillomavirus · Condom use self-efficacy
Health locus of control · Perceived behavioral control · Expected result

## 1 Introduction

The main utility of using condoms for the health care of adolescents includes preventing unwanted pregnancies and preventing sexually transmitted infections (STIs). Human papillomavirus (HPV) is the most important risk factor for genital warts and cervical cancer. Approximately 99.7% of cervical cancer patients have had HPV [1, 2]. HPV transmission occurs via skin-to-skin contact, usually during sexual intercourse, and is often transmitted unknowingly, because most infections are asymptomatic. The peak time for HPV acquiring infection for both women and men is shortly after becoming sexually active [2, 3]. Prophylactic vaccines have been approved against oncogenic HPV genotypes 16 and 18, which are responsible for approximately 70% of cervical cancer cases,

© Springer International Publishing AG, part of Springer Nature 2019
N. J. Lightner (Ed.): AHFE 2018, AISC 779, pp. 283–293, 2019.
https://doi.org/10.1007/978-3-319-94373-2_32

and it is recommended that the vaccine series be initiated before sexual activity begins [2, 4, 5]. As such, HPV vaccination is routinely recommended for adolescents, with 33.4% of females having completed their HPV vaccine series in the USA [6] and 49% in Canada [7], and contributes to an HPV vaccine inoculation rate of less than 4% in the countries that vaccines are not mandatory are not publicly funded [8–10]. Therefore, other factors, such as condom use as a precautionary measure against adolescent HPV infection, should not be neglected in preventing adolescent HPV-related diseases. Thus, the use of condoms to prevent STIs among adolescents is unsatisfactory. Statistics indicate that 58.7% of adolescent boys use condoms during their first time having sex, compared with 55.1% of girls [11]. Therefore, it is worth discussing the factors that affect the self-efficacy of condom use in young girls to prevent the HPV infection and the effects of self-efficacy condom use.

Persistent infection with sexually transmitted high-risk genotypes of HPV is a cause of cervical cancer [1]. Currently, cervical cancer is the fourth most frequent cancer in women worldwide. It takes 15 to 20 years for cervical cancer to develop in women with normal immune systems [2]. HPV infections are transmitted through contact with infected genital skin or mucosal surfaces/secretions. HPV infection can occur in male or female genital areas that are covered (protected by the condom) as well as those areas that are not [6]. Prospective studies have demonstrated a protective effect of condoms on the acquisition of genital HPV. Condom use may reduce the risk for genital HPV infection and HPV-associated diseases, e.g., genital warts and cervical cancer.

HPV infection is considered a STI. The main method of STI prevention, i.e., safe sex, includes three principles (ABC principles) in Taiwan: abstinence, being faithful to your sole partner (monogamy), and using condoms for the entirety of intercourse [6]. Based on the survey data, the mean age of first sexual activity is getting lower; with 25% of people have sex for the first time before the age of 19 years [12]. Condoms can reduce the risk of most STDs as well as the risk for pregnancy [12]. Condoms, when used correctly and consistently, have an 80% or greater protective effect against the sexual transmission of HIV and other STIs [13], including diminishing HPV acquisition [14, 15], accelerating the regression of HPV-associated penile lesions in male sexual partners of women with cervical intraepithelial neoplasia, and clearance of the HPV infection in women [16, 17]. Consistent condom use has been associated with a decreased likelihood of HPV acquisition among young women [15]. Some cross-sectional studies have demonstrated protective associations between condom use and prevalence of genital HPV infection [14, 18]. One Taiwanese study indicated that 61.5% of people who had their first sexual encounter did not use a condom, and among people with sexual experience, 52.21% used condoms less frequently, and only 25.71% consistently used condoms [19]. Thus, condom use prevalence among adolescents is unsatisfactory.

Self-efficacy is one's belief in their ability to succeed in specific situations or accomplish a task [20]. Previous studies have shown that the high perceived self-efficacy of condom use is associated with habitual condom use [21, 22]. The study also indicated that familiarity with the use of condoms, self-efficacy of condom proficiency, and perception of condom users positively affected condom use by adolescents with positive experiences in the future [23]. The current study investigated the associated factors of self-efficacy of condom use among adolescent girls to prevent HPV acquisition. The construct of the health locus of control assumes that people with an internal health locus of control are more likely to engage in positive and protective health behaviors and take control of their own health. People with an external health locus of control view their health as out of their control, and thus, engage in less positive and protective health behaviors while believing that others are responsible for their health [24]. A study regarding health locus of control and risky sexual behavior of African American adolescents found that adolescents with an internal locus of control were more likely to use condoms than adolescents with an external locus of control [25]. In a similar study of adolescents in England, Mendolia and Walker [26] found that adolescents with an external locus of control had a 15–16% higher risk of an unprotected sexual intercourse history and were younger than 16 years at their first sexual intercourse than adolescents with an internal locus of control. Burnett [27] found that university adolescents in the United States with an external locus of control were more likely to adopt unsafe sexual behavior. The purpose of this study is to investigate the related factors for self-efficacy of condom use among adolescent girls to prevent HPV acquisition.

## 2   Methods

### 2.1   Design and Sampling

This study used a cross-sectional and descriptive design. Participants were recruited first-year students of five senior high schools in southern Taiwan using the convenience sampling method. For this study, each eligible participant (1) was an adolescent girl in the ten years of senior high school, (2) had never been married, (3) had not have taken any medicine or nursing courses, and (4) was willing to participate in the study. Prior to data collection, meetings with administrators at the participating schools were arranged to present the study. Agreement from homeroom teachers was also obtained in order for the principal investigator to explain the study to students in first-year classes. Questionnaires were administered to participants in their classrooms and were completed at the time of distribution. The total numbers of eligible participant who attended classes on the designated days and times of recruitment completed the questionnaires was 598. Data were collected from September of 2016 to February of 2017.

### 2.2   Measures

Data of this study was collected using the self-administered questionnaires, including the general characteristics questionnaire, condom use self-efficacy scale, perceived condom use control scale, health locus of control scale, and expected result of condom use scale. Questionnaires used previous relevant published studies and survey instruments [28, 29] as references. Content validity was verified by six experts in nursing, public health, obstetrics (ob) and gynecology (gyn), and education. The questionnaire was pre-tested on six adolescent girls for clarity and ease of reading to evaluate face validity. Forty participants were invited to examine the test-retest reliability of the questionnaire after a two-week interval. The intraclass correlation coefficient for condom use self-efficacy scale, perceived condom use control scale, health locus of control scale, and expected result of condom use scale were 0.87, 0.75, 0.78, and 0.80, and Cronbach's alpha coefficients of internal consistency were 0.92, 0.82, 0.80, and 0.92, respectively.

# 3 Results

## 3.1 Participant Demographics

A total of 598 participants were surveyed. The mean age for the participants was 15.98 (SD = 0.88) years. The majority of the participants were sexually inexperienced (n = 573, 95.88%). Sixty-four percent of participants were aware of HPV (n = 383), and 96.92% of participants were unvaccinated against HPV-related disease (n = 580). About 30.25% (n = 181) reported previous obstetrics/gynecology visits for gynecologic problems. Participants who had sexually experienced 4.60 (SD = 0.87) and had a significantly higher self-efficacy score for condom use than those who had not 4.09 (SD = 0.70) (t = −2.565, p = .011) (Table 1).

**Table 1.** Demographic data of participants and ANOVA of their self-efficacy on condom use (N = 598)

| Variables | Condom use self-efficacy for HPV prevention | | | |
|---|---|---|---|---|
| | n [%] | Mean (SD) | F/t value | p |
| Sexual experience | | | | |
| No | 573 [95.88] | 4.09 (0.70) | −2.565 | .011 |
| Yes | 25 [4.12] | 4.60 (0.87) | | |
| Have you ever heard of the HPV | | | | |
| No | 215 [35.89] | 4.14 (0.79) | 0.732 | .464 |
| Yes | 383 [64.11] | 4.09 (0.67) | | |
| Have HPV vaccinated | | | | |
| No | 580 [96.92] | 4.11 (0.71) | 0.691 | .490 |
| Yes | 18 [3.08] | 3.95 (0.40) | | |
| Have you ever discussed sexual issues with adult family members | | | | |
| No | 280 [46.86] | 4.04 (0.66) | −1.866 | .063 |
| Yes | 318 [53.14] | 4.20 (0.74) | | |
| History of obstetrics/gynecology visits | | | | |
| No | 417 [69.75] | 4.08 (0.69) | −0.981 | .327 |
| Yes[a] | 181 [30.25] | 4.15 (0.75) | | |
| Religious beliefs | | | | |
| Buddhist/Taoist/I Kuan Tao | 386 [64.56] | 4.14 (0.70) | 1.311 | .271 |
| Christian/Catholic | 43 [7.15] | 3.95 (0.65) | | |
| None/Other | 1169 [28.29] | 4.07 (0.76) | | |
| Relationship with parents | | | | |
| Harmonious | 373 [62.35] | 4.08 (0.70) | 0.833 | .435 |
| Ordinary | 183 [30.60] | 4.16 (0.69) | | |
| Standoffish/Conflicting | 42 [7.05] | 4.03 (0.84) | | |

[a] Integrated dysmenorrhea, menstrual disorder, vaginal excretion, pruritus, and others.

## 3.2    Self-efficacy to Use Condom for HPV Prevention

The mean score of self-efficacy to use condom for HPV prevention was 4.11 (SD = 0.71) out of a total possible score of 6 (Table 2). The mean score for sexually inexperienced and sexually experienced had significantly difference in self-efficacy to use condom scale in several items, including "Carry on a condom, I may feel embarrassed (t = −2.107, p = .036)", "I will be worried about being rejected to use condoms by partner (t = −4.127, p < .001)", "I wouldn't feel confident to suggest using condoms because I would be afraid the partner with bad thinking (t = −1.962, p = .05)", "I will feel embarrassed if wearing a condom in the process cannot be completely (t = −3.051, p = .002)", "I feel confident that I could use a condom with a partner without "breaking the mood." (t = −2.539, p = .011)" and "It is difficult to ask partner to put on a condom (t = −2.565, p = .011)" (Table 2). Among sexually inexperienced participants, the higher mean score item was "Even I know the request of using condom might upset partner, I would still insist on my request"; the lower mean score items were "Carry on a condom, I may feel embarrassed", "I will feel embarrassed if wearing a condom in the process cannot be completely", "I wouldn't feel embarrassed to buy condoms". Among sexually experienced participants", the higher mean score item was "I will be worried about being rejected to use condoms by partner"; the lower mean score items were "I wouldn't feel embarrassed to buy condoms", "Carry on a condom, I may feel embarrassed", and "I feel confident that I could use a condom successfully" (Table 2).

## 3.3    Factors Associated with Self-efficacy to Use Condom for HPV Prevention

In Table 3, the results of the regression analysis were presented. Model 1 used the data of all participants to figure out which factors affect self-efficacy to use condoms for HPV prevention. The result pointed out that perceived condom use control, health locus of control, and expected result of condom were all significant and the R2 equals to 30.00%. It means that all the three factors were effective factors. Sexually experienced participants were analyzed in Model 2. Only the perceived condom use control was not significant. The R2 equals to 78.49%. Obviously, for participants who had sexual experiences using condom was a common sense and did not affect the self-efficacy to use condom for HPV prevention. It was not a critical factor for them. In Model 3, all the three factors were significant in the analysis for sexually inexperienced participants, too. The R2 only equals to 29.22%. That was to say, these three factors were all considered to the self-efficacy to use condoms for HPV prevention in this group.

Comparing the results of Model 2 and 3, the self-efficacy to use condom for HPV prevention was mostly affected by health locus of control, and expected result of condom for sexually experienced participants, however, the inexperienced participants considered more than the three factors used in this research only about one third reasons were found. It also can be observed that the biggest difference was the effect of health locus of control and this factor will be seen as the most important factor of self-efficacy to use condom for HPV prevention.

**Table 2.** Comparison of self-efficacy to use condom on sexually experienced (N = 598)

| Items | Mean (SD) | | $t$ | $p$ |
|---|---|---|---|---|
| | Sexually inexperienced ($n$ = 573) | Sexually experienced ($n$ = 25) | | |
| | 4.11 (0.71) | | | |
| | 4.09 (0.70) | 4.60 (0.87) | −2.565 | .011 |
| 1. I wouldn't feel embarrassed to buy condoms | 3.29 (1.40) | 3.69 (2.14) | −0.678 | .511 |
| 2. Carry on a condom, I may feel embarrassed® | 2.89 (1.34) | 3.69 (1.80) | −2.107 | .036 |
| 3. I will be worried about being rejected to use condoms by partner® | 3.62 (1.46) | 5.31 (1.18) | −4.127 | <.001 |
| 4. I wouldn't feel confident to suggest using condoms because I would be afraid the partner with bad thinking® | 4.34 (1.33) | 5.08 (1.44) | −1.962 | .050 |
| 5. I will feel embarrassed if wearing a condom in the process cannot be completely® | 3.01 (1.32) | 4.15 (1.72) | −3.051 | .002 |
| 6. I feel confident that I could use a condom successfully | 3.64 (1.26) | 3.92 (2.02) | −0.501 | .626 |
| 7. I feel confident in my ability to persuade a partner to accept using a condom when we have intercourse | 4.40 (1.15) | 4.85 (1.82) | −0.889 | .392 |
| 8. I feel confident I could gracefully dispose of a condom when we have intercourse | 4.41 (1.21) | 4.85 (1.52) | −1.266 | .206 |
| 9. I feel confident that I could use a condom with a partner without "breaking the mood" | 4.42 (1.13) | 5.23 (1.36) | −2.539 | .011 |
| 10. I feel confident that I would remember to use a condom even after I have been drinking | 4.28 (1.19) | 4.69 (1.25) | −1.235 | .218 |
| 11. I feel confident that I would remember to use condom even if I were high | 4.33 (1.18) | 4.46 (1.27) | −0.394 | .694 |
| 12. I feel confident I could use a condom during intercourse without reducing any sexual sensations | 4.39 (1.12) | 4.77 (1.42) | −1.196 | .232 |
| 13. It is difficult to ask partner to put on a condom® | 3.90 (1.31) | 4.85 (1.21) | −2.565 | .011 |
| 14. If partner cannot use the condom, I believe I will resolutely stop sex | 4.66 (1.15) | 4.46 (1.20) | 0.620 | .536 |
| 15. If party asked not to use condoms, I think I would obedience® | 4.62 (1.22) | 4.54 (1.39) | 0.223 | .824 |
| 16. To avoid embarrassment, I wouldn't feel confident to suggest using condoms® | 4.57 (1.25) | 5.23 (1.17) | −1.880 | .061 |
| 17. Even I know the request of using condom might upset partner, I would still insist on my request | 4.80 (1.00) | 4.46 (1.56) | 0.776 | .453 |

® These items were averaged questions.

**Table 3.** Multiple linear regression analyses of factors related to self-efficacy to use condom for HPV prevention

| Variables | B | SD | t | p | R² |
|---|---|---|---|---|---|
| Model 1 | | | | | |
| Constant | 16.932 | 4.12 | 4.111 | <.001 | 30.00% |
| Perceived condom use control | 1.139 | 0.17 | 6.896 | <.001 | |
| Health locus of control | 0.420 | 0.12 | 3.544 | <.001 | |
| Expected result of condom use | 1.021 | 0.18 | 5.799 | <.001 | |
| Model 2 | | | | | |
| Constant | −40.477 | 21.03 | −1.925 | .086 | 78.49% |
| Perceived condom use control | −0.472 | 1.15 | −0.410 | .692 | |
| Health locus of control | 2.608 | 0.74 | 3.548 | .006 | |
| Expected result of condom use | 2.420 | 0.94 | 2.583 | .030 | |
| Model 3 | | | | | |
| Constant | 18.438 | 4.14 | 4.450 | <.001 | 29.22% |
| Perceived condom use control | 1.119 | 0.17 | 6.768 | <.001 | |
| Health locus of control | 0.383 | 0.12 | 3.224 | .001 | |
| Expected result of condom use | 1.008 | 0.18 | 5.690 | <.001 | |

# 4  Discussion

The current study revealed that perceived behavioral control, health locus of control, and expected results were important factors that affected adolescent girls' condom use self-efficacy to prevent HPV acquisition. It also can be observed that the biggest difference is the effect of health locus of control and this factor will be seen as the most important factor of self-efficacy to use condom for HPV prevention. Compared with past studies, this study shows that most adolescent girls are aware of HPV [30, 31], and adolescent girls showed more knowledge regarding HPV. Another, the current result was consistent with the belief that having control over one's own health was associated with healthier behavior [32]. Condoms are the only device that both reduce the transmission of HIV and other STIs and prevent unintended pregnancy. The use of condoms to prevent STIs has been mostly focused on the prevention of HIV transmission [33–35]. Although condoms cannot completely protect against HPV acquisition, empirical results point indicate consistent and correct use of condoms also reduces the risk of acquiring other STIs and associated conditions, including genital warts and cervical cancer [36]. However, the issue of how condoms are used to prevent HPV infection has not been given much attention worldwide.

Both sexually inexperienced and sexually experienced participants had mean score of less than 4 for these items (out of a total possible score of 6): "I wouldn't feel embarrassed to buy condoms" "Carry on a condom, I may feel embarrassed" "I will feel embarrassed if wearing a condom in the process cannot be completely". Young girls not only need knowledge about condom use but also need the proper skills for condom use. The results on one previous study indicated that condom-related embarrassment extends beyond condom use to pre- and post-use situations. The embarrassment associated with purchasing condoms exceeds that of using condoms, and purchase-related condom embarrassment significantly and negatively impacts the frequency of condom use [37]. Another study among young men in Sweden found that the main barriers to safe sex were interference with spontaneity, pleasure reduction, embarrassment or distrust, and difficulties in communicating about safe sex [38, 39]. This showed that embarrassment and difficulties in communicating about safe sex were the main barriers to safe sex among young women and men.

The current result indicated that sexual experience is significantly higher for condom use self-efficacy than asexual experience (t = −2.565; p = .011). It justifies Bandura's argument; personal direct experience has a very important influence on self-efficacy [25, 40]. The current study showed perceived control, health locus of control, and the expected result of condom use were important predictors of condom use self-efficacy. However, the obviously variances between sexual experience or not, for those who have no sexual experience, to enhance the effectiveness of their use of condoms, there is still a need to actively explore the influence of condom use self-efficacy and other impact factors. Young girls should be encouraged to use condoms during their first sexual intercourse to protect themselves against STIs and to maintain their sexual health. Another previous study found that certain aspects of sexual communication mediated the effect of self-efficacy on condom use [35]. In the future, based on the findings of this study, we can design the basis for health education and actively involve adolescents.

# 5    Conclusions and Application

The current study showed that perceived of control, health locus of control, and the expected result of condom use were important predictors of condom use self-efficacy. The health locus of control was seen as the most important factor of self-efficacy to use condom for HPV prevention among adolescent girls. Therefore, it is necessary to strengthen the awareness of adolescent girls on self-health management. To prevent HPV acquisition, adolescent girls are willing to use condoms, but are not confident in using it correctly, and might feel embarrassed when unable to put it on correctly. To overcome these issues, healthcare workers should emphasize the practical use of condoms to ensure the sexual health of adolescent girls. Simulated films should be made in demonstrating how to put on and take off condoms correctly. A checklist could also be designed for evaluation of the practical simulation training. With these, we can strengthen adolescent girls' condom use self-efficacy and provide a reference to prevent the acquisition of sexual-related diseases.

# References

1. Walboomers, J.M., Jacobs, M.V., Manos, M.M., Bosch, F.X., Kummer, J.A., Shah, K.V., Snijders, P.J., Peto, J., Meijer, C.J., Munoz, N.: Human papillomavirus is a necessary cause of invasive cervical cancer worldwide. J. Pathol. 189(1), 12–19 (1999). https://doi.org/10. 1002/(SICI)1096-9896(199909)189:1<12::AID-PATH431>3.0.CO;2-F
2. World Health Organization (2016). http://www.who.int/mediacentre/factsheets/fs380/en/
3. Adams, M., Jasani, B., Fiander, A.: Human papilloma virus (HPV) prophylactic vaccination: challenges for public health and implications for screening. Vaccine 25(16), 3007–3013 (2007). https://doi.org/10.1016/j.vaccine.2007.01.016
4. Clifford, G., Franceschi, S., Diaz, M., Munoz, N., Villa, L.L.: Chapter 3: HPV type-distribution in women with and without cervical neoplastic diseases. Vaccine 24(Suppl 3: S3/26–34) (2006). https://doi.org/10.1016/j.vaccine.2006.05.026
5. Dunne, E.F., Datta, S.D., Markowitz, L.E.: A review of prophylactic human papillomavirus vaccines: recommendations and monitoring in the US. Cancer 113(10 Suppl), 2995–3003 (2008). https://doi.org/10.1002/cncr.23763
6. Centers for Disease Control Taiwan: Safe sex (2013). http://www.cdc.gov.tw/professional/info. aspx?treeid=beac9c103df952c4&nowtreeid=3a380faf26d530d6&tid=F9393FF1D6981B85
7. Graveland, B.: HPV vaccine tough sell in parts of Canada. The Toronto Star, 3 March 2009
8. Chow, S.N., Soon, R., Park, J.S., Pancharoen, C., Qiao, Y.L., Basu, P., Ngan, H.Y.: Knowledge, attitudes, and communication around human papillomavirus (HPV) vaccination amongst urban Asian mothers and physicians. Vaccine 28(22), 3809–3817 (2010). https:// doi.org/10.1016/j.vaccine.2010.03.027
9. Kang, H.S., Moneyham, L.: Attitudes toward and intention to receive the human papilloma virus (HPV) vaccination and intention to use condoms among female Korean college students. Vaccine 28(3), 811–816 (2010). https://doi.org/10.1016/j.vaccine.2009.10.052
10. Tu, Y.C., Wang, H.H., Lin, Y.J., Chan, T.F.: HPV knowledge and factors associated with intention to use condoms for reducing HPV infection risk among adolescent women in Taiwan. Women Health 55(2), 187–202 (2015). https://doi.org/10.1080/03630242.2014. 979970
11. Health Promotion Administration Ministry of Health and Welfare Taiwan (2016). http:// social.tainan.gov.tw/dvsa/page.asp?id={FF55CF8C-D053-46E5-9535-F1F20351836F}
12. Centers for Disease Control Taiwan (2016). http://www.cdc.gov.tw/professional/info.aspx? treeid=cf7f90dcbcd5718d&nowtreeid=f94e6af8daa9fc01&tid=2C4A7EB431FC2797
13. World Health Organization (2009). http://www.who.int/hiv/topics/condoms/en/
14. Nielson, C.M., Harris, R.B., Nyitray, A.G., Dunne, E.F., Stone, K.M., Giuliano, A.R.: Consistent condom use is associated with lower prevalence of human papillomavirus infection in men. J. Infect. Dis. 202(3), 445–451 (2010). https://doi.org/10.1086/653708
15. Winer, R.L., Hughes, J.P., Feng, Q., O'Reilly, S., Kiviat, N.B., Holmes, K.K., Koutsky, L. A.: Condom use and the risk of genital human papillomavirus infection in young women. N. Engl. J. Med. 354(25), 2645–2654 (2006). https://doi.org/10.1056/NEJMoa053284
16. Bleeker, M.C., Hogewoning, C.J., Voorhorst, F.J., van den Brule, A.J., Snijders, P.J., Starink, T.M., Berkhof, J., Meijer, C.J.: Condom use promotes regression of human papillomavirus-associated penile lesions in male sexual partners of women with cervical intraepithelial neoplasia. Int. J. Cancer 107(5), 804–810 (2003). https://doi.org/10.1002/ijc. 11473

17. Centers for Disease Control and Prevention: National and state vaccination coverage among adolescents aged 13–17 years–United States, 2012. MMWR Morb. Mortal. Wkly Rep. **62** (34), 685–693 (2013)

18. Repp, K.K., Nielson, C.M., Fu, R., Schafer, S., Lazcano-Ponce, E., Salmeron, J., Quiterio, M., Villa, L.L., Giuliano, A.R.: Male human papillomavirus prevalence and association with condom use in Brazil, Mexico, and the United States. J. Infect. Dis. **205**(8), 1287–1293 (2012). https://doi.org/10.1093/infdis/jis181

19. Lin, Y.C., Chu, Y.H.: An analysis of adolescent's condom-using through trans theoretical model. Stud. Sex. **1**(1), 67–85 (2010). (in Chinese)

20. Bandura, A.: Self-efficacy - toward a unifying theory of behavioral change. Psychol. Rev. **84** (2), 191–215 (1977). https://doi.org/10.1037//0033-295x.84.2.191

21. Marin, B.V., Gomez, C.A., Tschann, J.M.: Condom use among Hispanic men with secondary female sexual partners. Public Health Rep. **108**(6), 742–750 (1993)

22. McConnaughy, E.A., DiClemente, C.C., Prochaska, J.Q., Velicer, W.F.: Stages of change in psychotherapy: a follow-up report. Psychotherapy **26**, 494–503 (1989)

23. Chen, T.H., Yen, H.W.: The influence of the consistent condom use of college senior students. Formos. J. Sex. **10**(1), 53–70 (2004)

24. Waller, K.V., Bates, R.C.: Health locus of control and self-efficacy beliefs in a healthy elderly sample. Am. J. Health Promot. **6**(4), 302–309 (1992). https://doi.org/10.4278/0890-1171-6.4.302

25. St Lawrence, J.S.: African-American adolescents' knowledge, health-related attitudes, sexual behavior, and contraceptive decisions: implications for the prevention of adolescent HIV infection. J. Consult. Clin. Psychol. **61**(1), 104–112 (1993)

26. Mendolia, S., Walker, I.: The effect of noncognitive traits on health behaviours in adolescence. Health Econ. **23**(9), 1146–1158 (2014). https://doi.org/10.1002/hec.3043

27. Burnett, A., Sabato, T., Wagner, L., Smith, A.: The influence of attributional style on substance use and risky sexual behavior among college students. Coll Stud J **48**(2), 325–336 (2014)

28. Asante, K.O., Doku, P.N.: Cultural adaptation of the condom use self efficacy scale (CUSES) in Ghana. BMC Public Health **10**, 227 (2010). https://doi.org/10.1186/1471-2458-10-227

29. Wallston, K.A.: The validity of the multidimensional health locus of control scales. J. Health Psychol. **10**(5), 623–631 (2005). https://doi.org/10.1177/1359105305055304

30. Hsu, Y.Y., Cheng, Y.M., Hsu, K.F., Fetzer, S.J., Chou, C.Y.: Knowledge and beliefs about cervical cancer and human papillomavirus among Taiwanese undergraduate women. Oncol. Nurs. Forum **38**(4), E297–E304 (2011). https://doi.org/10.1188/11.ONF.E297-E304

31. Lin, Y.J., Fan, L.W., Tu, Y.C.: Perceived risk of human papillomavirus infection and cervical cancer among adolescent women in Taiwan. Asian Nurs. Res. **10**(1), 45–50 (2016). https://doi.org/10.1016/j.anr.2016.01.001

32. Helmer, S.M., Kramer, A., Mikolajczyk, R.T.: Health-related locus of control and health behaviour among university students in North Rhine Westphalia, Germany. BMC Res. Notes **5**, 703 (2012). https://doi.org/10.1186/1756-0500-5-703

33. Smith, D.K., Herbst, J.H., Zhang, X., Rose, C.E.: Condom effectiveness for HIV prevention by consistency of use among men who have sex with men in the United States. J. Acquir. Immune Defic. Syndr. **68**(3), 337–344 (2015). https://doi.org/10.1097/QAI.0000000000000461

34. World Health Organization (2015). http://www.who.int/hiv/mediacentre/news/condoms-joint-positionpaper/en/

35. Xiao, Z., Li, X., Lin, D., Jiang, S., Liu, Y., Li, S.: Sexual communication, safer sex self-efficacy, and condom use among young Chinese migrants in Beijing, China. AIDS Educ. Prev. **25**(6), 480–494 (2013). https://doi.org/10.1521/aeap.2013.25.6.480

36. Centers for Disease Control and Prevention: Condom fact sheet in brief (2013). https://www.cdc.gov/condomeffectiveness/docs/condomfactsheetinbrief.pdf

37. Moore, S.G., Dahl, D.W., Gorn, G.J., Weinberg, C.B., Park, J., Jiang, Y.: Condom embarrassment: coping and consequences for condom use in three countries. AIDS Care **20** (5), 553–559 (2008). https://doi.org/10.1080/09540120701867214

38. Ekstrand, M., Tyden, T., Larsson, M.: Exposing oneself and one's partner to sexual risk-taking as perceived by young Swedish men who requested a Chlamydia test. Eur. J. Contracept. Reprod. Health Care **16**(2), 100–107 (2011). https://doi.org/10.3109/13625187.2010.549253

39. Tung, W.C., Cook, D.M., Lu, M.: Sexual behaviors, decisional balance, and self-efficacy among a sample of Chinese college students in the United States. J. Am. Coll. Health **60**(5), 367–373 (2012). https://doi.org/10.1080/07448481.2012.663839

40. Bandura, A.: Self-efficacy the Exercise of Control. W.H. Freeman and Company, New York (1997)

# Human Factors for Aging: Innovation for Enhanced Quality of Life

# Requirements for Assisting Senior Cyclists - An Integrative Approach

Annika Johnsen[✉] and Walter Funk

Institute for Empirical Sociology, Marienstraße 2, 90402 Nuremberg, Germany
{Annika.Johnsen,Walter.H.Funk}@ifes.uni-erlangen.de

**Abstract.** Due to their sensory, cognitive and motor preconditions, senior cyclists represent a group of road users who are particularly at risk in road traffic. Knowing that senior cyclists were rarely in the focus of technical developments so far, the present paper explores the potential for assistance systems taking into account their preconditions and needs. The described research is part of a requirements analysis, based on desk research, a review of accident data and qualitative assessments. The results can contribute to a better understanding of situational factors and age-related declines with a possible impact on the safety of senior cyclists. Furthermore, they can be used as a basis for technical developments that aim at improving the safety of senior cyclists.

**Keywords:** Vulnerable road users · Senior cyclists
Cycling assistance systems · Age-related declines

## 1   Introduction

Between the years 1980 and 2015, the accident risk of German cyclists older than 65 years had risen by more than 60% [1]. In Germany, senior cyclists also represented more than half of all cycling fatalities (57.8%) in 2016 [2]. On the one hand, this can be explained by their physical frailty, which makes them prone to a high risk of injuries in the case of an accident [3, 4]. On the other hand, (uncompensated) sensory impairments were found to be positively linked to the occurrence of senior bicycle accidents in the past [5]. Despite their overrepresentation in fatalities and their age-related declines of physical and sensory nature, senior cyclists are yet rarely at the focus of technical developments bearing the potential to improve their safety. Only recently, a project commissioned by the Dutch Ministry of Infrastructure and Environment has addressed this issue, focusing on the development of an advisory system [6]. The present paper reports the results of research on the preconditions and requirements of senior cyclists. The research is embedded within the project Safety4Bikes - a project funded by the German Federal Ministry of Education and Research with the objective of improving the safety of cycling children and senior cyclists. The described results refer to findings on senior cyclists and are based on desk research, a review of German accident data and qualitative assessments.

N. J. Lightner (Ed.): AHFE 2018, AISC 779, pp. 297–307, 2019.
https://doi.org/10.1007/978-3-319-94373-2_33

# 2   Methods

## 2.1   Review of Literature

It was emphasized that riding a bike is a combination of perceptual-motor and cognitive tasks of which the mastering not least depends on developmental aspects and practice [7]. The described literature review aimed at describing age-related preconditions of senior cyclists from a developmental perspective and discussing them in the light of their possible meaning for cycling skills. Thereby, recent findings on (1) vision, (2) hearing, (3) attention, and (4) specific motor skills, i.e. reaction time, physical strength, mobility and balance, were included, assuming that impairments of these abilities have an impact on the safety of senior cyclists.

## 2.2   Review of Accident Data

The review of accident data was conducted on the basis of GIDAS-data (German In-Depth Accident Study) [8] including accidents of senior cyclists aged 60 years and older during the timeframe 2012–2017. The analysis comprised 568 accidents which were analyzed by frequency and crosstabs procedures using the software SPSS (version 24). Accordingly, the six most frequent accident situations were ranked and examined in more detail to identify situational factors with the strongest hazard potential. In the analysis of collisions, situations caused by the cyclists were distinguished from situations caused by other road users. The consideration of single accidents served the purpose of getting a further insight into dangerous situations that could possibly represent an overstrain to senior cyclists.

## 2.3   Focus Group Sessions and Expert Interviews

The aim of the focus group sessions and expert interviews was to explore the view of senior cyclists and road safety trainers regarding age-related problems during cycling, perceptions on dangers in traffic and the potential of assistance systems improving the safety of senior cyclists. Each of the focus groups (n = 2) consisted of five participants who cycled regularly and were at least 60 years old. The sessions lasted 70 and 115 min and took place at the Institute for Empirical Sociology in Nuremberg and at the facilities of the German Cyclist's Association (ADFC) in Munich. The expert interviews (n = 2) aimed at obtaining further insight into the stated aspects from a more objective view. In this context, two referents[1] of a training program for senior cyclists (initiated by the German Insurers Accident Research) participated in a telephone interview, which lasted 70/105 min. The statements of the focus group sessions and interviews were recorded and transcribed using the clean read method [9]. For analysis of data qualitative content analysis according to Mayring (2010) was used, following the procedure of deductive category formation [10]. The transcripts were processed in

---

[1] Members of the German Road Patrol (Deutsche Verkehrswacht, abbr. DVW).

MAXQDA (version 12.2.1.), a software tool for the analysis of text material enabling the user to manage multiple transcriptions within a project and assign text segments to a category. The assignment of the statements to categories allows counting how often the individual categories appear in the text material.

# 3 Results

## 3.1 Preconditions of Senior Cyclists with a Possible Impact on Safety

Aging is associated with a decrease in several areas of sensory, cognitive and motor functioning. The following sections describe age-related declines of which an impact on safe cycling is assumed.

### 3.1.1 Vision

Declines in the sensory perception manifest themselves in an impaired vision and hearing ability. Age-related, visual declines have an impact on visual acuity, contrast sensitivity, peripheral vision, accommodation, scotopic vision and the adaptation to changing light conditions [11]. Visual acuity, the ability to perceive contours and patterns in detail and with high contrast, can refer to stationary elements (static acuity) or moving objects (dynamic acuity). By the age of 65–74, 4.7% of persons show static visual acuity of 20/60 or worse. This figure rises to 12.7% for persons aged 75 or older [12]. Even stronger decreases were reported for dynamic acuity [11]. Visual acuity is important in situations where the distance and speed of other road users must be estimated. Examples of this are overtaking maneuvers, turning maneuvers, as well as driving into roads where right-of way rules are applicable [13]. A further characteristic of the vision in old age is an increased need for light, which is caused by a clouding of the eye lens [14]. Accordingly, low luminance is associated with losses in visual performance. The reason for this is that the ability of the eye to adjust to light-deprived conditions (dark adaptation) becomes worse with increasing age. The declines are manifested in a reduced sensitivity of the perception threshold [11] and a slower adaptation process compared to young adults [15]. The contrast sensitivity, which is involved with the recognition of shapes and gradations, also decreases with advancing age [16]. First losses occur between age 40 and 50 [17]. It was stated that a 60-year-old needs about three times the object contrast to achieve the same visual performance as a 20-year-old [18]. Accommodation, the ability of the eye to focus clearly on close objects, already starts to decline in early adolescence. Whilst at the age of 20 the human eye can focus clearly on objects as near as at 10 cm (3.94 in.), the average near point distance of 60-year olds increases to 100 cm (39.4 in.) [19]. Furthermore, the timespan required by the accommodation-process is extended. A comparison of accommodation times of 40 year olds (0.5–0.8 s) to 60 year olds (2.0 and 2.7 s) suggested increases between 1.2 and 2.2 s [20]. The extension of accommodation time is critical as during this time span seniors cannot rely on their vision safely.

### 3.1.2    Hearing

Besides vision, the auditory perception is also affected by ageing. Age-related hearing losses (presbyacusis) occur gradually, between the 5th and 6th decade of life [21]. The symptomatology includes ear noises (tinnitus), impairments in spatial hearing, a diminished perception of high-pitched sounds and deficits in the filtering of auditory stimuli [22, 23]. Declines in hearing might affect the safety of senior cyclists in terms of being unable to spatially allocate approaching vehicles or difficulties in hearing safety-relevant traffic noises, such as the ringing of a high-pitched bicycle bell. The negative effects of hearing loss can be reduced by using a hearing aid. The early fitting of the hearing aid plays a particularly important role, especially in the prevention of declines in speech processing [24]. However, only few of those affected by hearing loss are actually equipped with hearing aids. In a study with seniors who were at least 60 years of age, only 51 out of 210 (24%) hearing-impaired participants were equipped with a hearing aid [25]. The relatively low supply with hearing aids may be due to the fact that people are often unaware of their increasing hearing loss. A finding suggesting this comes from Holube and Gablenz (2013) [26]. In their study among a sample from Northern Germany one-third of the seniors, who had previously been diagnosed as hearing-impaired, rated themselves as normal hearing.

### 3.1.3    Attention

Attention declines can have a negative impact on the ability to detect dangers in good time - another skill that is crucial for safe cycling. The impact of ageing is mostly investigated in the context of selective and divided attention. Declines in selective attention were suggested for visual search tasks, in which older adults took longer than younger adults for responding to targets. Further findings suggested an increased difficulty in suppressing irrelevant (auditory) stimuli during a selective hearing task [27]. Furthermore, the parallel processing of two or more sources of information, referred to as divided attention, is impaired. This was suggested by a comparative study using a simulated driving task. The dual-task consisted of lane tracking and responding to a self-paced visual task (dot counting) manually or by speech. Age-related effects became apparent in the quality of lane tracking and the accuracy of visual analysis. Interestingly, those effects were less pronounced in the vocal condition than in the manual one. The authors interpreted this finding as an age-related difficulty in integrating responses [28].

### 3.1.4    Specific Motor Skills

Besides attention, the physical strength and the reaction speed can also have a critical impact on safety during situations in which the cyclist is required to react quickly or even perform emergency braking. The muscular strength already starts to decrease at the age of 30. After 50 years of age, the losses are accelerated amounting to approximately 12–15% per decade [29]. For reaction time, it was suggested that the brake reaction/movement time increases by approximately 2% for each successive five-year age range, beginning at age 15 and ending with the group aged 75 years and older [30]. The keeping of balance, as well as physical mobility represent further important prerequisites for safe cycling. Both have an impact on safety-relevant behaviours such as the hand signal and shoulder checking (e.g. in turning situations). In the context of balance, it was stated that the rates of falls and their associated complications rise steadily with age [31]. During studies investigating the impact of platform disturbances, older adults not only took longer than their younger peers to correct the destabilization of their posture, but also became unstable during small perturbations from which younger adults could easily recover [32]. With regard to cycling, these decreases are particularly dangerous in situations in which abrupt changes of bicycle's posture (caused by strong steering or braking) require a quick shifting of balance to avoid falls. The decreases in physical mobility occur already as early as age 25 and amount to 5% per decade [33, 34]. Particularly concerned are the head, neck and trunk areas, as well as joints that are hardly used in the everyday life (e.g. hip and shoulder joints) [34]. The mobility of the head and neck areas is important for safety when cycling, as the cyclist must be able to check the rear of the bicycle in situations where other road users approach from behind (e.g. overtaking or turning situations).

## 3.2    Review of Accident Data

Of the 568 reviewed accidents involving senior cyclists, 426 were collisions and 142 were single-bicycle accidents. Over 90% of the accidents (including collisions and single bicycle accidents) occurred during daytime. Less than 10% took place at night (5%) or at dawn (4%). The severity of injury was rated according to the Abbreviated Injury Scale (AIS). It was shown that only in 3.9% of the cases the seniors were not injured. The other accidents resulted in injuries classified as minor (67.5%), moderate (20.8%) or even worse (1.2%).

In the collisions, car drivers (314 out of 426) caused the majority. The senior cyclists were only responsible for a quarter of them (107 out of 426). In Table 1, the most frequent car-to-cyclist crashes involving senior cyclists can be viewed. Those crashes were documented as a three-digit code number in the reviewed data set. The first digit represents one out of seven categories that can be assigned to the accident, whilst the other two key figures indicate detailed characteristics. As can be seen, especially crossing scenarios at intersections seem to play a dominant role (accident types 342, 341, 301 and 321). Accident type 342 (83 accidents) is the most common type of accident among senior citizens, who, despite the motorist's main fault, are partly to blame for using the cycle path incorrectly. In accident type 341 (39 accidents) the cycle path is used in the direction of travel, again with the car driver denying the right of way to the cyclist. In the accident types 301 (21 accidents) and 321 (19 accidents) the cyclist violates the right of way of the car when entering the intersection from the road. Accident types 211 and 243 occur at intersections and involve cars performing turning maneuvers. In type 211, the car is turning left whilst the cyclist approaches from across the road. In accident type 243, a turning vehicle collides with a crossing cyclist who enters the street from a pedestrian track. In accident type 581 ("dooring") the cyclist collides with the opening door of a car parked on the right side of the road. The fault in this type of accident is exclusively at the car driver.

Of the registered single-bicycle accidents, many occurred in the context of abrupt changes in the horizontal/vertical orientation of the bicycle. Those accidents referred to switching between road and pavement/cycling track (20 accidents), strong braking (20 accidents), sudden swerving to avoid collisions with other road users or animals (8 accidents) and unfavorable road conditions, including slippery roads (9 accidents) or gradients (5 accidents). Further accidents were linked to the consumption of alcohol

(11 accidents), medical/physical conditions (9 accidents) or a loss of balance (10 accidents). Also, startling at the sudden perception of animals, persons or vehicles (10 accidents) was among the accident causes.

**Table 1.** Most frequent car-to-cyclist crashes involving senior cyclists (>60 years) in GIDAS (2012–2017) (Graphics adapted from [35])

| Situation | Description | Main cause |
|---|---|---|
| 342 | Cyclist enters the intersection from a cycle path opposite the direction of travel whilst vehicle approaches from left | Car driver (98%) ignored traffic signs regulating right of way (70%) |
| 341 | Cyclist enters the intersection from a cycle path in the direction of travel, whilst the vehicle approaches from right | Car driver (100%) ignored traffic signs regulating right of way (74%), |
| 301 | Cyclist and car approach each other on an intersection without cycle path | Cyclist (71%) ignored traffic signs regulating right of way (57%) |
| 321 | Cyclist and car approach each other on an intersection without cycle path | Cyclist (68%) ignored priority of vehicles approaching from right (47%) |
| 211 | Cyclist approaches intersection from across the road whilst the car is turning left | Car driver (83%) committed error while turning left (72%) |
| 243 | Cyclist enters the street from a pedestrian track and, whilst the vehicle is turning left | Car driver (88%) committed error while turning right (71%) |
| 581 | Cyclist collides with an opening door of a car parked on the right side of the road | Car driver (100%) causes dooring accident (94%) |

## 3.3    Focus Group Sessions and Expert Interviews

The first topic of the qualitative assessments addressed declining skills of the older target group with an impact on safe cycling. As can be seen in Table 1, the most frequently mentioned decline was the keeping of balance. It was pointed out by one of the road safety trainers that in order to check the rear area of the bicycle, seniors sometimes turn their entire trunk to compensate for limited mobility in the neck area. This would lead to involuntary steering movements, resulting in losses of balance. In this context, one of the focus group participants even suggested complete waiver of shoulder checking in order to avoid losses of balance. Besides the keeping of balance sensory losses were also discussed, especially with regard to vision. Some of the cyclists reported declines in physical endurance, indicating that these were particularly pronounced during cycling on routes with gradients or after the winter break.

In the context of dangerous situations, the danger of being overlooked by the car driver was often brought up. Statements on this topic referred to cycling next to trucks or SUVs (blind spots) as well as vehicles performing turning maneuvers and overseeing the approaching cyclist. A road safety trainer explained that, as part of the "Fit for the Bicycle" program, he often advised the participants to establish eye contact with the driver and to wait until the latter responds before crossing a road (where the driver might turn right). A further topic brought up by the cyclists was overtaking by other road users, which was often associated with unpleasant feelings like fear or discomfort. A road safety trainer criticized that vehicles often keep to little distance when overtaking.

In the context of unsafe routes bicycle paths, with high proximity to other road users were often brought up. Participants describe cycle paths that are marked on the road, narrow cycle paths, cycle paths with two directions of travel, sealed walking and cycle paths, as well as cycle paths leading into the road. Furthermore, unsafe routes were described with regard to soil conditions, including uneven floors, with stones, roots and/or bumps. In this context, also slippery roads (especially in winter) were mentioned. On the question of how to support older cyclists with technical systems, several ideas were generated. Both the older cyclists as well as the road safety instructors, expressed a desire for a self-standing bicycle, i.e. a bicycle that does not fall and also remains stable during strong braking. When it comes to distance regulation, some of the focus group participants expressed desire for an overtaking warning function referring to overtaking by other cyclists, who would not announce the over-taking maneuver in advance. Further ideas referred to a blind spot detection that issues warnings to the cyclists about his/her blind spot risk (Table 2).

**Table 2.** Frequency of the categories derived from the focus groups and interviews

| Topics | Statements | Focus groups | Expert interviews |
|---|---|---|---|
| Declining skills | Balance | 13 | 12 |
| | Vision | 19 | 1 |
| | Physical endurance | 14 | 1 |
| | Mobility | 9 | 5 |
| | Shoulder checking | 3 | 7 |
| | Reaction speed | 4 | 5 |
| | Hearing | 2 | 6 |
| | Getting on- off the bike | 3 | 4 |
| | Concentration | 3 | 3 |
| Dangerous situations | Blind spots | 10 | 3 |
| | Turning vehicles | 7 | 2 |
| | Overtaking | 5 | 1 |
| | Car parked on the cycle path | 8 | 0 |
| | Strong braking | 1 | 2 |
| Unsafe routes | Cycle tracks with high proximity to other road users | 16 | 13 |
| | Unfavorable road conditions | 9 | 10 |
| | Highly frequented tracks | 4 | 1 |
| | Intersections | 0 | 5 |
| | Road | 3 | 0 |
| Technical improvements | Stable bicycle | 8 | 7 |
| | Rear view extension | 8 | 7 |
| | Distance warning function | 7 | 5 |
| | Blind spot detection | 5 | 4 |
| | Direction indicator | 6 | 0 |

# 4 Discussion

In the previous section, backgrounds on dangers posed to older cyclists were presented. It became clear, that the development of appropriate safety systems must not only take into account situational factors but also consider the impacts of age-related declines. The majority of the reviewed accident situations occurred in the context of crossing at intersections and were caused by motorists. This suggests that there is an increased need to raise the awareness of motorists on the vulnerability of older cyclists and to inform them about their presence in the respective situations. In this context, the development of adapted Car2X communication could have a beneficial impact on the safety of senior cyclists.

Furthermore, systems that specifically address age-related declines could help the cyclists to become aware of potential dangers posed by other road users before it is too late. As could be seen, older cyclists are particularly vulnerable at intersections when motorists approach them from the side or from behind. It is unclear to what extent age-related declines are involved here. On the one hand, it can be assumed that already the perception of collision opponents is affected by declines in the peripheral vision, shoulder gazing and spatial hearing. On the other hand, the cyclists might have remarked the other road user, but simply were not able to react in time, as a result of decreased reaction speed. Systems that address age-related declines must compensate for such difficulties. In the focus group, an interest in such functions was clearly stated. The distance warning function or the rear view extension are examples for desired functions, helping senior cyclists to detect other road users more easily.

However not only the detection of other road users seems to be critical to the safety of senior cyclists, but also the maintenance of postural stability during changes of the bicycle's orientation. This became clear in the context of single-bicycle accidents relating to unexpected changes in posture or position, which were induced by sudden swerving, strong braking, switching between road and pavement/cycling track or uneven roads. The analysis of the qualitative assessments showed that the senior cyclists are aware of their balance declines. As a result, the keeping of balance was often stated as a declining skill, affecting the safety of senior cyclists. In this context, strong braking or cycling on uneven floors or slippery roads were apprehended as critical, whilst a desire for a stable bicycle or a sort of stabilization function was frequently expressed.

Another approach to improving the safety of senior cyclist could be the reduction or avoidance of such situations by providing alternative routes considering the needs of senior cyclists in terms of soil conditions, space, traffic density, and their particular vulnerability at intersections.

# 5   Conclusion

The presented research aimed at describing the hazards faced by senior cyclists on the basis of declining abilities, as well as accident-specific characteristics. The results can be taken into account as a first starting point in the development of systems or functions that aim at improving the safety of older cyclists. However, it must be emphasized at this point that the presented approach is purely explorative and cannot provide reliable statements on concrete influences and causes of the accident situations described. Furthermore, it remains questionable to what extent the results can be transferred to other countries or populations. This is partly because the accident data review is based on German data and partly because the members of the German Cycling Federation (ADFC) who participated in the focus groups may not represent the average senior cyclist. As a consequence, further experimental research is necessary in order to clarify the role of age-related declines in accidents involving senior cyclists.

# References

1. Johnsen, A., Funk, W.: Safety4Bikes: Arbeitspaket 1: Nutzerstudien. Analyse der Ziel- und Anspruchsgruppen. Technical report, Institute for empirical Sociology (2017)
2. Statistisches Bundesamt: Verkehrsunfälle: Unfälle von Senioren im Straßenverkehr 2016. Technical report, German Federal Statistical Office (2017)
3. Von Below, A.: Verkehrssicherheit von Radfahrern: Analyse sicherheitsrelevanter Motive, Einstellungen und Verhaltensweisen. A report of the German Federal Highway Research Institute, vol. M 264. BASt (2016)
4. Spolander, K.: Better cycles: an analysis of the needs and requirements of older cyclists. A Vinnova report, Vinnova (2007)
5. Hagemeister, C., Tegen-Klebingat, A.: Cycling habits and accident risk of older cyclists in Germany. In: Proceedings of the International Cycling Safety Conference, pp. 20–21. Helmond (2012)
6. De Hair, S., Engbers, C., Dubbeldam, R., Zeegers, T.: Safe & aware on the bicycle: an advisory system for elderly cyclists for improving safety and comfort. In: Ageing and Safe Mobility. BASt, Bergisch Gladbach (2014)
7. Wierda, M., Brookhuis, K.A.: Analysis of cycling skill: a cognitive approach. Appl. Cogn. Psychol. **5**(2), 113–122 (1991)
8. Brüning, E., Otte, D., Pastor, C.: 30 Jahre wissenschaftliche Erhebungen am Unfallort für mehr Verkehrssicherheit. Zeitschrift für Verkehrssicherheit **51**(4), 175–181 (2005)
9. Mayring, P.: Qualitative content analysis: theoretical foundation, basic procedures and software solution. In: Monograph, SSOAR (2014)
10. Mayring, P.: Qualitative Inhaltsanalyse. In: Mey, G., Muck, K. (eds.) Handbuch qualitative Forschung in der Psychologie. Verlag für Sozialwissenschaften, Wiesbaden (2010)
11. Hilz, R., Cavonius, C.R.: Psychophysik des Sehens im Alter. In: Tesch-Römer, C., Wahl, H.W. (eds.) Seh-und Höreinbußen älterer Menschen. Dietrich Steinkopff Verlag, Darmstadt (1996)
12. Reuben, D.B., Stillman, R.A., Traines, M.: The aging driver. Am. Geriatr. Soc. **36**, 1135–1142 (1988)
13. Lachenmayr, B.: Anforderungen an das Sehvermögen des Kraftfahrers. Deutsches Ärzteblatt **100**(10), A624–A634 (2003)
14. Cohen, A.S.: Wahrnehmung als Grundlage der Verkehrsorientierung bei nachlassender Sensorik während der Alterung. In: Schlag, B. (ed.) Leistungsfähigkeit und Mobilität im Alter. TÜV Media, Köln (2008)
15. Bockelmann, W.D.: Auge-Brille-Auto. Springer, Heidelberg (1987)
16. Wahl, H.W., Heyl, V.: Sensorik und Sensumotorik. In: Brandstädter, J., Lindenberger, U. (eds.) Entwicklungspsychologie der Lebensspanne: ein Lehrbuch. Kohlhammer, Stuttgart (2007)
17. Owsley, C., Sekuler, R., Siemsen, D.: Contrast sensitivity throughout adulthood. Vis. Res. **23**(7), 689–699 (1983)
18. Berke, A.: Visuelle Wahrnehmung im Straßenverkehr in den verschiedenen Lebensaltern (2017). https://sbao.ch/dbFile/817/9a96/1.%20Dr.%20Andreas%20Berke_Visuelle%20Wahrnemung_19.03.2017.pdf1.pdf
19. Rensing, L., Rippe, V.: Altern. Springer, Heidelberg (2014)
20. Ernst, R.: Mobilitätsverhalten und Verkehrsteilnahme älterer Menschen. Auswirkungen auf Kompetenz und Lebensgestaltung. Peter Lang Europäischer Verlag der Wissenschaften, Frankfurt (1999)

21. Zahnert, T.: Differenzialdiagnose der Schwerhörigkeit. Deutsches Ärzteblatt **108**(25), 433–444 (2011)
22. Gebhardt, C.: Hören mit Hirn: Wirksamkeit eines Trainings der auditiven Differenzierungsfähigkeit bei Schwerhörigen im Alter von 55 bis 70 Jahren. Doctoral thesis, Albert Ludwig University of Freiburg (2006)
23. Schaade, G.: Wahrnehmung. In: Schaade, G., Wojnar, J. (eds.) Ergotherapeutische Behandlungsansätze bei Demenz und dem Korsakow-Syndrom. Springer, Heidelberg (2016)
24. Misoch, S.: Hören im Alter: Eine Übersicht im Auftrag von Pro Senectute Schweiz (2016). https://www.prosenectute.ch/dam/jcr:818b4e16-14fb-4242-bc27-629274ec81c0/Hören-imAlter_Bericht_FHS-St.Gallen_IKOA.pdf
25. Hesse, G.: Hörgeräte im Alter. HNO **52**(4), 321–328 (2004)
26. Holube, I., Gablenz, P.: Wie schlecht hört Deutschland im Alter? Conference Paper, 16. Jahrestagung der Deutschen Gesellschaft für Audiologie in Oldenburg (2013)
27. McDowd, J.M., Filion, D.L.: Aging, selective attention, and inhibitory processes: a psychophysiological approach. Psychol. Aging **7**(1), 65 (1992)
28. Brouwer, W.H., Waterink, W., Van Wolffelaar, P.C., Rothengatter, T.: Divided attention in experienced young and older drivers: lane tracking and visual analysis in a dynamic driving simulator. Hum. Factors **33**(5), 573–582 (1991)
29. Rinkenauer, G.: Motorische Leistungsfähigkeit im Alter. In: Schlag, B. (ed.) Leistungsfähigkeit und Mobilität im Alter. TÜV Media GmbH, Köln (2008)
30. Shaheen, S.A., Niemeier, D.A.: Integrating vehicle design and human factors: minimizing elderly driving constraints. Transp. Res. Part C Emerg. Technol. **9**(3), 155–174 (2001)
31. Bridenbaugh, S.A., Kressig, R.W., Gschwind, Y.J.: Sturz im Alter. In: Pinter, G., Likar, R., Schippinger, W., Janig, H., Kada, O., Cernic, K. (eds.) Geriatrische Notfallversorgung: Strategien und Konzepte. Springer, Wien (2013)
32. Ketcham, C.J., Stelmach, G.E.: Movement control in the older adult. In: Pew, R.W., Hemel, S.B. (eds.) Technology for Adaptive Aging. National Academies Press, Washington DC (2004)
33. Tittlbach, S.: Entwicklung der körperlichen Leistungsfähigkeit. Eine prospektive Längsschnittstudie mit Personen im mittleren und späteren Erwachsenenalter. Hofmann Verlag, Schorndorf (2002)
34. Illig, C.: Körperliche Aktivität im Alter: Einfluss auf die psychische Gesundheit, die kognitiven Funktionen und die körperliche Leistungsfähigkeit. Doctoral thesis, Leipzig University (2012)
35. Poschadel, S.: Prototypische Kinderunfälle im innerstädtischen Straßenverkehr: Von Unfallanalysen über Präventionsmöglichkeiten zur Entwicklung eines Unfallmodells. Faculty of Psychology, Ruhr-University Bochum (2006)

# Aging and Functional Changes in Polymorphonuclear Leukocytes

Jawahar(Jay) Kalra[1,2(✉)], Avani Saxena[1], Nasim Rostampour[1],
and Erik Vantomme[1]

[1] Department of Pathology and Laboratory Medicine, College of Medicine,
University of Saskatchewan, Saskatoon, Canada
jay.kalra@usask.ca
[2] Royal University Hospital, Saskatoon Health Region,
103 Hospital Drive, Saksatoon, SK S7N 0W8, Canada

**Abstract.** Polymorphonuclear (PMN) leukocytes are one of the most important defenses against bacterial infections. The reports of age related functional changes in PMN leukocyte have been conflicting in the literature. We measured the luminol-dependent chemiluminescence (LDCL) activity for reactive oxygen species (ROSs) and superoxide anion ($O_2$-) production in vitro, to study the age related functional changes in PMN leukocyte. Luminol-dependent chemiluminescence activity for ROSs and superoxide anion generation by PMN leukocyte from different age groups did not change significantly. There were no significant differences in total white blood cells and PMN counts in subjects of various ages. These results suggest that there were no significant functional alterations in PMN leukocyte with aging with respect to ROSs and superoxide anion production.

**Keywords:** Polymorphonuclear (PMN) leukocytes
Reactive oxygen species (ROSs) · Aging · Functional changes

## 1 Introduction

Immunosenescence refers to the gradual declining in immune system brought by natural age advancement [1]. This usually happens with a state of low-grade chronic inflammation known as 'inflammaging' [2]. Inflammaging is marked by an increase in the levels of inflammatory cytokines, including tumor necrosis factor alpha (TNF-α), interleukin (IL)-1β and IL-6 [3, 4]. Moreover, during healthy aging, anti-inflammatory factors, mediate the pro-inflammatory condition [5–7]. Other studies suggested that epigenetic processes which are regulating the aging of immune system also cause the immunosenescence and inflammaging [8–10]. Interestingly, dysregulation in epigenetic responses might have an impact on age-related diseases such as atherosclerosis, Alzheimer's, osteoporosis, diabetes, and cancer [11, 12]. Moreover, it may be suggested that during aging failing in innate immunity leads to problems in adaptive immunity.

Polymorphonuclear (PMN) leukocytes are phagocytic granulocyte immune cells, which are the first responder of the innate immune system and are coordinators of the adaptive immune response [13]. PMN leukocytes are one of the innate defense

© Springer International Publishing AG, part of Springer Nature 2019
N. J. Lightner (Ed.): AHFE 2018, AISC 779, pp. 308–318, 2019.
https://doi.org/10.1007/978-3-319-94373-2_34

mechanisms and combat infections by phagocytosing and destroying the microorganisms. PMN leukocytes kill the microorganisms (bacteria, fungi and some enveloped viruses) by producing and releasing many chemicals including reactive oxygen species (ROSs), proteases, and phospholipases.

Several studies have investigated the connection between PMN leukocyte functional changes and aging. In an earlier report, slightly increased ability of PMN leukocytes for host defense was reported in elderly hospitalized subjects [14]. However, other investigators have demonstrated no relationship between PMN leukocytes' functions and aging in non-hospitalized subjects [15, 16]. Further Epps et al. (1978) reported depressed activity of PMN leukocytes in very young and very old human subjects using chemiluminescence (CL) method [17]. Charpentier et al. [18] demonstrated a dramatic decrease in the phagocytic activities of leukocytes of healthy elderly humans over the age of 70 years [18]. In hospitalized geriatric patients and healthy elderly people over 70 years, PMN leukocytes have shown decreased chemotactic response, increased adherence, decreased nitroblue-tetrazolium (NBT) dye reduction capability and diminished Candida-killing activity [19, 20]. However, contrary to the former report [20] later adopting prescribed protocol, Corberand et al. [21] demonstrated that PMN leukocytes are intrinsically normal in aged subjects. Nagel et al. [22] in healthy individuals of various ages, using the quantitative NBT dye reduction test and production of superoxide in response to stimulation with latex particles, suggested a heterogeneity in any age-associated defect in PMN function. However, later Nagel et al. [23] observed lower phagocytic activity of PMN leukocyte in healthy elders and debilitated elders of the domiciliary facility. In addition, phagocytosis was not impaired with age when opsonized yeast cell was incorporated into normal PMN leukocyte [24]. In other investigation PMN leukocytes' chemotaxis, phagocytosis and NBT reduction capacity was significantly depressed by aging process [25]. Also, reduced phagocytosis with aging have been suggested to be associated with psychological stress or life events [26]. Fulop et al. [27] suggested oxidative metabolism producing free radicals and antibody-dependent cellular cytotoxicity (ADCC) diminished in PMN leukocyte of aged healthy subjects of both sexes. Furthermore, it has been reported that basic level of luminol-dependent chemiluminescence (LDCL) was increased and this enhancement of LDCL was more significant by PMN leukocytes of aged males than of females, while no comparison was made with young/middle-aged subject [28]. Moreover, it has been demonstrated that phagocytic activity of opsonized particle by PMN leukocyte was impaired with aging in healthy subjects [29]. However, during a study of oxygen metabolite generation, CL response of PMN leukocytes after stimulation with opsonized Zymosan was similar to controls in healthy elderly subjects [30]. Herrero et al. [31] revealed that PMN leukocytes' reactive oxygen species production decreased during aging. In addition, this study showed PMN leukocytes phagocytosis activity reduced in response to formyl-methionyl leucyl- phenylalanine (FMLP) stimulation in elderly subjects. During aging the production of ROS in basal level increased in elderly individuals compared to young subjects [32]. Fulop et al. [33] demonstrated increased susceptibility of PMN leukocytes to death by apoptosis with increasing age. Moreover, impaired function of PMN leukocytes in aging was associated with increased apoptosis [34]. Some of other studies reflecting age-related functional changes in PMN leukocytes are summarized in Table 1.

**Table 1.** Functional changes in polymorphonuclear leukocytes with aging

| PMNs function | Year | Study | Changes with aging |
|---|---|---|---|
| Apoptosis | 2007 | Fortin et al. [35] | Decreased |
|  | 1997 | Fulop et al. [33] | Increased |
| Migration and chemotaxis | 2016 | Nikolich-Zugich and Davies [36] | Unchanged |
|  | 2000 | Wenisch et al. [37] | Decreased chemotaxis |
|  | 2014 | Chen et al. [38] | Inaccurate migration |
| Phagocytosis and intracellular killing | 2010 | Christy et al. [39] | Decrease in phagocytic activity |
|  | 1981 | Charpentier et al. [18] | |
|  | 1984 | Fulop et al. [24] | Unchanged phagocytosis |
|  | 2005 | Gocer et al. [40] | Decreased killing |
|  | 1982 | Nagel et al. [22] | Unchanged bactericidal activity |
| Products | 2015 | Baehl et al. [41] | Decreased cytokine/chemokines |
|  | 2015 | Baehl et al. [41] | Increased cytokine/chemokines |
|  | 2016 | Nogueira-Neto et al. [42] | Increased production of ROS |
|  | 1982 | Nagel et al. [22] | Diminished superoxide generation |
|  | 1985 | Fulop et al. [27] | The antibody-dependent cellular cytotoxicity (ADCC) decrease |
|  | 1989 | Fulop et al. [43] | Decrease in inositol phosphate formation |
|  | 2014 | Sapey et al. [44] | Increased elastase |

In view of conflicting reports in the literature on the function of PMN leukocyte, we investigated whether there were any alterations in the function of PMN leukocyte with aging, by studying the production of reactive oxygen species (ROSs) and superoxide anion ($O_2$-) *in vitro*. In this regard we studied the activation of PMN leukocytes in blood and measured LDCL from the normal subjects of various ages. PMN leukocyte yields a CL following phagocytosis that can be correlated with metabolic activation of hexose monophosphate shunt and is also oxygen dependent [45]. Phagocytosis by PMN leukocyte elicits a burst of oxidative metabolism that is intimately associated with the bactericidal activity of the cell [46]. Cyclic hydrazides, such as luminol (5-amino 2, 3-dihydro-1, 4 phthalazinedionel produce CL when reacted with a variety of oxidizing agents. In this reaction luminol oxidized to the electronically aminophthalate ion, that relaxes to ground state by photon emission [47]. LDCL provides a sensitive indicator of the rate of production of reactive oxygen species (ROSs) by resting and stimulated phagocytes *in vitro* [48]. Therefore, reactive oxygen species (ROSs) production of activated PMN leukocyte can be measured by LDCL.

# 2 Materials and Methods

## 2.1 Subjects

The study included 55 normal healthy human subjects (26 males and 29 females, age range 3–89, mean age 45, 5 years). These subjects were grouped into decades for comparison purposes. All subjects in the study were healthy volunteers recruited from hospital employees or their friends and acquaintances. Informed consent was obtained from all subjects. These subjects were not suffering from any disease and were not on any medications including oral contraceptives.

## 2.2 Preparation of Opsonized Zymosan

Opsonized Zymosan was prepared for chemiluminescence by the method of Prasad et al. [49] and Kalra et al. [50]. In short, Zymosan (Sigma Chemical Company) was opsonized by addition of Zymosan suspension in Hank's balanced salt solution (HBSS) containing human serum. The mixture was incubated, centrifuged and the pellet was suspended in HBSS to make the final concentration of Zymosan 10 mg/ml.

## 2.3 White Blood Cells (WBC) and PMN Leukocyte Counts

Peripheral venous blood collected in ethylene diaminetetra acetic acid (EDTA) containing tubes. Total white cell and PMN leukocyte counts were performed with the use of a Technicon H 6000 and by microscopic differential from smears with Wright's Giemsa stain.

## 2.4 Chemiluminescence Studies

The method of chemiluminescence (CL) measurement was essentially similar to that of Prasad et al. (1989) [49] and Kalra et al. [50]. In short, for luminol dependent CL, 0.05 ml (approximately $2.0 \times 10^5$ PMN leukocyte) of blood was added to a counting vial that contained Hank's balanced salt solution (HBSS) at pH 7.4 and luminol at a final concentration of $10^4$ mol/l. Samples were placed in a Luminometer (LKB-1251) for 5–10 min and phagocytosis was initiated by opsonized Zymosan. Chemiluminescence was monitored for 60 min in the presence and absence of superoxide dismutase (SOD). The counts were made for 5 s for every 5 min for a period of 60 min.

## 2.5 Quantitation of Superoxide Anion Production

Superoxide anion ($O_2$-) production was measured, which was quantitated by the reduction of ferricytochrome-C using a spectrometer at a wavelength of 550 nm. Results are expressed as nmoles of $O_2$- produced per 30 min per $10^6$ PMN leukocytes.

## 2.6    Data Analysis

The results are expressed as Mean ± SD. Statistical analysis of the results was performed with the use of repeated measures analysis of variance (BMDP Statistical Software, University of California, Berkely). Student test was done for comparisons at $p < 0.05$.

# 3    Results

### 3.1    Chemiluminescence (CL) Activity of PMN Leukocytes

Luminol-dependent chemiluminescence (CL) for each sample was determined (a) without activation by Zymosan (resting), (b) with activation by Zymosan in the absence of superoxide dismutase, and (c) with activation by Zymosan in the presence of superoxide dismutase. The area under each curve was integrated to give the total CL response during the period of monitoring. The difference in areas under Zymosan-activated and resting curves is designated as reactive oxygen species CL, while the difference between the area under Zymosan-activated and Zymosan-activated in the presence of SOD is designated as SOD-inhibitable reactive oxygen species CL. The integrated area under the curve is in mV × min (mV. min). The absolute values are expressed as mV min per $10^6$ PMN leucocytes.

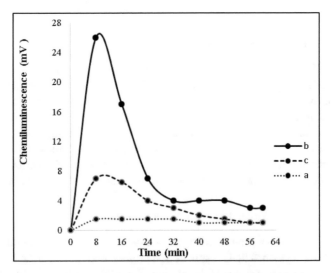

**Fig. 1.** Typical tracing of Zymosan activated chemiluminescence of PMN leukocytes in the presence and absence of superoxide dismutase (SOD). (....a....), Resting chemiluminescence (without Zymosan activations); (—b—), Zymosan activated chemiluminescence in the absence of SOD; (---c---), Zymosan activated chemiluminescence in the presence of SOD. Area under b – area under a = reactive oxygen species CL; Area under b – area under c = SOD inhibitable reactive oxygen species CL.

A typical time response of CL activity from PMN leukocytes of subjects of various ages is shown in Fig. 1. The peak CL activity of PMN leukocytes from the blood in the absence of SOD occurred between 4 and 15 min after the addition of Zymosan and thereafter a gradual decline was seen (b). However, in the presence SOD there is an inhibition of CL because SOD destroys the superoxide anion (c). These results suggest that most of the CL activity was related to the production of ROS.

Total chemiluminescence activity results are expressed as the percent stimulation of Zymosan activated chemiluminescence of PMN leukocytes which is representative of ROSs production (Fig. 2). There were no significant differences in the total CL activity from PMN leukocyte in subjects of various ages grouped as decades.

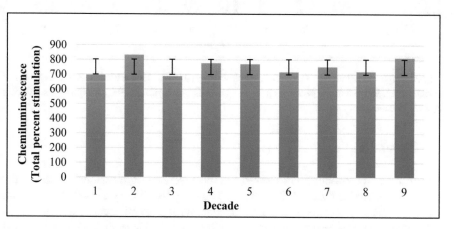

**Fig. 2.** Total percent of stimulated chemiluminescence activity of PMN leukocytes. Results are expressed as Mean ± SD. Each bar represents the average of at least six subjects in each decade group.

### 3.2  Rates of Superoxide Anion Production by PMN Leukocytes

There were no significant differences in the rate of production of superoxide anion by PMN leukocytes of subjects of various ages grouped as decades (Fig. 3).

### 3.3  White Blood Cell and PMN Leukocyte Counts

The mean total absolute count of circulating WBC and PMN leukocyte in decade 2 were 7.30 ± 0.80, 4.24 ± 0.75 giga-cells/l and in decade 3 were 6.59 ± 0.51, 3.77 ± 0.41 giga-cells/l respectively. There were no statistically significant differences in total WBC and PMN leukocyte counts in the blood of healthy subjects of various ages grouped as decades.

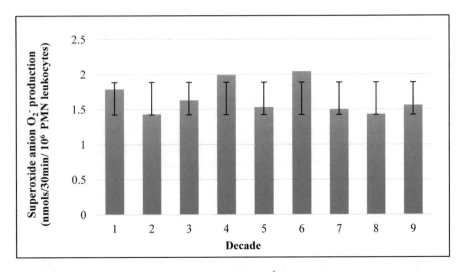

**Fig. 3.** Superoxide anion production in nmol/30 min/$10^6$ PMN leukocytes in healthy subjects of various ages. Results are expressed Mean ± SD. Each bar represents the average of six subjects in each decade group.

## 4  Discussion

The results of the present study showed that there were no significant differences in the chemiluminescent activity of Zymosan-activated PMN leucocytes with aging. With regards to rates of superoxide anion production, no significant changes were observed with aging in normal healthy subjects. In addition, no significant differences in the total WBC and PMN leucocyte counts were observed with aging. In this study opsonized Zymosan was used to activate PMN leucocytes that has been used by other investigators [49, 51]. Whole blood was used to investigate the PMN leucocyte chemiluminescence in this study. No attempt was made to isolate PMN leucocytes. However, the chemiluminescence of blood was expressed in terms of the PMN leucocyte count. Whole blood has been used by us and various investigators in the past for chemiluminescent studies [49, 52]. Polymorphonuclear leucocyte stimulation is accompanied by increased oxygen consumption [53] leading to the production of various reactive oxygen species. PMN leucocytes play a major role in the inflammatory state, where PMN leucocytes invade the area and phagocytose the foreign agents and debris [54]. Activation of PMN leucocytes initiates a respiratory burst with a sudden and large increase in ROSs which can be released into external tissue environment [55]. In the present investigation opsonized Zymosan activated the PMN leucocytes and this activity was measured as ROS production through the LDCL. Luminol-dependent chemiluminescence provides a sensitive indicator of the rate of production of reactive oxygen species by resting and stimulated PMN leucocytes *in vitro*.

It is clear that there are conflicting reports in the literature regarding the changes in the function of PMN leukocytes with aging. We have accumulated the results of many reports into two broad categories: (A), where no changes were reported in the function of PMN leukocyte with aging that included bactericidal activity, oxidative metabolism, and phagocytosis, up regulation of beta-2- adrenergic receptors [15, 16, 22, 24]. This group of reports support our results and are consistent with our findings where no changes were observed in ROSs production measured as LDCL. (B), where there were changes reported in the function of PMN leukocytes with aging that included decrease or increase in phagocytic activity, diminished superoxide generation, free radicals and ADCC, increased LDCL (more in males), but without comparison to other ages, diminished respiratory burst and decline in other functions [17, 18, 22, 25, 27, 43]. This discrepancy may be due to a variety of reasons (differences in tissue sites, sample collections, lack of quality control, ethnicity, sex, race and possible socioeconomic status) which might have affected the outcomes of different investigations. Nagel et al. have reported lowered phagocytic ability of PMN leukocytes in "healthy elders". However, many of these subject might had geriatric diseases such as arteriosclerosis or osteoarthritis with no symptoms or some may have had subclinical pathologies [23]. In addition, there may be some variations due to the methods employed to assess PMN leukocyte function, as luminol-dependent chemiluminescence measurement is sensitive to several interferences [56]. It is worth to mention that different studies measured different aspects of PMN leukocytes function and may not be comparable. Hence it should be emphasized that a common methodology be adopted with good lab practices and consideration to other factors. In conclusion, in the present investigation there was no significant functional changes in PMN leukocytes with aging at least in the reactive oxygen species and superoxide anion production activity as measured by luminol-dependent chemiluminescence.

# References

1. Pawelec, G., Solana, R.: Immunosenescence. Immunol. Today **18**, 514–516 (1997)
2. Franceschi, C., Bonafe, M., Valensin, S., et al.: Inflamm-aging: an evolutionary perspective onimmunosenescence. Ann. N. Y. Acad. Sci. **908**, 244–254 (2000)
3. Castelo-Branco, C., Soveral, I.: The immune system and aging: a review. Gynecol. Endocrinol. **30**, 16–22 (2014)
4. Franceschi, C., Capri, M., Monti, D., et al.: Inflammaging and anti-inflammaging: a systemic perspective on aging and longevity emerged from studies in humans. Mech. Ageing Dev. **128**, 92–105 (2007)
5. Carrieri, G., Marzi, E., Olivieri, F., et al.: The G/C915 polymorphism of transforming growth factor beta1 is associated with human longevity: a study in Italian centenarians. Aging Cell **3**(6), 443–448 (2004)
6. Lio, D., Candore, G., Crivello, A., et al.: Opposite effects of interleukin 10 common gene polymorphisms in cardiovascular diseases and in successful ageing: genetic background of male centenarians is protective against coronary heart disease. J. Med. Genet. **41**, 790–794 (2004)
7. Morrisette-Thomas, V., Cohen, A.A., Fulop, T., et al.: Inflamm-aging does not simply reflect increases in pro-inflammatory markers. Mech. Ageing Dev. **139**, 49–57 (2014)
8. Dorshkind, K., Montecino-Rodriguez, E., Signer, R.A.: The ageing immune system: is it ever too old to become young again? Nat. Rev. Immunol. **9**, 57–62 (2009)

9. Sidler, C., Woycicki, R., Ilnytskyy, Y., et al.: Immunosenescence is associated with altered gene expression and epigenetic regulation in primary and secondary immune organs. Front. Genet. **4**, 211 (2013)

10. Szarc vel Szic, K., Declerck, K., Vidakovic, M., et al.: From inflammaging to healthy aging by dietary lifestyle choices: is epigenetics the key to personalized nutrition? Clin. Epigenet. **7**, 33 (2015)

11. Fulop, T., Kotb, R., Fortin, C.F., et al.: Potentialrole of immunosenescence in cancer development. Ann. N. Y. Acad. Sci. **1197**, 158–165 (2010)

12. Licastro, F., Candore, G., Lio, D., et al.: Innate immunity and inflammation in ageing: a key forunderstanding age-related diseases. Immun. Ageing **2**, 8 (2005)

13. Agrawal, A., Khan, M.J., Graugnard, D.E., et al.: Prepartal energy intake alters blood polymorphonuclear leukocyte transcriptome during the peripartal period in holstein cows. Bioinform Biol. Insights **11** (2017). https://doi.org/10.1177/1177932217704667

14. Phair, J.P., Kauffman, C.A., Bjornson, A.: Investigations of host defense mechanisms in the aged as determinants of nosocomial colonization and pneumonia. J Reticuloendothel Soc. **23**, 397–405 (1978)

15. Palmblad, J., Haak, A.: Ageing does not change blood granulocyte bactericidal capacity and levels of complement factors 3 and 4. Gerontology **24**(5), 381–385 (1978)

16. Phair, J.P., Kauffman, C.A., Bjornson, A.: Host defenses in the aged: evaluation of components of the inflammatory and immune responses. J. Infect. Dis. **138**, 67–73 (1978)

17. Epps, D.E., Goodwin, J.S., Murphy, S.: Age-dependent variations in polymorphonuclear leukocyte chemiluminescence. Infec. Immunol. **22**, 57–61 (1978)

18. Charpentier, B., Fournier, C., Fries, D.L., et al.: Immunological studies in human ageing. I. In vitro functions of T cells and polymorphs. J. Clin. Lab. Immunol. **5**, 87–93 (1981)

19. Laharragne, P.F., Corberand, J.X., Fillola, G., et al.: Impairment of polymorphonuclear functions in hospitalized geriatric patients. Gerontology **29**, 325–331 (1983)

20. Corberand, J.X., Nguyen, F., Laharragne, P.F., et al.: Polymorphonuclear functions and ageing in humans. J. Am. Geriatr. Soc. **29**, 391–397 (1981)

21. Corberand, J.X., Laharragne, P.F., Fillola, G.: Neutrophils of healthy aged humans are normal. Mech. Ageing Dev. **36**, 57–63 (1986)

22. Nagel, J.E., Pyle, R.S., Chrest, F.J., Adler, W.H.: Oxidative metabolism and bactericidal capacity of polymorphonuclear leukocytes from normal young and aged adults. J Gerontol. **37**, 529–534 (1982)

23. Nagel, J.E., Han, K., Coon, P.J., et al.: Age differences in phagocytosis by polymorphonuclear leukocytes measured by flow cytometry. J. Leuko. Biol. **39**, 399–407 (1986)

24. Fulop, T., Foris, G., Leovey, A.: Age-related changes in CAMP and CGMP levels during phagocytosis in human polymorphonuclear leukocytes. Mech. Ageing Dev. **27**, 233–237 (1984)

25. Antonaci, S., Jirillo, E., Ventura, M.T.: Non-specific immunity in ageing: deficiency of monocyte and polymorphonuclear cell mediated functions. Mech. Ageing Dev. **24**, 367–751 (1984)

26. Tsukamoto, K., Machida, K.: Effects of life events and stress on neutrophil functions in elderly men. Immun. Ageing **9**(1), 13 (2012). https://doi.org/10.1186/1742-4933-9-13

27. Fulop Jr., T., Foris, G., Worum, I., et al.: Age-dependent alterations of Fc gamma receptor-mediated effector function of human polymorphonuclear leukocytes. Clin. Exp. Immunol. **61**, 425–432 (1985)

28. Fulop Jr., T., Foris, G., Worum, I., et al.: Age elated variations of some polymorphonuclear leukocyte functions. Mech. Ageing Dev. **29**(1), 1–8 (1985)

29. Emannelli, G., Lamzio, M., Anfossi, T., et al.: Influence of age on polymorphonuclear leukocytes in vitro: phagocytic activity in healthy human subjects. Gerontology **32**, 308–316 (1986)

30. Kuriowa, A., Miyamoto, O.N., Shibuya, T.: Re-evaluation of the phagocytic respiratory burst in the physiological or inflammatory state and in ageing. J. Clin. Lab. Immunol. **29**, 189–191 (1989)

31. Herrero, C., Marques, L., Lloberas, J., et al.: IFN-gamma-dependent transcription of MHC class II IA is impaired in macrophages from aged mice. J. Clin. Invest. **107**, 485–493 (2001)

32. Tortorella, C., Piazzolla, G., Spaccavento, F., et al.: Regulatory role of extracellular matrix proteins in neutrophil respiratory burst during aging. Mech. Ageing Dev. **119**, 69–82 (2000)

33. Fulop Jr., T., Fouquet, C., Allaire, P., et al.: Changes in apoptosis of human polymorphonuclear granulocytes with aging. Mech. Ageing Dev. **96**(1–3), 15–34 (1997)

34. Whyte, M.K., Meagher, L.C., MacDermot, J., et al.: Impairment of function in aging neutrophils is associated with apoptosis. J. Immunol. **150**(11), 5124–5134 (1993)

35. Fortin, C.F., Larbi, A., Dupuis, G., et al.: GM-CSF activates the Jak/STAT pathway to rescue polymorphonuclear neutrophils from spontaneous apoptosis in young but not elderly individuals. Biogerontology **8**, 173–187 (2007)

36. Nikolich-Zugich, J., Davies, J.S.: Homeostatic migration and distribution ofinnate immune cells in primary and secondary lymphoid organs with aging. Clin. Exp. Immunol. **187**(3), 237–244 (2016)

37. Wenisch, C., Patruta, S., Daxbock, F., et al.: Effect of age on human neutrophil function. J. Leukoc. Biol. **67**, 40–45 (2000)

38. Chen, M.M., Palmer, J.L., Plackett, T.P., et al.: Age-related differences in the neutrophil response to pulmonary pseudomonas infection. Exp. Gerontol. **54**, 42–46 (2014)

39. Christy, R.M., Baskurt, O.K., Gass, G.C., et al.: Erythrocyte aggregation and neutrophil function in an aging population. Gerontology **56**(2), 175–180 (2010). https://doi.org/10.1159/000242461

40. Gocer, P., Gurer, U.S., Erten, N., et al.: Comparison of polymorphonuclear leukocyte functions in elderly patients and healthy young volunteers. Med. Princ. Pract. Int. J. Kuwait Univ. Health Sci. Centre **14**, 382–385 (2005)

41. Baehl, S., Garneau, H., Le Page, A., et al.: Altered neutrophil functions in elderly patients during a 6-month follow-up period after a hipf racture. Exp. Gerontol. **65**, 58–68 (2015)

42. Nogueira-Neto, J., Cardoso, A.S., Monteiro, H.P., et al.: Basal neutrophil function in human aging: implications in endothelial cell adhesion. Cell Biol. Int. **40**, 796–802 (2016)

43. Fulop Jr., T., Varga, Z., Csongor, J., et al.: Age related impairment in phosphatidylinositol breakdown of polymorphonuclear granulocytes. FEBS-Lett. **245**, 249–252 (1989)

44. Sapey, E., Greenwood, H., Walton, G., et al.: Phosphoinositide 3-kinase inhibition restores neutrophil accuracy in the elderly: toward targeted treatments for immunosenescence. Blood **123**, 239–248 (2014)

45. Allen, R.C., Yevich, S.J., Orth, R.A., et al.: The superoxide anion and singlet molecular oxygen: their role in the microbial activity of polymorphonuclear leukocyte. Biochem. Biophys. Res. Commun. **60**, 909–917 (1974)

46. Babior, B.M.: Oxygen dependent microbial lolling by phagocytes. N. Engl. J. Med. **298**, 659–688, 721–725 (1972)

47. Roswell, O.F., White, E.H.: The chemiluminescence of luminol and related hydrazides. In: Deluca, M. (ed.) Methods of Enzymology, pp. 409–423. Academic Press, New York (1978)

48. Allen, R.C., Loose, L.O.: Phagocytic activation of a luminol dependent chemiluminescence in rabbit alveolar and peritoneal macrophages. Biochem. Biophys. Res. Commun. **69**, 245–252 (1976)

49. Prasad, K., Kalra, J., Bharadwaj, B.: Increased chemiluminescence of polymorphonuclear leucocytes in dogs with volume overload heart failure. Br. J. Exp. Path. **70**, 463–468 (1989)
50. Kalra, J., Chaudhary, A.K., Prasad, K.: Increased production of oxygen free radicals in cigarette smokers. Int. J. Exp. Int. J. Exp. Path. **72**, 1–7 (1991)
51. Holt, M.E., Ryall, M.E.T., Campbell, A.K.: Albumin inhibits human polymorphonuclear leucocyte luminol-dependent chemiluminescence: evidence for oxygen free radical scavenging. Br. J. Exp. Path. **65**, 231–241 (1984)
52. Selvaraj, R.J., Sbarra, A.J., Thomas, G.B., et al.: A microtechnique for studying chemiluminescence response of phagocytes using whole blood and its application to the evaluation of phagocytes in pregnancy. J. Reticuloendothel. Soc. **3**, 3–16 (1982)
53. Dewald, B., Baggiolini, M., Curnutte, J.T., et al.: Subcellular localization of the superoxide forming system in human neutrophils. J. Clin. Invest. **63**, 2I–29 (1979)
54. Weissman, G.: Leukocytes as secretory organs of inflammation. Hosp. Pract. **13**, 53–62 (1978)
55. Babior, B.M.: The respiratory burst of phagocytes. J. Clin. Invest. **73**, 561–599 (1986)
56. Vilim, V., Wilhelm, J.: What do we measure by a luminol-dependent chemiluminescence of phagocytes? Free Radic. Biol. Med. **6**(6), 623–629 (1989)

# Human Factors in Aging Consumers

Gianni Montagna[1](✉), Laura Piccinini[1], Sílvia Pereira[2],
and Cristina Carvalho[1]

[1] Lisbon School of Architecture, CIAUD,
Rua Sá Nogueira, Alto da Ajuda, 1349-063 Lisbon, Portugal
g.montagna@gmail.com, laurapiccinini@uol.com.br,
cristifig@gmail.com
[2] Lisbon School of Architecture,
Rua Sá Nogueira, Alto da Ajuda, 1349-063 Lisbon, Portugal
aivlisilvia@gmail.com

**Abstract.** Human factors are a big issue when we talk about the general population and even more if talking about specific groups of users, as in the case of senior. These kinds of users are a group in great expansion with numerous associated specific needs that compete for the development of their well-being and maintenance of a high standard of comfort and health. Identifying the biggest changes seniors find in their bodies over time, how they view these changes, how they adapt to it, is a frequent issue for this type of users, who in many cases do not yet have clothing and equipment specifically adapted to their daily tasks and needs. A bibliographic review and analysis of some case studies will be conducted in order to obtain a more complete picture of the reality that surrounds this group of users and their needs in the choice of clothing.

**Keywords:** Human factors · Elder users · Aging consumers · Inclusive design

## 1 Introduction

Human factors are fundamental elements of the product design discipline because they help in identifying and characterizing the structural elements that make up the human needs of the user and help in approximation and study of problem solving between product and who uses it.

Senior users are a rapidly expanding group that is expected to grow further in the coming years. The projections of the United Nations, in its World Population Aging 2017 report [1], states that by 2050, more than 35% of the population in Europe and 28% in Northern America, will be 60 years of age or older. The advancement of research in the area of science and technology in relation to the aging of the population has created new paradigms of studies on the physical and psychological health of the elderly. The longevity of human existence rests on scientific development and technological advances, which greatly extend the average age of the population's life. According to the United Nations (UN), in 2006, the citizen is considered elderly in developed countries, from the age of 65 years. In developing countries this age has already declined to 60 years. This difference is directly related to the quality of life in each of the two groups of countries.

Senior users and the elderly population have specific needs for the use of design products that are associated with their physical and psychological state, but which may not be considered to be aged, but only different in terms of well-being and maintenance of a high standard of comfort and health.

The human factors involved into the different life plans of these users are very different, complex and hierarchical so that together they can form the net of integrated needs that can respond in a concrete, dynamic and effective way. This connection of different needs that come from very different areas, such as social, material, psychological, physical, etc., should, as a whole, be able to respond effectively to the different levels of need of users that over time they see their body transform and change.

If there is any case there is a stigma for the creation of products aimed at this age group and economic, the inclusion of the needs of this type of users in the production of design products, whether objects or clothing or any other type of experience, will undoubtedly be a great value for users and for this fast growing area.

Adapting to new realities is a frequent issue for this type of users, who in many cases do not yet have clothing and equipment specifically adapted to their daily tasks and needs.

The identification, analysis and organization of the main aspects that can contribute to an improvement of the day-to-day of this group of users, together with the possibility of obtaining data that allow the development of new products adapted for this group, is one of the objectives of this study that intends to be the starting point for different studies about this group of users/consumers.

## 2   Human Factors Observations

Human factors are defined [2] as "the scientific discipline concerned with understanding interactions among humans and other elements of a system". In this context, and taking into account that the human body is the interface that manages all the relations between the individual and the system, there are multiple elements that, depending on different variables, human, environmental, psychological, etc., that may influence the management ecosystem in a different way. Human Factors [3] is the scientific discipline concerned with the understanding of interactions among humans and other elements of the system to optimize human well-being, and overall system performance. In this sense [2], ergonomists contribute to the design and evaluation of tasks, jobs, environments and systems in order to make them compatible with the needs, abilities and limitations of people.

Designers and users observe, experience and perceive the different factors and variables of design differently and can value different decision-making: if on the one hand the designer is concerned with the aesthetics and functionality of the product, the end user, for on the other hand, it is concerned with its identification with the product, the use of the product in specific environments, its personal aesthetics, etc., and may or may not develop an affective relationship with the object.

Montagna [4], cited other authors, refers that human factors could be resumed into three main groups: the first one refers to the individual, the second one refers to the organization, and a third one is the fringe between the first and the second (Fig. 1).

**Human/ Individual:**
- Physiology
- Psychology
- Age/ Experience/ Motivation
- Ergonomics factors

**Interaction/ Interface:**
- Procedures
- Physical Environment (Light, noise, temperature, etc.,)
- Quality and contents of work
- Equipments

**Management/ Organization:**
- Cultural environment
- Services
- Interfaces design
- Communications

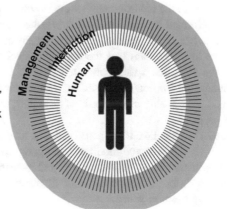

**Fig. 1.** Domains of human factors. From the author, adapted from [5–9], are shown the three levels in which the majority of the human factors are organized

The three areas in which human factors that interfere in the use and experience of objects with the user by [4] can be classified, organized and described as follows:

- The Human level is the first area specially dedicated to the user, and involves areas of human anatomy, anthropometry, biomechanics and physiology, factors related with race, age, background but also motivation, experience and psychological issues. From an inclusive point of view, we consider this level as the fundamental part of any analysis of the project as well as in relation to the object of study and the environment in which it operates. For fashion field, we consider its values and its involvement in fashion, both depending on their personal variables and lifestyles preferences [10].
- The Interaction level is intended to take into account the synergy of the user/individual with the environment/actuating space. In this area the human actuates as an interface with the work/background, taking into account the work procedures, the physical environment, but also equipment, software, medical devices, information technology, quality of work, safety, etc. This area of intervention identifies mental processes such as perceptual processes, memory, reasoning, etc., but also processes such as decision making, human-machine interaction and human-environment.
- The Management level is the third area of intervention of human factors concerning the area of organization, more usually called management or systems. This area is concerned with the relationship of the individual/user with the social or professional organization. The main issues are related with the cultural environment, units cooperation, Communications, local procedures, work life quality, and also interfaces design, leadership, resources, responsibilities, morale, psychological pressure, work systems and design, teamwork, participatory design, cooperative work, virtual organizations teleworking, retail services, post purchase services, etc.

The classification of human factors should be understood as a flexible and adaptable adaptation to users' needs, allowing users not only to be permeable and their interaction with the environment but also to consider how this interaction develops and can be interpreted by the user. In fact [4], the interaction level is to be intended as the medium between the human and the organization, and the mediator between the subjective level (human) and the objective level (organization). The interaction area, that is the interface space between the tangible and the intangible levels aims to reformulate the information from the designer and from the user, and respond positively and with quality of the needs of each part, users and designers, inside the fashion design project.

Human factors have to be perceived as a mix of personal and public meanings that changes with the time and modifies itself geographically. Each human factor involved into the project making, should be read and interpreted in the light of different realities, adapting to different factors in order to respond to a common ground code understandable by users in general.

# 3  The Senior User

The aging process [11] is inherent to the human being and the degree and that its effects will vary according to genetic factors, quality of life and social environment. In reality, age categories and all meanings attached to them are creations of society and imposed on the individual to determine their social position [12]. It is socially expected that the elderly person is a fragile and helpless person, who constantly cares for his health and who is very limited by his/her disadvantaged physical condition. If individuals who socially fall into the category of old age are not depressed or have any physical limitations, [12], they are considered an exception to the rule, since they do not follow the pattern of social behavior expected for this group.

The aging process is responsible for substantial changes in the physiology and psychology of the human being, limiting it often in performing basic tasks that it has always developed without any kind of support.

"Functional disability can be modulated by cognitive, psychological status, age, gender, number of chronic-degenerative diseases, educational level, social support, lifestyle and environmental factors [13]. Functional incapacity, or disability, is a dynamic and progressive process, a consequence of chronic degenerative diseases and physiological changes associated with aging, which can occur acutely, such as in cerebrovascular accident and femoral fracture, which cause functional limitations".

With aging, the basal metabolic rate decreases, loss of adipose tissue occurs in the layer of hypodermis and the sparse and exhausted microvasculature interfere with the effective regulation of heat loss, that is, the body decreases its own temperature regulation capacity, making the elderly feel colder than young people, making it difficult to exchange heat [14].

For example, visual acuity, hearing, touch, temperature and humidity are factors that directly affect human performance but there are other factors also considered such sports or diet [15]. According to this thinking, the way each individual dresses or also understands the clothing, affects each other in an individualized and differentiated way.

Throughout the 20th century, popular knowledge, demography and the social sciences contributed to establishing gerontology as a scientific discipline and configuring it as a multidisciplinary area of knowledge. Sociology and psychology have also collaborated in their formation, by directing the specialized view to the psychosocial aspects of old age."

But not all seniors have health problems or special features that require design objects or tailored attire to meet their personal and interaction needs with the environment and with others. If on the one hand this particular group of consumers needs design objects and clothing with some adaptations that relate to the normal transformation of body shape throughout life and increasing levels of physical and psychological comfort, on the other hand also need clothing that does not classify them as an insignificant and insignificant market range but requires integration into the fashion products markets.

## 4 Human Factors and Garment Design

The creation of clothing products always depends on the needs of the end user and also the support of a multidisciplinary team that helps in product development. Design professionals look for differentiated products, adding more value to the brands for which they develop the product, seeking to place them in a privileged position in the market. To better achieve these results, a good auscultation and understanding of the target public is required, an adequate choice of materials and creative resources, be they conceptual or technological development of raw materials, colours and shapes, but also the choice of the best production method for the type of product to be developed. If, on the one hand, this versatility of creative resources adds important quality to clothing, it also makes the process more complex, as it requires the integration of knowledge and professionals from different areas such as fabric manufacturing technologies, materials choice, patternmaking, surveys with user needs, production process and many other factors that influence the process of product development of clothing. Given the ageing of population, these understandings is necessary in order to improve the products intended to this segment, Besides that, these considerations may contribute to the advancements of the textile and apparel industry, once the needs and expectation of a large portion of population can be satisfied [16].

In this sense, human factors prove to be a fundamental tool for identifying the elements that can produce greater knowledge to be applied to design and fashion design, allowing the maximization of comfort and the improvement of the functionality of design objects.

## 5 Something Is Changing

Consumption plays an important role in building the identities of individuals, as they seek to express and confirm who they are through their possessions [12]. We can take into account, [12], that goods are classified into cultural categories that, for example, determine what is appropriate to the consumption of men and women in terms of clothing colour, shape, size, and also determine what and how we should dress or eat. It is from this appropriation of meanings attributed to consumer goods that individuals can construct and communicate their identity [17]. Identity [18], is the result of social interactions between individuals and groups and the mechanisms of differentiation and identification established between them, I identify identity, then a way to categorize them.

By observing the cultural manifestations of those who grow old in the contemporary world, we identify significant changes in habits, images, beliefs, and terms used to characterize this period of life. The emergence of the category "old age" is considered, by specialized literature, one of the major transformations that have passed the history of old age. In fact, the modification of the sensibility invested in old age ended up generating a deep inversion of the values attributed to it: previously understood as physical decay and disability, a moment of rest and stillness in which solitude and affective isolation prevailed, it came to mean the moment leisure, hobbies and skills and to the cultivation of affective and loving ties as alternatives to the family [19].

From the nineteenth century onwards, gradually, differentiations between ages and specialization of functions, habits and spaces related to each age group emerge. In the twentieth century, one can observe uniformity within the age groups, markings of interests and positions between different ages, such as admission to school and university and retirement. The psychological and cultural needs of this new growing group stimulated the emergence of universities of the third age and the spaces of coexistence specific for the third age. The practice of sports, tourism and old-age clubs are essential means for socializing and forming interpersonal ties at this stage of life [12]. Fashion designers currently perceiving this emerging demand of this new public of the elderly has been showing in their collections pieces more adapted to this public. One of the examples is the Iris Apfel, businesswoman and interior designer who at 97 still remains an icon of fashion and very present figure of the American society (Fig. 2).

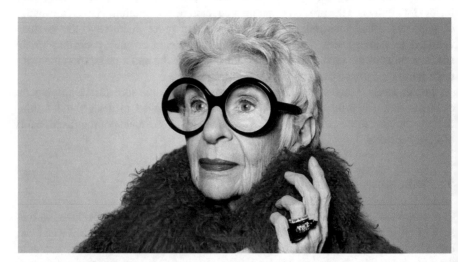

**Fig. 2.** Iris Apfel. Retrived on 26 February 2018 from http://the-talks.com/interview/iris-apfel/

Maysles, the director of "Grey Gardens" and "Gimme Shelter," is no stranger to stories about eccentric female characters. Iris Apfel is a 93-year-old interior designer, business woman, and style maven whose influence on the New York style scene can be traced back decades. The documentary offers a unique perspective into the delightful life of a living legend.

"Iris' is an exceptionally charming and moving film about a life well-lived," said Magnolia President Eamonn Bowles in a press release. "I was completely taken by Iris Apfel watching it, and I'm confident audiences will fall for her too."

# 6   Conclusions

It is important to identifying the biggest changes seniors users may find in their bodies over time and how they perceive these changes, how they adapt to it. Seniors should be able to respond to these new realities in order to feel better, more autonomous, self-sufficient, more confident and secure at different levels, be they material or immaterial, may help to make these issues holistic and enable an integrated response.

In the very near future we may witness a growing awareness of the needs of the elderly. There is already strong evidence that the elderly are potentially the fast-moving consumer market in the developed world. The industry together with the designers should keep in mind, as a priority, which can be supported in design methodologies such as in the case of inclusive design, the conduction of analysis and research, having end users as representative groups at all stages of the design process and in particularly psychological stress. Psychological stress has often been described as a feeling overwhelmed by the need for constant adjustment for an individual's changing environment, yet stress affects people of all ages, but the lives of the elderly may be particularly affected. Major changes can cause anxiety that lead to feelings of insecurity and/or loss of self-esteem and depression. Thus, the physical and molecular consequences of the psychological stress associated with the aging process should be taken into particularly as the molecular changes induced by psychological stress can compromise healthy aging, and thus the consumption habits of the elderly population.

Considering the key goal of a public relations, campaign, targeting, behavioral attitudes and intentions for the elderly, future studies may examine factors that raise possible long-term effects of future-related technologies, such as identifying ways to address the situation of older people through future technologies related to their condition, health and well-being.

**Acknowledgments.** The authors of this paper wish to thanks the Centre for Research in Architecture, Urbanism and Design (CIAUD) of the Lisbon School of Architecture of the University of Lisbon and FCT for founding this project.

# References

1. UN World Population Ageing 2017 Report
2. https://www.un.org/development/desa/ageing/wp-content/uploads/sites/24/2017/05/WPA-2017-Launch-to-the-IDOP-5-October-2017.pdf
3. Zink, K.J.: Human factors, management and society. Theor. Issues Ergon. Sci. **7**(4), 437–445 (2007). https://doi.org/10.1080/14639220500077346
4. Village, J., Searcy, C., Salustri, F., Patrick Neumann, W.: Design for human factors (DfHF): a grounded theory for integrating human factors into production design processes. Ergonomics **58**(9), 1529–1546 (2015). https://doi.org/10.1080/00140139.2015.1022232
5. Montagna, G.: Multi-dimensional consumers: fashion and human factors. Procedia Manuf. **3**, 6550–6556 (2015)
6. Mellamy, L., Geyer, T.: RR543 - development of a working model of how human factors, safety management systems and wider organizational issues fit together (2007). http://www.hse.gov.uk/research/rrpdf/rr543.pdf
7. Hughes, R.G., Henriksen, K., Dayton, E., Keyes, M.A., Carayon, P., Hughes, R.: Understanding adverse events: a human factors framework (2008)
8. Teperi, A.-M.: Improving the mastery of human factors in a safety critical ATM organisation. Unpublished Master Dissertation, Faculty of Behavioural Sciences at the University of Helsinki, Helsinki (2012)
9. OGP: Human factors engineering in projects. The International Association of Oil & gas Producers, London (2011)
10. FAA: Addendum: Chapter 14, Human Factors (PDF). Federal Aviation Administration, Washington (2011)
11. Solomon, M.: Os segredos da mente dos consumidores (C. M. e. P. Cotrim, Trans. 1ª ed.). V. N. Famalicão: Centro Atlântico, Lda. (2009)
12. Menegucci, M., Santos Filho, A.: Profeção e conforto: a relação entre os tecidos e o design ergonómico do vestuário para idosos. In: 9º Congresso Brasileiro de pesquisa e desenvolvimento em design, São Paulo (2010)
13. Cordeiro, R.P., Pereira, S.J.N.: Beyond appearances: a study about women age identity in old age. BJM **15**(5) (2016)
14. Bonardi, G., Souza, V.B.A., Moraes, J.F.D.; Incapacidade funcional e idosos: um desafio para os profissionaisde saúde; Curso de Pós-Graduação Gerontologia Biomédica do Instituto de Geriatria e Gerontologia da PUCRS; Scientia Medica, Porto Alegre **17**(3), 138–144 (2007)
15. Varnier, T., Merino, E.A.D.: Fatores humanos aplicados a produtos de moda: materiais têxteis com termorregulação voltados ao público idoso. Hum. Factors Des. **6**(11), 072–089 (2017)
16. Tilley, A.R., Dreyfuss, H.: The Measure of Man and Women: Human Factors in Design. Wiley, New York (2001)
17. das Neves, É.P., et al.: Biomechanics and fashion: contributions for the design of clothing for the elderly. Procedia Manuf. **3**, 6337–6344 (2015)
18. McCracken, G.: Cultura & Consumo. Mauad Editora Ltda (2003)
19. Cuche, D., Mahler, P.: La noción de cultura en las ciencias sociales. Ediciones Nueva Visión (1999)
20. Silva. L.R.F.: From old age to third age. Hist. Sci. Health Manguinhos Rio de Janeiro **15**(1), 155–168 (2008)

# Research Based on the Design of Personalized Exercise Program for Community Elderly

Yuting Lin[✉] and Delai Men

South China University of Technology,
Guangzhou University City, Panyu District, Guangzhou, China
447138290@qq.com, mendelai@scut.edu.cn

**Abstract.** The purpose of this study is to find the psychological and physiological characteristics of the elderly in the community, as well as the existing problems in daily exercise, actual needs and potential needs. So as to truly scientifically and effectively improve the effect of exercise and provide the basis for the implementation of the design of programs for personalized and customized sports for the elderly in the community. Through the research methods of literature, interview, mathematical statistics, logical analysis and 5W2H design methods, this study further explores and probes into the fact that there is a blind obedience to the majority of community elders during exercise, lack of fitness guidance, lack of supervision and effectiveness evaluation and other issues. According to the data analysis of the survey, this study designed to plan how to implement the program of personalized customization for the elderly in the community in the future.

**Keywords:** Community elderly · Exercise program · Personalized
5W2H method

## 1 Research Background

This paper studies how to carry out the campaign to implement personalized customization for the elderly in the social context of urbanization and aging population.

### 1.1 Urbanization

The trend of urbanization in China has continued, and the community life style has been popular.

Urbanization is an inevitable stage of national development. As the population and resources are concentrated in major cities. According to the 2016–2020 Forecast Report on Urbanization Growth in China, the urban resident population in China will reach 810 million in 2018, and the urbanization rate in China will reach 63.4% by 2020. Nowadays, China vigorously promotes the reform of a new type of urbanization. The trend of sustained urbanization during the 13th Five-Year Plan period will not change [1]. With the development of urbanization, the labor force inflows. Based on the traditional Chinese family pattern, parents will follow their children into urban community life. Since children have long been working in the company and have few days of living in

© Springer International Publishing AG, part of Springer Nature 2019
N. J. Lightner (Ed.): AHFE 2018, AISC 779, pp. 327–337, 2019.
https://doi.org/10.1007/978-3-319-94373-2_36

urban communities on a daily basis, the elderly have become the main activity groups in urban communities. At the same time, community life has also become a major way of living for the elderly in the contemporary age.

Communities are the organizational unit essence of social groups that break through the space constraints of the traditional unit compound and gradually give priority to the community in living and living functions. Under the new situation of China's new urbanization, it pays attention to improving the quality of life of urban people and providing services to convenience people and people to promote social harmony. Nowadays, the major cities in our country have entered the stage of smart urbanization. The community is the key point of the construction of intelligence and a breakthrough in information management. The construction of community management and service informatization is a good foundation for the elderly to design and provide service system.

## 1.2 Population Aging

However, nowadays, China is not ready to deal with the trend of aging. Measures are inadequate in all aspects: infrastructure, service system, medical insurance and so on.

Between 2015 and 2050, the proportion of the world's population over the age of 60 will almost double from 12% to 22%, and population aging will accelerate much faster than in the past [2]. Many countries in the world face major challenges and must ensure that their health and social systems are well prepared. Especially in China, the population of China will still maintain its momentum of inertia over the next 10 years, with an annual average net increase of about 4 million. In 2050, the population of the elderly will peak, and aging will surely bring about a tremendous impact. At the same time, the aging population has become the major consumer service group in the society. Urban development and development need to be based on this. Therefore, the trend of aging has also become a propeller of the design and study of the elderly service system.

## 1.3 The Research Significance

With the aging and the extension of human life expectancy, changing the pattern of elderly life, emphasizing the importance of health promotion and health promotion.

Improving the level of disease treatment and improving medical security are just expeditious measures and emergency measures. To truly tackle the challenge of aging, we must take the initiative to implement measures to achieve healthy aging instead of inability to wait for others to take care of them Afterlife. Promoting health management throughout the life cycle and changing old-age medical models and concepts. The goal is to promote health rather than disease treatment.

Based on the trend of urbanization and community management, this study designs a service system to study how the elderly can promote self-development in order to meet the challenge of aging.

## 1.4    Research Object

The study is aimed at elderly people over the age of 60 in Guangzhou. Due to the differences in the geographical location of Guangzhou's urban areas, some communities covering the main urban area to remote areas were selected during the survey. Literature, data, investigation, The method of statistics carries on the investigation and study to the elders to participate in the community physical exercise.

## 1.5    Research Methods

Through the research methods of literature, interview, mathematical statistics, logical analysis and 5W2H design methods, this study further explores and probes into the fact that there is a blind obedience to the majority of community elders during exercise, Lack of fitness guidance, lack of supervision and effectiveness evaluation and other issues. According to the survey data analysis for the future implementation of community planning program of personalized customization of the elderly concept.

### 1.5.1    Literature Method

By referring to the CNKI and other electronic databases and the WHO reports, I have read and understood the theoretical basis of the elderly fitness and the development of the elderly fitness in China, providing more detailed and comprehensive literature for the study of the topic and facilitating the implementation of the Research and Analysis on the Custom Design of Senior Citizens in China Community [3].

According to the World Health Organization's report, Global Recommendations for Healthy Physical Activity, which targets movement-goal recommendations for all healthy people 65 and over and patients with chronic NCDs in this age group. People need to develop exercise methods based on the amount of exercise goals, combined with their own physical condition.

Relative to foreign countries, China's elderly fitness is developing at a slower pace. Although the fitness square dance in China is widely popular in the world, its lack of pertinence in sports itself and its sports effects are not guaranteed. Taken together, China's elderly sports and fitness is still a problem. In China, there is a lack of systematic education on the knowledge of the elderly health movement. At the same time, there is a problem of non-popularization and lack of pertinence in the dissemination of knowledge about the elderly's exercise and fitness.

### 1.5.2    Expert Interview Method

Through interviewing or telephone interviews with the planning and organizing personnel of the community sports activities and the relevant management personnel of the community, the general situation is known. Then the interviews with the elderly in the community are conducted to fully understand the development of the community aged fitness activities.

### 1.5.3    Questionnaire Method

The elderly in the community as the main survey object, set the survey content and print out to fill in, the survey can be related to the implementation of sports and fitness programs, weekly participation, exercise and health knowledge of the degree of understanding and so on. After completing the questionnaire, collect statistics and analysis.

### 1.5.4    Mathematical Statistics

The survey data obtained using statistical software to calculate the corresponding results.

### 1.5.5    Logic Analysis

Using induction, deduction, analysis, synthesis and other logical analysis, a variety of information carried out in-depth discussion.

### 1.5.6    5W2H Analysis

WHAT, WHY, WHO, WHEN, WHERE, HOW, HOW MUCH five words set questions, find the clues to solve the problem, find ideas for the design, the design concept, so as to create a new invention project [4].

WHAT - what is it? What is the purpose? What kind of work?

The program of customized sports for the elderly is a service system aimed at guiding elderly people to carry out physical exercises in a targeted and scientific manner and providing a full range of systematic services through personalized customization, instructional teaching and monitoring and evaluation.

WHY - Why do? Cannot do? Is there any alternative?

Address the challenges of population aging, effectively improve the physical fitness of the elderly, and promote healthy aging. Since China has entered the stage of population aging, it is an inevitable issue. Therefore, measures to improve the physical quality of the elderly are an inevitable move. This program is the most fundamental way to solve the problem, but also the most effective.

WHO - who? Who will do it?

The elderly are the center of the service system and the actual operators. The community managers are responsible for coordinating the organization and layout of community public spaces and setting up basic fitness facilities. The medical institutions are responsible for providing professional medical guidance.

WHEN - when? What time to do? What time is the most appropriate?

Elderly people wear exercise-related products to detect physical data, exercise assessment every 2 to 4 weeks

WHERE - where? Where to do it?

Due to urbanization and modern community management, the service system is based on the community.

HOW - what to do? How to improve efficiency? How to implement? What is the method?

The elderly upload relevant body data, wear products for monitoring, data upload to a unified management platform. The community management agency is responsible for organizing the exercise assessment and communicating with the relevant medical institutions for regular physical examination.

HOW MUCH - how much? To what extent? How many? Quality level? What is the cost output?

Wear the monitoring product is the sensor as the main device, the cost is not high, the basic can afford. In response to the challenge of population aging, the government will also give strong support to the community infrastructure to purchase according to demand, co-funded by the community government.

## 2 Findings and Analysis

The survey sent a total of 168 questionnaires, the actual recovery of 147 questionnaires, of which 122 valid questionnaires.

According to the survey we can see:

### 2.1 Community Physiological Characteristics of the Elderly

The proportion of elderly people participating in physical fitness activities in Guangzhou community is very high. Among them, most of the women who participate in community physical fitness activities are 9.66% of the total number of the aged people aged 55–60. As the elderly in this age group have just retired They are in the stage of adapting to roles and need to take care of their grandchildren. Therefore, they do not have sufficient time to participate in sports activities. People aged 61 to 65 account for 36.7% of the total number of the elderly and people aged 66 to 70 years of age The total number of people is 37.2%. As can be seen from the survey results, the majority of the elderly aged 60 to 70 are as a result of the elderly having adapted to their roles and their grandchildren have gone to school. Therefore, they have plenty of time to participate in physical fitness activities. Aged 10.8% of the total number of the elderly, over the age of 75 accounted for 5.64%, 75 years of age or older less, due to physical conditions, mobility, illness, fear of injury is not to participate in sports activities.

### 2.2 Community Elderly Psychological Characteristics

The survey shows that the seniors in the community have a positive understanding of the role of physical exercise in physical fitness. They think that physical exercise and physical fitness are very good for 67.4% of the respondents, 19.2% are good for their health and well-being, Some 11.4% of the respondents reported that physical and psychological health benefits, and 2.6% of the respondents considered it to be of no benefit. The survey found that while recognizing the benefits of exercise health, seldom or even not participating in physical exercise, conscious but not acting.

Some of them think that doing manual work such as housework and farm work does not require additional participation in physical exercise. According to the report of "BMC Public Health", people often overestimate the amount of housework done. Any kind of manual work has its limitations and the activities of some organizations and organs. However, it does not consider whether the role of the human body is Comprehensive and reasonable.

In recent years, China has swept the world with square dance. During the course of the investigation, most people, especially females, were also found to choose square dance as the main form of physical exercise [5]. The vast majority of people think that dancing can exercise and increase body coordination, and that collective activities can bring delight in body and mind. However, studies have found that the square dance is aerobic exercise, many people will focus on aerobic exercise and neglected strength training. Many older people mistakenly believe that strength training is a matter for young people. In fact, strength, balance, reaction and endurance can provide strong protection to the elderly and can even delay the effects of aging.

## 2.3    The Choice of Daily Fitness Exercise: The Type of Exercise, the Choice of Exercise Duration, the Choice of Place

### 2.3.1    Way of Exercise

Survey shows that the elderly choose a variety of fitness programs, like to choose from the venue, equipment, restrictions on the project. Elderly fitness programs in Guangzhou mainly include running classes (jogging and walking), dance classes (square dance, ballroom dancing, etc.), chess games (chess, mahjong, etc.), balls (croquet, table tennis, etc.) Climbing, exercise in community fitness equipment, etc.) [6]. Among them, runners have less requirements on the venue, equipment, and personal skills, and their activity intensity is small. They can not only keep fit but also cultivate their body and mind, which are suitable for the physical and mental needs of the elderly. The elderly men and women show different characteristics, older women are more inclined to choose dance items, such as square dance, both to exercise and make friends, very much loved by older women.

The survey showed that 13.1% of the surveyed elderly participated in the activities of community organizations, and that 37.2% of the surveyed persons participated in free-form activities (mainly those who exercised alone or accompanied their friends and family members) Of the elderly accounted for 33.1% of the surveyed population. Visible Guangzhou community elderly participate in fitness activities mainly individual and independent organization of exercise. Personal spontaneous exercise, only by their own preferences and experience to choose sports, from the perspective of scientific movement, this choice has some blindness and randomness, fitness science, health is poor, and the durability of fitness is not easy to stabilize, Not easy to exchange with others, to a certain extent, weakened the effectiveness of physical fitness. However, the way of self-organizing exercise, although it can promote communication, but the collective project is poorly targeted, the effectiveness of the exercise based on personal physical condition. The participation of community organizations less exercise, mainly due to the lack of community venues today, the lack of guidance of sports instructor.

### 2.3.2    Exercise Time

WHO has issued the Elderly Goal, which targets all healthy people over the age of 65 and is also suitable for those with chronic NCDs in this age group: the elderly should complete at least 150 min of moderate-intensity aerobic physical activity weekly, Or at least 75 min per week of high-intensity aerobic physical activity, or a combination of moderate and high-intensity activities of comparable magnitude.

The survey shows that the elderly in Guangzhou take part in physical exercise for 3 to 4 times a week is the most (62.3%), exercise duration 30–60 min/times the most

(66.2%). It shows that there are some enthusiasm and initiative in elder community participation in physical exercise in Guangzhou community, but it is not clear whether the exercise intensity and sports effectiveness meet the standard.

### 2.3.3 Sports Venues

The sports and physical exercise places for the elderly in the urban areas of Guangzhou are mainly located in the vicinity of residential quarters, the Park Square, the sports venues of nearby schools, the roadside, etc. The places are relatively fixed. Many communities have some basic fitness facilities for the elderly Physical fitness, but such outdoor places by external interference factors (such as the weather). In the residential area near 37.1% of exercise, parks and plazas accounted for 32.5%, to the venues for only 3.8%. The survey results show that the charging venues, whether it is charging standards or equipment and equipment, are not suitable for the elderly, in addition to less expensive private venues for consumer groups targeted at the elderly, and the concept of consumption of the elderly did not Physical exercise included.

Due to the densely-populated buildings in Guangzhou and the limited land use in public places, the layout of public spaces needs to be fully taken into account in the development of the community. In urban construction, community distribution should be taken into consideration to establish public activity venues. Governments and agencies need to make relevant considerations to better cope with aging challenge.

## 3 Existing Issues (Elderly Individuals, Sports Associations, Community Management), Actual Needs and Potential Needs

The vast majority of the elderly take a proactive and proactive attitude toward the exercise of physical exercise. However, due to personal preference and experience, the manner and duration of exercising their choice of exercise have a certain degree of blindness and the effect of exercise has not been guaranteed. Most of the elderly have non-communicable chronic diseases. They need to formulate related exercises according to their individual conditions. However, the vast majority of the elderly lack of targeted and scientific sports instruction. There are some potential safety problems during exercise, which have not reached the expected exercise Effect, but not worth the candle. And at present, many elderly people lack the actual test recording equipment and evaluation system after exercising, so the actual effect of exercise is unknown.

Under the background of the current aging population, China's pension system has gradually shifted to "home-based, community-based and institutional support." The survey found that in the process of promoting home-based care services in an all-round way, the living conditions of the elderly are being extended to all kinds of community-based home-care service institutions. Most of the home-based and non-disabled elderly people's daily leisure sports activities have become an important part of old-age care. Therefore, the daily exercise of the elderly need to establish a system of connecting individuals, communities, medical institutions, in order to better promote healthy aging.

Elderly physical exercise should be based on personal physical condition, combined with the doctor's professional guidance and exercise of scientific guidance for the development of sports programs. Exercise records at any time to observe changes in body function, regular physical examination, assessment of the actual effect of exercise to see whether the standard.

# 4 Existing Product Service System Concept

## 4.1 Elderly Personalized Custom Sports Program Service System

Based on the above analysis, due to the new urbanization stage and community management, the service system designed and researched in this paper is based on the urban community as the basic unit of the service system and plays an important role in connecting the elderly and related organizations (community management, government, Medical institutions) the role of the link. The service system consists of three main elements: the elderly, community management agencies, medical institutions.

### 4.1.1   Community Elderly

Community elders serve as service targets. Firstly, they actively take the initiative to actively manage the community-based management of urban communities. Under the organization of community managers, they perform the first full-body checkup at community health stations and enter body-related data into the community management system. APP to obtain customized sports program, exercise programs according to the program of exercise and its video instruction; wear monitoring tools (sports bracelet) during exercise to monitor and record changes in the personal physical data of the elderly; regularly cooperate with the community management agencies for physical examination, To assess whether the effect of exercise standards.

### 4.1.2   Community Management Agency

Community management agencies serve as management roles in the service system. They plan the layout of public spaces in the community and acquire relevant sports infrastructure. They also establish community health databases for aged people, contact medical institutions and organize the elderly for physical examination. The community bodies of the elderly Data entry database; issue of exercise monitoring tool (sports bracelet) to guide the elderly proper use of monitoring tools and APP; set up community health service stations, regularly organize the elderly for physical examination, upload relevant data, contact medical institutions for data analysis, evaluation the effect of community elder's exercise and give relevant suggestions.

### 4.1.3   Medical Institutions

Medical institutions in the service system is mainly responsible for providing professional guidance in the field of medicine. The medical organization dispatches the doctor to communicate with the elderly in the community and make suggestions with the customized sports program according to the sports APP, which is mainly to adjust the recommended sports data in the APP control system. Based on the physical data uploaded from monitoring products and the physical data of the elderly who are regularly checked by community agencies, the effect of their exercise is evaluated.

## 4.2   Sports Monitoring Products

To ensure safer exercise and better exercise results, elderly people in the community wear sports monitoring products during exercise to monitor and record the physical condition of the body.

The sports monitoring product uses sports bracelet as a carrier, which mainly monitors and records related data of the elderly and uploads it to the cloud to create a sports diary. Monitoring recorded data include: exercise time (min), the number of movements (times/week), heart rate (bpm), blood pressure (mmHg), oxygen content and so on.

## 4.3   Sports APP

### 4.3.1   Design Concept

The main concept of the design is around the customization of individual sports programs, which have a professional terminology in the world, called exercise prescription. 1969 World Health Organization has begun to use exercise prescription terminology. The complete concept of exercise prescription is: Rehabilitation Physician or physical therapist, in physical exercise or patient, according to medical examination data (including exercise test and physical test), according to their health, physical and cardiovascular function, in the form of prescription Prescribed the type of exercise, exercise intensity, exercise time and exercise frequency, put forward the precautions in exercise.

Today in the information age, the concept of exercise prescription and information management technology are combined, so the design concept of the sports APP is proposed.

### 4.3.2   Functional Classification

This sports APP function is divided into: Exercise program customization, data monitoring, video teaching.

#### Sports Programs Customized

According to the health database established by the community, the physical data of elderly people in the community provided by the community are combined with the data adjustment made by the doctor to recommend the content and exercise amount of elderly people's physical exercise. Uploaded to the community health database through a medical examination of the whole body, and the doctor adjusts the user's exercise program in the APP control system through face-to-face communication with the user and body data to adjust exercise content and limit exercise amount.

Exercise content includes the type of exercise, exercise intensity, exercise time, exercise frequency, exercise schedule and precautions and so on. Which sports are divided into three categories: endurance (aerobic) exercise, strength exercise and stretching exercises and aerobics. The amount of exercise is based on data such as heart rate index.

Sports According to the user's personal preferences of choice, you can recommend the user favorite sports, according to the time of the exercise and sports to develop programs in line with sports goals.

**Data Monitoring**

Sports bracelet for physical activity related to the elderly in real-time monitoring data uploaded to the APP to determine the appropriate exercise intensity. By directly measuring heart rate, blood pressure, blood oxygen and other data, and record the exercise time, can be calculated by formula (exercise intensity = exercise/exercise time), indirectly determine the exercise intensity.

Through the data monitoring function, accurately determine the amount of exercise, the effective implementation of exercise programs. Second, with this function, the elderly trigger an automatic alarm function (automatic call to relatives and friends, contact with a medical station, etc.) if they have an over body reaction (abnormal body data) during exercise.

**Video Teaching**

APP sports video teaching, including sports teaching videos, text pictures of a detailed description of the elderly under the guidance of the video scientifically and efficiently exercise.

### 4.3.3    Use Process

Upload data → customization → recommended sports → select sports → sports according to the video guide → real-time monitoring data.

### 4.3.4    Features

The app is based on the intelligent management of community information and is designed specifically for the community's health campaign for the elderly. The APP, in conjunction with the monitoring product (sports bracelet), provides real-time monitoring of users, recording of body-related data, uploading to the cloud and building exercise diaries for the convenience of doctors, relatives and friends and helps in the treatment of some conditions. Second, APP is not only a fixed recommendation sports program, but according to the user's personal preferences to recommend sports, thereby enhancing the user's interest. In addition, the sports APP has an abnormal automatic alarm system. When the user wears the bracelet, the body data is too abnormal and an automatic alarm function is triggered, such as automatically calling friends and relatives and the Medical Station.

## 5   Summary

At present, the scale and development of the aged sports in our country are still at the primary stage. Elderly physical education is a weak link in the sports for all. In this paper, the physical and psychological characteristics of elders physical exercise in Guangzhou community physical and psychological characteristics, sports patterns, sports venues and other factors were analyzed and analyzed: Guangzhou community elders in the process of physical fitness to participate in physical fitness relatively high, but the lack of fitness knowledge And scientific guidance, there is a certain degree of blindness in physical exercise and fitness, resulting in the lack of protection of sports effects and sports safety. The community management agencies mainly show that the institutions are not sound enough, the community layout and facilities management are not perfect,

Based on the above research results, according to the actual situation in Guangzhou, this paper puts forward the concept of personalized customized sports program service for the elderly: that the service system of personalized customized sports programs for the elderly is based on the aging population, To maintain social stability and build a harmonious society, based on the general health needs of the elderly based on the elderly individuals, community management agencies and medical institutions as the main force to work together for the elderly in urban communities to provide better sports Service system: 1. Combining information management technology to establish the community health database for the elderly; 2. According to the health data, medical institutions to conduct management analysis, given professional medical guidance, custom recommended personalized exercise program; 3. Design monitoring products, Physical activity monitoring of the elderly in real time; 4. Design sports APP, recommended sports programs and video teaching and detailed text captions, recording physical data to create a sports diary. 5. Record and analyze body data to assess the quality and effectiveness of exercise.

The service system of Guangzhou elderly personal customized sports program is a huge system that involves all aspects of social organization. Due to its limited ability and time, limited resources such as manpower, material resources and research funding, it can be examined. The limited number of respondents limited the final research results. In future research, I will expand the sample size and improve the effectiveness and scientificness of the research.

This study mainly researches and puts forward the design concept from the problems that appeared in the elderly community fitness movement in Guangzhou City. However, there is no complete and detailed design for the system, product and APP. In this regard, I will work hard in the future to further study.

# References

1. Zhang, J.: Park elderly fitness crowd basic knowledge of sports fitness grasp the status quo. Hebei Normal University (2017)
2. Li, R.: The legalization of elderly fitness clubs from the perspective of new institutionalism - a case study of SAMQ. J. Guangxi Univ. (Philos. Soc. Sci.) 36(04), 67–71 (2014)
3. Shang, S.: Chongqing old city elderly sports fitness activities survey and development strategies. Chongqing University (2012)
4. Huang, S., Zheng, H., Li, X., Zhang, X., Xue, P.: Study and analysis on the current situation of elderly physical fitness in urban community in Anhui Province. J. Shandong Inst. Phys. Educ. 26(11), 16 (2010)
5. Li, L.-G., Jiang, Z.-D., Liu, Y.-C., Ma, G.-H.: Complement of diversified elderly fitness service system in national fitness center. Sports Res. 31(02), 74–77 (2010)
6. Wang, W.: Study on current situation and improvement of elderly physical fitness service system in community of Xiamen City. Xiamen University (2009)

# Colors of Handrails Considering the Visibility of Elderly People: An Experimental Evaluation Using Handrail Photographs

Takashi Sakamoto[1]([✉]), Yuki Yoshizawa[2], and Yasuyo G. Ichihara[2]

[1] National Institute of Advanced Industrial Science and Technology,
AIST Central-2, 1-1-1 Umezono, Tsukuba, Ibaraki 305-8568, Japan
takashi-sakamoto@aist.go.jp
[2] Kogakuin University,
1-24-2 Nishi-shinjuku, Shinjuku, Tokyo 163-8677, Japan
ichihara@cc.kogakuin.ac.jp

**Abstract.** We investigated visibility in the elderly for the color combinations of handrails and walls that were often seen in places such as general houses, railway stations, hospitals, and elderly facilities. The experimental evaluation was done using 10 photographs (representative from a total of 147 photographs), showing color combinations of handrails and walls. Twenty elderly participants (aged 63 to 86 years old) evaluated the visibility of handrails based on the seven-point Likert scale. This study reveals the colors of handrails and walls with better visibility for elderly people based on the experimental evaluation.

**Keywords:** Color · Railing · Handrail · Visibility · Elderly · Visual evaluation

## 1 Introduction

Do the handrails that we see in our daily lives consider the elderly's visibility? Handrails are important facilities for the elderly to walk safely. The handrails are almost always installed, whether indoors or outdoors, in places where stairs are located. However, handrails are rarely installed considering visibility in elderly people, as we found in our preliminary survey on handrails. Visibility of the handrails depends not only on their colors, but also on the colors of the walls. Nevertheless, the color combinations and contrast between handrails and walls are not taken into account at the product design stage, because handrails and walls are supplied by separate manufacturers. To make matters worse, almost all customers and contractors only emphasize the beautiful and satisfactory appearance of handrails harmonized with the architectural design.

The visibility of the handrails, as well as their physical design, is a subject to be considered. Physical elements such as railing height, thickness, and slipperiness of the surface should be considered to prevent falls in the elderly. A lot of studies have been reported from the viewpoint of these physical elements [1–4]. Of course, such physical elements are important; but it is also necessary to consider the visibility of handrails. If this point is not emphasized, not a few elderly people will fail to notice and grasp the handrails.

© Springer International Publishing AG, part of Springer Nature 2019
N. J. Lightner (Ed.): AHFE 2018, AISC 779, pp. 338–343, 2019.
https://doi.org/10.1007/978-3-319-94373-2_37

This study focuses on an experimental evaluation on handrails visibility. The experimental evaluation was done using 10 photographs of handrails and walls, selected by classifying 147 pictures that were taken in general houses, stations, hospitals, etc. 20 elderly participants evaluated the visibility of handrails in the 10 photographs based on the seven-point Likert scale.

## 2 Related Studies

Several reports have emphasized the range of physical elements of handrails appropriate for elderly people [1–4]. Some of them argued that their original mechanism and ideas are effective to prevent falls in the elderly [5–9], etc. In addition, there are many guidelines on handrails that suggest a contrasting color to the wall [10–13], etc. Nevertheless, we could not find any study that actually examined the visibility of handrails for the elderly.

It is known that color vision changes along with the progression of aging. Blue and violet appear to be darker for the elderly, because spectral luminous efficiency for the short wavelengths such as blue and violet becomes worse with aging [14].

## 3 Methods

The experimental participants were 20 Japanese individuals: 12 males and 8 females aged from 63 to 86 years old. We used the seven-point Likert scale as a measure to determine the degrees of visibility.

Before the experiment, we collected 147 photographs of handrail-wall combinations installed in general houses, hospitals, railway stations, public facilities, and elderly facilities. According to the color combinations of handrails and walls, the 147 photographs could be classified into eight patterns (see Table 1).

**Table 1.** Eight patterns of color combination of handrails and walls.

| Patterns | Handrail colors | Wall colors | Installation locations |
|----------|-----------------|-------------|------------------------|
| 1 | Green | White | Public facility |
| 2 | Silver | Gray | Public facility |
| 3 | White | Dark brown | Public facility |
| 4 | Light orange | White | General house |
| 5 | Dark brown | White | General house |
| 6 | White | White | General house |
| 7 | Red | White | Elderly facility |
| 8 | Silver | White | Railway station |

We selected 10 sample photographs (Fig. 1) as visual stimuli that consisted of eight photographs that represented the eight color-combination patterns as shown in Table 1, and two photographs of handrails with LED lightings. These 10 photographs were used

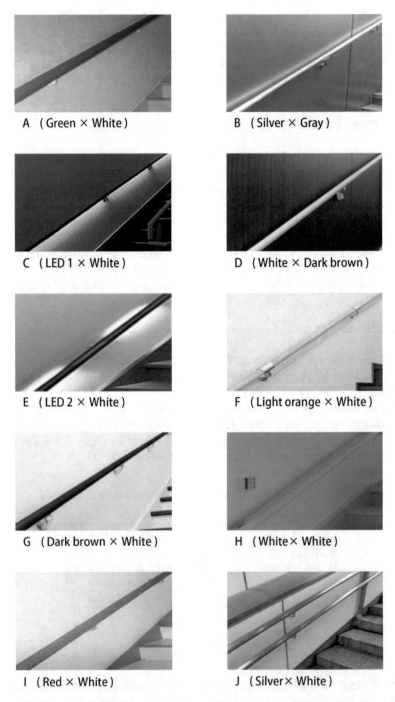

**Fig. 1.** Ten photographs present color combinations of handrail and wall.

for the visibility experiment on elderly people: We printed the photographs on the questionnaire sheets with Likert scales and presented them to the participants.

## 4  Results

The Visibility evaluations for 10 sample photographs were collected from 19 elderly participants. Incomplete evaluation data from one old man was excluded. Cluster analysis revealed that 10 sample photographs could be divided into largely four groups, as shown in a dendrogram (Fig. 2). Figure 3 shows the results of the statistical test based on analysis of variance (ANOVA) and multiple comparison analysis, and the above mentioned four groups were represented with the colors of the bar in orange, pale orange, purple, and blue respectively. These four groups illustrated good, somewhat good, neither good nor bad, and somewhat-bad visibility, respectively. There was a statistically significant difference between these four groups.

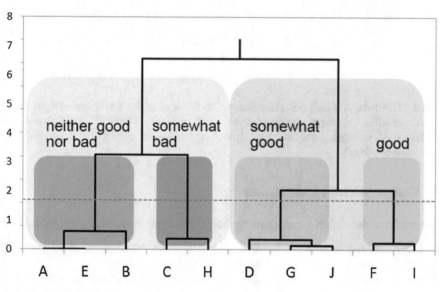

**Fig. 2.** Dendrogram illustrates that 10 photographs can be divided into four groups largely.

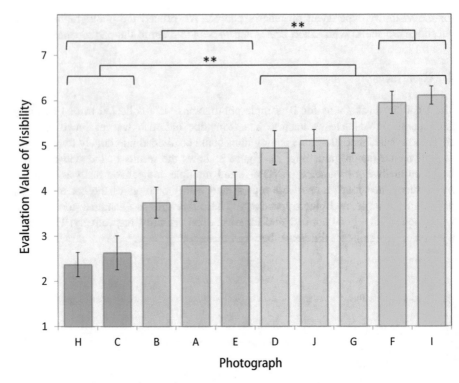

**Fig. 3.** This bar-graph indicates evaluation values of visibility for the 10 photographs (A–J). Double asterisks (**) mean significant at 1% level ($p < 0.01$). Colors of bars illustrate four groups: good (orange), somewhat good (pale orange), neither good nor bad (purple), and somewhat bad (blue).

## 5    Discussion and Conclusion

The results of the visibility evaluation for the 10 photographs (A–J) suggest followings:

1. Clear contrast between a handrail-color and background-color enables elderly people to see handrails clearly, such as in D, F, G, and I.
2. Handrails with the high conspicuity color such as red and orange are evaluated as good visibility, such as in F and I.
3. Although handrail and wall colors are clearly separated, handrails with poor conspicuity color such as green as in A are not evaluated as having good visibility.
4. If the handrail and the background wall have same colors, they will be evaluated as bad, such as in H.
5. Silver (metal) handrails are evaluated as somewhat good or not so bad, in spite of poor contrast to the background wall colors, such as in B and J.
6. Handrails installed in a dark place are evaluated as poorly visible even though the LED light was on, such as in C and E.

Under the existing experimental conditions, we cannot control various variables affecting the visibility evaluation properly. Our next tasks will be to control them and to confirm the visibility of handrails installed in the real space and under the real light.

# References

1. Maki, B.E.: Influence of handrail shape, size and surface texture on the ability of young and elderly users to generate stabilizing forces and moments. National Research Council of Canada, Division of Electrical Engineering (1988)
2. Maki, B.E., Bartlett, S.A., Fernie, G.R.: Research note effect of stairway pitch on optimal handrail height. Hum. Factors **27**(3), 355–359 (1985)
3. Fernie, G.: Biomechanical Assessment of Handrail Parameters: with Special Consideration to the Needs of Elderly Users. National Research Council Canada, Division of Electrical Engineering (1988)
4. Ishihara, K., Nagamachi, M., Komatsu, K., Ishihara, S., Ichitsubo, M., Mikami, F., Osuga, Y., Imamura, K., Osaki, H.: Handrails for the elderly: a survey of the need for handrails and experiments to determine the optimal size of staircase handrails. Gerontechnology **1**(3), 175–189 (2002)
5. O'brien, J.L., Thomas, E.M., Donald, A.N.: Support pole with a pivoting and locking handrail for elderly and disabled persons. U.S. Patent No. 5,586,352 (1996)
6. O'brien, J.L., Thomas, E.M., Donald, A.N.: Multi-level trapeze handle and support system for elderly and disabled persons. U.S. Patent No. 6,068,225 (2000)
7. O'brien, J.L., Thomas, E.M., Donald, A.N.: Pivoting and locking wall mounted support rail for elderly and disabled persons. U.S. Patent No. 7,823,229 (2010)
8. Lacey, G., Dawson-Howe, K.M.: The application of robotics to a mobility aid for the elderly blind. Rob. Auton. Syst. **23**(4), 245–252 (1998)
9. Nitta, O., Hashimoto, M., Inoue, K., Takahashi, Y.: developmental research of a power assistance type handrail. J. Jpn. Acad. Health Sci. **7**(3), 164–168 (2004)
10. Accessibility for the Disabled - A Design Manual for a Barrier Free Environment. http://www.un.org/esa/socdev/enable/designm/AD2-05.htm. Accessed 1 Mar 2018
11. Colour and Contrast. http://dementia.stir.ac.uk/design/good-practice-guidelines/colour-and-contrast. Accessed 1 Mar 2018
12. Public Consultation on the Review of the "Design Manual: Barrier Free Access 1997", The Government of the Hong Kong Special Administrative Region (2006). http://www.lwb.gov.hk/eng/consult_paper/bfa.htm. Accessed 1 Mar 2018
13. Lighting and colour for hospital design, R&D Report B(01)02, NHS Wales (2004)
14. ISO 24502:2010: Ergonomics – Accessible design – Specification of age-related luminance contrast for coloured light (2010)

# Robotic Shopping Trolley for Supporting the Elderly

Yoshinori Kobayashi$^{(\boxtimes)}$, Seiji Yamazaki, Hidekazu Takahashi,
Hisato Fukuda, and Yoshinori Kuno

Guraduate School of Science and Engineering, Saitama University,
255 Shimo-Okubo, Sakura Ward, Saitama City, Japan
{yosinori,yamazaki,takahashi,fukuda,
kuno}@cv.ics.saitama-u.ac.jp

**Abstract.** As the advance of an aging society in Japan, along with the lack of caregivers, the elderly care has become a crucial social problem. To cope with this problem, we are focusing on shopping. Shopping is one of the important daily activities and expected to be effective for the elderly rehabilitation because it feels easier than walking rehabilitation and it can give the positive effect for the cognitive functions by memorizing and checking out items to buy. The current shopping rehabilitation is carried out with a caregiver accompanied by the elderly one by one for guiding inside the store, carrying shopping basket, monitoring, etc. Consequently, the caregivers' load is very high. In this paper, we propose a robotic shopping trolley that can reduce the caregivers' load in shopping rehabilitation. We evaluate its effectiveness through experiments at an actual supermarket.

**Keywords:** Autonomous mobile robot · Elderly care · Shopping trolley

## 1 Introduction

In current shopping rehabilitation, caregivers need to accompany the elderly one by one for guiding inside the store, carrying shopping basket, monitoring, etc. Consequently, the caregivers' load is very high. On the contrary, elderly people want to enjoy shopping more freely without time limitations, if possible. According to the staff of care facilities, shopping rehabilitation is done daily by consuming almost the whole working time of one caregiver (8 h/day), and if it is possible for one caregiver to watch two or three elderly people, it will lead to significant cost reduction. In addition, the elderly also want to select shopping items slowly and they want to buy bargains without worrying about the caregiver watching them. In this paper, we propose a robotic shopping trolley which is responsible for "in-store guide", "baggage transportation", "walking support", which was the role of caregivers, by applying mobile robot technology to robotic shopping carts (Fig. 1). We develop robotic shopping trolley with these functions and evaluate its effectiveness by conducting experiments in cooperation with the care facility and supermarket.

Several shopping assistance robots have been proposed, some of which have been commercialized. However, for example RT.2 [1] is specialized in the function to

© Springer International Publishing AG, part of Springer Nature 2019
N. J. Lightner (Ed.): AHFE 2018, AISC 779, pp. 344–353, 2019.
https://doi.org/10.1007/978-3-319-94373-2_38

support walking, so it cannot provide users directions to the destination. Navii [2], ShopBot [3], and TOOMAS [4] are robots that provide guiding inside the shop, but it cannot transport baggage. DASH [5] can carry baggage but it does not possess the function to support walking. On the contrary, our robotic shopping trolley is intended for elderly people with the ability to guide them inside stores, carry baggage, and support his/her walking. There are few examples of shopping support robots that combine these functions for elderly support.

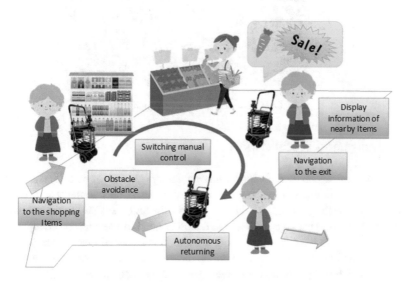

**Fig. 1.** Features of our robotic shopping trolley.

## 2  Robotic Shopping Trolley

Our robotic shopping trolley consists of an elderly shopping trolley in which the section for the wheels are converted to a mobile robot platform [6], a PC and LiDAR (Fig. 2). The PC performs localization estimation using measurement data from the LiDAR and generates a control command to the mobile robot platform at each time sequence. Based on the command, the mobile robot generates the angular velocity of the wheels to control the motors. A touch panel screen is provided as an interface for inputting instructions to the robot such as destinations. We use ROS [7] as a software framework. Programs that run on the PC, such as retrieving sensor data and controlling mobile robot, are divided into independent processes for each function. ROS is utilized as a framework of inter-process communications.

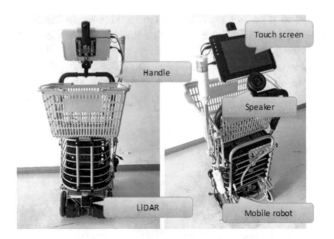

**Fig. 2.** Overview of our robotic shopping trolley.

# 3    Mapping and Localization

The system estimates its own position using odometry (rotation of wheels) and LiDAR, and performs autonomous movement. Localization based on odometry is a low cost calculation but estimation errors due to wheel slip and road surface distortion are accumulated with the passage of time. On the other hand, if there are no changes in the environment and the position of the robot is same, it is expected that the measured data from LiDAR will be identical even when the measurement time is different. In the scan matching algorithm, a previously generated environment map is compared with LiDAR scan data at each time to estimate the location of the robot. In our system, localization estimation by odometry is performed at each time sequence, and accumulated error is recovered by scan matching every 0.5 s.

## 3.1    Environment Map

The observation likelihood is derived based on the statistics of scan data measured when the robot moves in the environment for generating the map. Here, the observation likelihood is the probability that a certain point is observed for a long time by LiDAR. The observation area is divided into cells of square size $a$, and the distribution of observation points in each cell is expressed by using one normal distribution. To avoid the discontinuity of distribution between neighborhood cells, the system calculates a normal distribution for each cell which boundary is shifted $a / 2$ (examples of shifted cells are indicated as the colored squares in Fig. 3) and map data is constructed by integrating them (Fig. 3). An example of the observed point cloud is shown in Fig. 4 (top). Figure 3 (bottom) shows this converted to observation likelihoods. Higher likelihoods can be found in the position where the observation points are dense in a narrow range such as walls (expressed in bright white in Fig. 4). In other words, the observation likelihood decreases when the observation points are sparse and unstable such as with pedestrians.

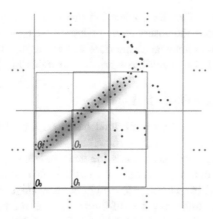

**Fig. 3.** Cells for calculating the distribution of the scan data.

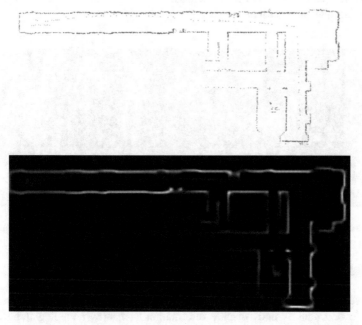

**Fig. 4.** An example of the observed point cloud (top) and converted observation likelihood (bottom).

## 3.2   Monte Carlo Localization

Scan matching is performed by the particle filter framework. The position of the robot is expressed as a set of samples, and each sample is moved based on odometry. The likelihood score of each sample is calculated by comparing the observation data from LiDAR with the map data. Specifically, observation data from LiDAR are projected onto the map. The sum of the observation likelihood of each projected point is used as the score of the sample. Therefore, when the many LiDAR points projected on the positions in the map where the observation likelihoods are high, the score of the sample becomes high. The environmental shape observed for a long time such as a wall is preferentially evaluated. This contributes robust and stable localization estimation.

### 3.3    Path Planning and Obstacle Avoidance

In our system, the traveling path is planned based on a preset route map. Figure 5 shows an example of the route map. A route map is represented by nodes and edges. The robot moves along the edge towards the goal node. By giving a rectangle area along the edge, we can define the available area of the robot movement (white rectangle in the figure). Therefore, in addition to the environmental shape, a route map can define the places that would ordinarily be off-limits for the robot. Therefore, avoiding obstacles can also be performed within the area. For avoiding the obstacle, our robot moves along the aisle, instead of selecting the route so as to maximize the distance to the obstacle. Because it is easy for the surrounding people such as pedestrians to predict the ongoing path of the robot.

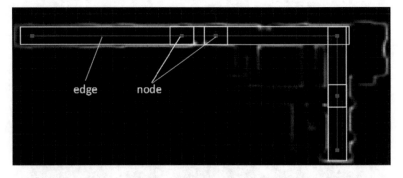

**Fig. 5.**  An example of a route map, which is represented by nodes and edges with rectangles.

## 4    Shopping Support Functions

In this section we describe the shopping support functions provided by our system. "guide to destination" and "display information of nearby shopping items" can be performed based on the information of robot location. In addition, our robotic shopping trolley is capable of hand-pushing, and this provide the function "walking support".

### 4.1    Guide to Destination

When the user inputs the shopping items to the robot, the robot guides the user to the specific locations of the items. Also, when shopping is completed and the "cash register" button is selected, guidance will be started to the cashier. Furthermore, when customers are in a large store, sometimes they get lost and cannot find the exit. Therefore, it is important for the elderly to be guided to the exit. After using the robotic shopping trolley, such as after unloading items into the user's car, the user can return the trolley to the store by automatically by pressing the "return" button.

These destinations are set on the touch panel screen (Fig. 6). First, the user touches the image of the place near the current location. Thereafter, the start point is set by touching the "Initial position" displayed at the lower right. Next, the user touches the image of the destination and finally touches the "Destination" button displayed in the lower right to set it as the destination. As a result, autonomous driving is started. The menu has a hierarchical structure. For example, when an image written as "vegetables" in the upper hierarchy is touched, lower hierarchical images classified as vegetables such as carrot and cabbage are displayed. If there are multiple destinations, the user can long press multiple images of items to be stopped before touching "Destination". Since the robot uses the node as the goal position, the system requires making a node for each item. Correspondence between nodes and items are stored in the data file. Therefore, when the planogram is frequently changed, it is necessary to update this data file.

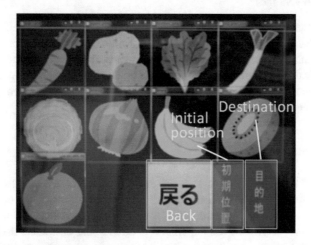

**Fig. 6.** Example of panel images. The user can choose the shopping items by tapping the illustration and input the command to start autonomous navigation.

## 4.2   Display Information of Nearby Shopping Items

The system presents information of nearby shopping items such as bargain sales on the screen when the robot is traveling in front of them. It is possible to obtain the current position of the robot from the localization system. Using this information, advertisement images are displayed while traversing a certain section on the map. As shown in Fig. 7, two points are selected from the map coordinate system, the rectangular area is generated to show the advertisement on the screen.

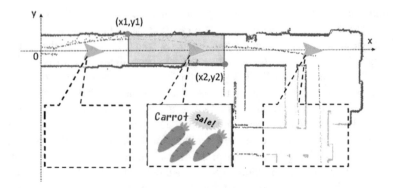

**Fig. 7.** Inside mechanism to display information of nearby shopping items.

## 4.3   Walking Support

By pushing the trolley by hand, the users can lean against the handle for supporting their body. By using the lever, the user can switch the mode between autonomous driving and hand pushing. When the lever is grasped, the wheel is unlocked and it can be hand-pushed. By pressing the button on the touch panel screen, autonomous driving can be restarted. This function can also be used when the users want to buy other items suddenly while they are guided to the preset target items.

## 5   Experiment

We conducted an experiment at an actual supermarket. The area for fresh foods and groceries is about $1400 \text{ m}^2$. Also, there is a care facility at about 60 m from the shopping area. In the experiment, we did not make any changes in the sales floor arrangement. We conducted the experiment while regular customers and clerks were present. Figure 8 shows a part of the result of the scanning data inside the store. The red line is a trajectory that the robot passed. The yellow green point is scan data. In the experiment, we asked three elderly people to use the robotic shopping trolley. Each participant performed shopping assuming (1) shopping items on the list, (2) choosing items to buy at any time, (3) window shopping. After the experiment, we interviewed each participant.

## 5.1   Result

Examples of the experimental scene are shown in Fig. 9. The senior participant selects the shopping items on the touch panel screen (1). Then the robotic shopping trolley guides them to the item's location. While moving in a corridor, information such as bargain sales of nearby shopping items is displayed on the screen (2). Since the elderly person chooses bananas, the robotic shopping trolley guides the person to the banana's sales spot (3), and then it goes to the checkout counter (4). Whenever the robot starts, stops or changes course, an arrow is displayed on the screen and an announcement such as "turning to the right" is made by sound. After returning to the original entrance, it automatically moves to the trolley storage area. The autonomous driving of the robotic shopping trolley was appreciated by the elderly subjects because they carry carts for oxygen therapy.

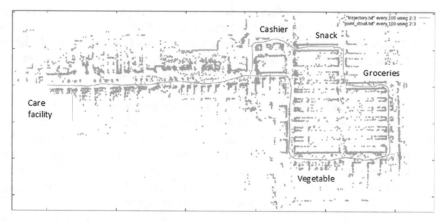

**Fig. 8.** Inside store point clouds data scanned by the robot to make the map.

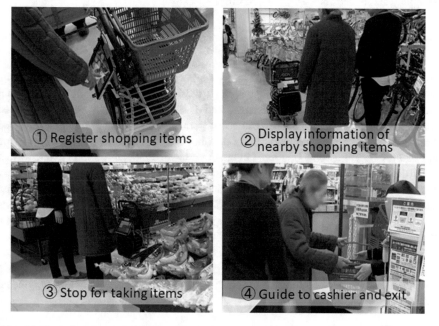

**Fig. 9.** Example scenes of shopping in an actual supermarket using robotic shopping trolley.

## 5.2    Discussion

Our proposed system received positive comments and evaluation results from the both the elderly and caregiver participants. However, when the participants recognized the position of the target item and the robotic shopping trolley could not stop exactly in front of it, they were not satisfied. Moreover, when the robotic shopping trolley was about 2 m apart from the user, they felt that they could leave it. In the narrow passage inside the shop, the robot stopped several times because there was not enough space to move. In this kind of situation, it was not easy for the elderly to know why the robot was stopped. No one took the action to switch to manual pushing and avoid obstacles. It seems that there were overly high expectations for the autonomous driving functions of the robotic trolley.

In this experiment, information of nearby shopping items was presented by images, but almost all participants do not see the displayed images. The participants seem to be focused on the shopping items rather than the touch panel screen while moving. We implemented the interface system using a touch panel screen, but no participants could smoothly operate the touch panel screen. A caregiver suggested that it is difficult for the elderly to find and select the shopping items on the touch panel screen. In the future, we will need to develop new interfaces such as speech recognition.

The participant who performed "window shopping" frequently used the hand pushing mode of our robotic shopping trolley. It is likely that the participant needed to move the robotic shopping trolley near the store shelves because he wanted to pick up shopping items and look at them carefully.

## 6    Conclusion

In this paper, we focus on shopping to support the elderly, developed a robotic shopping trolley that provides autonomous guidance and presents information about shopping items. Experiments were conducted at an actual supermarket. We confirmed that our system can localize its position and perform autonomous driving to assigned destinations. Moreover, we found that our robotic shopping trolley is able to provide support for shopping rehabilitation. On the other hand, although it is effective to switch between the autonomous driving and the hand-pushing, we found that it is necessary for the robot to move with the elderly collaboratively to be able to use the switching function. In addition, it was found that there was some difficulty for the elderly subjects to operate the touch panel. Our study suggests that product information should be displayed not only on the screen but also indicated by sound.

In the future, we plan to develop cooperative driving capabilities with users. Also, we are going to develop the ability to suggest shopping items according to the user's shopping history. Furthermore, we are considering developing a system that can update the map and planograms easily.

**Acknowledgments.** This work was supported partly by JSPS KAKENHI Grant Number 26330186 and Saitama Leading Edge Project.

# References

1. RT.2. https://www.rtworks.co.jp/eng/index.html
2. NAVii. http://www.fellowrobots.com
3. Gross, H.M., Boehme, H., Schroeter, C., Mueller, S., Koenig, A., Martin, Ch., Merten, M., Bley, A.: ShopBot: progress in developing an interactive mobile shopping assistant for everyday use. In: Proceedings of the SMC, pp. 3471–3478 (2008)
4. Gross, H.M., Boehme, H., Schroeter, C., Mueller, S., Koenig, A., Einhorn, E., Martin, Ch., Merten, M., Bley, A.: TOOMAS: interactive shopping guide robots in everyday use - final implementation and experiences from long-term field trials. In: Proceedings IROS, pp. 2005–2012 (2009)
5. DASH. http://5elementsrobotics.com/dash-robotic-shopping-cart/
6. T-frog Project: i-cart mini. http://t-frog.com/products/icartmini/
7. ROS: Robot operating system. http://www.ros.org/

# The New Concept of Aging: Fitness and Leisure Sporting Apparel Adequacy for the "Ageless" Generation

Ekaterina Emmanuil Inglesis Barcellos[1]($\boxtimes$), Galdenoro Botura Jr.[1],
Ana Cristina Broega[2], Lívia Inglesis Barcellos[1], and Monica Moura[1]

[1] Universidade Estadual Paulista - UNESP/FAAC - Campus de Bauru,
Av. Engenheiro Luiz Edmundo Carrijo Coube, 14-01,
Bauru, SP 17033-360, Brazil
ekaterina@faac.unesp.br, galdenoro@sorocaba.unesp.br,
livia.barcellos@gmail.com,
monicamora.design@gmail.com
[2] University of Minho, Campus de Azurém, 4804-533 Guimarães, Portugal
cbroega@det.uminho.pt

**Abstract.** Predictions about increasing longevity in the world indicate we will live with more than 40% of the population over 45 years. Composed of proactive and active individuals, this "mature" society is focused on healthy habits, disease prevention and the practice of physical activities. These individuals will be exercising increasingly and require a garment suitable for the purpose, within their physiological, sensorial, and emotional demands. This brief study, conducted in Brazil, analyzed a specific group of users and their expectations, with respect to the perception of comfort, style, performance, and suitability of sportive/fitness apparel. The research identified that this segment over 45 years, demonstrate greater interest in comfort, quality, technology, and practicality, rather than fashion details. These characteristics are not recognized yet by the productive market. There is a gap in the targeted supply, and the available clothing is restricted to offer items adapted with a focus on the younger target audience, not meeting the specificity and belonging expected by users.

**Keywords:** Comfort perception · Specific comfort · Design
Sportswear and fitness apparel · Longevity

## 1 Introduction

The similarities between the apparel of a determined social group reveal similar behaviors and essential interpretations of customs, cultures, hierarchies, and origins, among other evolutionary anthropological aspects. Social behavioral, and cultural changes associated with the search for more favorable living conditions have significantly altered the lifestyle as it concerns the fashion and the way of dressing of contemporary society during the last 50 years, especially in urban centers. In these places, sport presents itself as a characteristically urban element, and its clothes and fashion express values that reflect urban culture [1, 2]. Nonexistent until the 1960s, sportive phenomenon was perceived exponentially as a

© Springer International Publishing AG, part of Springer Nature 2019
N. J. Lightner (Ed.): AHFE 2018, AISC 779, pp. 354–366, 2019.
https://doi.org/10.1007/978-3-319-94373-2_39

determining factor in society's behavior and cultural language, where body culture and sporting products keeps increasing prominence, in addition to approaching genres and notions of comfort [2]. According to [1] "when the sports lifestyle appeared, it became clear that a sports outfit also gave a mark to whoever wore it. This outfit showed someone tuned to time, speed, audacity and all those values that sports brought" [1]. This culture became universal at the end of the 20th century, and at the beginning of the 21st century, as a form of dress code, a social indicator of belonging and contemporaneity.

Nowadays, well-being and health care were added to the cultural priorities within the lifestyle adopted by most people. Medicine, in turn, developed studies and preventive concepts of health, increasing the life expectancy and reducing mortality. Access to information increased knowledge about sports and ways of maintaining healthy routines and habits, [3] demystifying the distance and subjectivity characterized by the Olympic games, which characterized the sport as unattainable fitness or art attributed to few [4].

At the end of the 60's, the Cooper methodology of physical evaluation with running and aerobic exercises, allowed physical improvements in the cardiorespiratory performance of amateur athletes [3, 4]. With the success of the method and the consolidation of its results, the exercises left the outdoor areas restricted for sports, creating the indoor aerobic practice in smaller spaces [3]. The variety of exercises and the socialization of them delineate the concept of "fitness center", and simplified the practice of individual or group exercises, in any place. From these changes, sport, gymnastics, dance, and sports fighting were characterized as variants of 'Body Culture'.

The evolution of sports practice has broadened the inclusion of numerous amateur practitioners by exponentially increasing the number of users of sportswear apparel worldwide. In Brazil, place of this study and research application, aerobic gymnastics was introduced in the 1980s, following the molding of 21st century world lifestyle, in which new habits and cultural patterns were introduced [3].

This scenario formed a new niche of companies focused on the sports sector, leveraging a segment of garment production appropriate to these activities. Relatively standardized products have occupied sportswear stores for decades, offering preestablished clothing for physical activity that has been gradually adapted for use outside of exercise space as well. The gym uniforms were also replaced by products that provided a better look and a more appropriate performance, being valued by the society's behavior and promoted to street style fashion [1]. In the transition from the 20th to 21st century, due to the lack of time and quite committed mobility in large urban centers on the daily agenda of individuals, the physical and bodily activities ended up being superimposed to mobility within the stressful daily routine. In attempt to obtain quality of life and well-being, a necessary routine practice of specific and complementary physical activities originated, extending democratically to all individuals without limitations of age groups. These activities overlapped with the usual choice of clothing for practicality, social attitude and perception of greater comfort, creating a segment of clothing and a specific form of dress incorporated into the customs of society. At the same time, the health generation of the 80 s and 90 s grew older, becoming aware of the physical benefits obtained, and thus set a new concept of aging, focused on the body care and well-being and health. Currently this concept is basically a worldwide trend [5].

In Brazil, the perspective of population aging has become an imminent reality of the era of quality longevity. [6] data indicate that people over 45 years old are responsible for about 1/3 of enrollments in various fitness, sport and physical activities centers. Numbers disclosed by [6, 7] confirm that walking, running and amateur cycling appear in an ascending scale, demonstrating a significant increase in the practice of exercise and sports among the segment of individuals in this age group, especially in the last decade.

In this sense, it is suggested the line of approach of this article, about the sporting and fitness apparel for a new concept of aging, formed by a type of ageless generation. This group which denotes a lapse in relation to the identification and construction of a specific adequacy for its sportswear products, representative of this emerging mature segment in the current population. It begins with the historical profile, which deals with influences and social changes until the contemporaneousness that brought the notion of need to opt for specific products, necessary as speeches and social indicators in the choice of appropriate clothes. It is essential to understand that the greater specialty of speech creates the greatest specialty for specific clothing, which indicates a product gap in this case for the analyzed segment. Based on this observation, the need to analyze the type of clothing and the expectations that fit into this population group was identified and presented.

## 2 Social Changes: Body Education and Sportswear Insertion in Everyday Life

Over time, society has identified social roles for athletes and sports, and has dressed its practitioners by interpreting and specifying their needs according to norms and rules [8]. In antiquity, as depicted in sculptures and paints, the exercises were practiced outdoors, usually with the naked body, which changed greatly over the centuries. During the Victorian period, brimming with overlapping clothing and modesty rules, pudency and discretion a new demand was formed in bourgeois society that began to long for welfare and accumulation of objects that could convey security, quality and provide a control of personal satisfaction and the desire for comfort sensation [9]. From this feeling and demand, the basic notion for comfort was expressed by aspects as functionality, protection and well-being [8]. This new attitude changed the costumes and clothes, especially with the end of the concept of armor that protected the body replaced by aspects that released the body and changed the silhouette received the first sports influences, with the popularization of cycling in 1890, that changed the posture of the women. In the second half of the 19th century, the first "alternative" suits, skirts, and knickerbockers, broke the rule of these customs. The "Bloomer" trousers, spread by Amelia Bloomer, for women since 1850, were seen and regarded as vulgar and immoral, being allowed only for the practice of exercises and uniforms. Cycling was a means of locomotion between rural and urban regions, and later became a much-appreciated sport, which became integrated into urban life. Bicycles were seen by many as an instrument of feminism, giving women a measure of increased mobility, redefining Victorian ideas about femininity, helped to reform habits and dresses, reduced Victorian restrictions on clothing and undergarments, and facilitated the practice of physical activities [9, 10]. Until this period, the activities were carried out with the daily dress.

According reports of [9, 10], from 1920 onwards, the notion of corporal education began. Cultural currents focused on care such as body, medicine and health have helped change customs. The new yearning idealized "(…) a strong and agile body that wanted to show itself this way. Then the clothing revealed it with the culture of an urban society that valued the physical, the corporal and the sport". "Society began to demand them, to specify them and to specialize their functions" [10].

From 1920 onwards, the big cities incorporated the lifestyle of sports fashion and the perception of body culture, sport, and physical education. Changes in the aristocratic desire influenced clothing. Special new fabrics emerged in this period (jersey, knitting, silk and wool) meeting specific performance and other requirements [10].

From 1940 onwards, the production of sports clothing proliferated, and industries, clothing and sports equipment stores were created. At this point, a form of improvisation of products began, which did not follow more classic Victorian rules and standards [2]. They emphasized strength, athletic body culture and physical vigor. The clothes acquired more specificities and practicality for this purpose.

## 3   Longevity with Comfort: Sports Leisure Wear

Health care, wellness and exercise are part of the routine of many individuals in most countries in the contemporary world. The sociocultural notion that physical activities contribute positively, preventing various diseases and providing greater quality of life has concrete scientific bases. Doctors caution the use of appropriate clothing and the hygienic condition, recommend lightweight, loose, and comfortable weaves. In addition, corporal sports practices have expressed a specialization of discourses, and the specialty of discourse leads to a specialty of dress. In specializing a function and purpose, one creates the need to create a specific garment to supply it [1, 10]. The suits that were considered adequate do not generally correspond to the expectations of the users in their evolution.

According to [1] it can be verified that the sports clothes went through several phases: identification; necessity (clothing that adapts to a new social behavior); specialization (of speech and dress code); improvisation (varied forms and models to increase consumption); hygiene functions and "health canon" (when physicians become active thinkers about the product, alerting to sweating risks of the excess of sun exposure, lightness and comfort of tissues regarding body × exercise × environment); aesthetics (the link between fashion and sportive fashion, and its tangency in terms of fashion, style, lifestyle and comfort); performance (technical, technological improvement and clothing potential, respecting the notion of comfort); specific comfort (directed to a certain group, profile or class of users). This latter joins the previous steps in its main aspects and adds a series of specificity and needs.

Appropriate clothing for the analyzed class of mature subjects, more active or more focused on "balance" and well-being, essentially seeking to become healthier and owning the longevity benefits has become a contingency and a necessity within this process. The fashion and costumes that serve these users involve performance characteristics, practicality, and comfort.

Harvard University studies show that the practice of activities, although moderate, helps longevity, and that "joining moments of leisure to physical exercises can add four and a half years to the life expectancy of a person" [11]. PLOS [11] identified an increase of up to seven years in life expectancy, according to the quality of life obtained with the exercises and habits (tested in 650 thousand individuals, majority over 40 years of age, with different levels of weight).

In Brazil, a country favored by climatic conditions that allow the practice of exercises throughout the year, the number of people practicing maintains a continuous rate of increase. The information of the reports of [12] made in 2014 and 2016, over the last two decades shows that: the total percentage of adults in the population who practice physical activities such as leisure is about 38%; the number of physical activity practitioners increased considerably in Brazil and there was an effective growth of 11% in the number of people performing exercises during leisure or leisure time from 2009 to 2013 and upgoing until 2017 [13]. It was also found in [6] data that Brazil is the second country of the world in terms of number of academies, where the growth rate of fitness segment (2009 to 2012) was 29%, behind only the USA (0.7%), assuming the world leadership in sports and physical activity businesses [6, 14].

This data also shows that the age group analyzed here is responsible for 30% of the total number of gyms in the academies, and about 1.5 million mature individuals (over 45 years old) enrolled in academies in 2012 [14]. Figure 1 shows that most of them opt for walking, fitness, cycling, running or swimming [13].

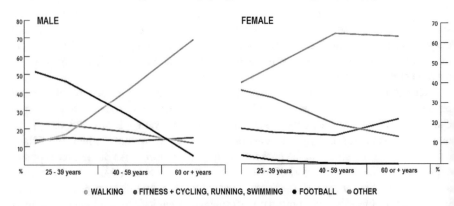

**Fig. 1.** Percentage of practitioners by age and physical activity - Brazil. Adapted from PNAD 2015 and IBGE 2017.

Projections indicate that the age group above 50 years will correspond to about 42% of the population by 2050. Further analyzes indicate that in the next five years this public will boost annual consumption in most fashion segments, and by the description of the increase of physical activities, especially in the consumption of sportswear, which will increase considerably to meet the segment. This perspective shows that by 2050, a contingent close to 100 million mature individuals with expectations of quality and comfort will need appropriate sportswear.

This new extract from the society called "ageless" people because they seem and feel that they are much younger than they really are, over the age of 45, and practice physical and sports activities like leisure, form a specific segment. Who have many specific expectations for comfort and style solutions for this sporting apparel in an elegant and appropriate manner.

## 4   Perception of Specific Comfort in Sportswear/Fitness

In the first half of the 20th century, routine clothing was considerate inappropriate for physical activity and sport, reflecting a first notion of lack of comfort. According [15] fashion expresses its cultural changes based on a specific tension to demonstrate a social condition in the dynamics of society [15] with interconnections and conflicts between users and their different origins and social expectations. [16] citing Rybczynski described comfort by comparing it to evolutionary values and a sense of peace.

The introduction of specific clothing for sporting practice occurred in the early decades of the 20th century due to the social changes of the 19th century by the introduction of yearnings for safety and comfort. With adaptations driven by the notion of acquired comfort, clothing made possible a more acute perception, an idea of specific comfort, already present in different human activities, as part of the sensitive history of things, objects, and their evolutionary design, and of the anthropological way to their uses over time [17], with transformations of human behavior. In the contemporary world, the cultural sporting trait has intensified as a social identity, including services and diverse products, in distinct fields of society that promote the sensation and/or perception of added comfort [8, 16].

Our body is an information center and on it clothes act as a declaration of freedom, of expression, of individuality. In this complex system, the brain processes sensory signals and formulates a subjective perception of individual sensations, based on past experiences and individual preferences, defined from physical, sociocultural, emotional, and environmental aspects [8]. These physical and psychophysiological sensations can determine the perception of comfort, which responds to "a pleasant state of physiological, psychological and physical harmony between the human being and the environment" [8].

On the other hand [8] defends the psychological dimension of comfort that values solutions in health area, aesthetics and beauty reinforce the cult of the body as a sociocultural process, [13] besides the cultural notion of health through care with the body that has intensified, and the number of academies that have multiplied, as well as the number of fans to the most active and accelerated lifestyle. The contemporary society is characterized by the intensified practice of physical activities and is adept to the "Fitness" style. This notion runs counter to the notion that "comfort, perceived as a mode of rest and even of laziness, tends to be regarded as a factor of action, thus avoiding the sterile dissipation of physical forces and subaltern activities, but favoring by this way a maximum activity of the properly human faculties" defended by [2].

However, in a broad analysis of the language of the body [18], affirm that "man is a highly perceptible being" (…), and that therefore "to live is to perceive." According to the authors, there are old perceptions and recent perceptions, and it can be concluded that contemporary man has developed his perception more acutely, culturally, throughout his evolution, distinguishing between what causes him discomfort, and what doesn't make you uncomfortable; between what gives him pleasure, and what causes him displeasure in the form of discomfort. They also complement that every change in the physiological state of an individual determines a change in the mental-emotional state, and the reciprocal one is equally valid. The human perception about the reactions of the body in its evolution demonstrates that "the human being is physiologically 'tuned' to distinguish between harmony and disharmony [18]. The rule serves to demonstrate, in a simplistic way, that the perception described by the authors, registers contrary the sensations, therefore there is a subjective identification of well-being or malaise, satisfaction or dissatisfaction. These descriptions define the original meaning of the word comfort, to strengthen, comfort, alleviate and soften, generating greater sense of satisfaction and protection against annoyances. In this way, the more or the less satisfactory welfare (in sports practice) reciprocates, that is, compensates for the perception of ultimate (psychological) comfort.

The authors referenced in [8], as well as [15], emphasize that the perception of comfort meets the harmonization of clothing and body, providing comfort, mobility, safety and welfare. The brain points to the final perception after the physical and physiological process add to the psychological/emotional, determining the relationship between object/clothing and environment × body and skin relationship, which finally indicates a situation of comfort or discomfort [8].

Considering the factors that involve the perception relationship of the ergonomic system created between the user-object-environment triangle, these aspects must be in a greater degree of agreement or disagreement with each other, not only in the relation between user and object, but also in the relation and interaction between them and the environment [19].

The internet allows for the diffusion of opinions without scientific or professional background, where bloggers, youtubers, personalities and social media users show their personal visions of comfort, style, security, and performance based on their lifestyle and products that complement this style. in most of the posts. In a way, the lack of groundwork of these influencers ignores the importance of comfort and well-being that are appropriate for the distinct biotype of each person. The practice immediately reaches a young and mass audience, which tends to assimilate information. In the case of the mature segment of users this does not occur. here is also a lack of specificity and adequacy of identity for this group of users, where functions such as utility, safety and purpose of each product proposal are not adapted to their physiological, physical limitations, body limitations, and skin sensitivity. As well as psychological and emotional expectations.

Based on this principle, a questionnaire study was proposed to delimit the expectation of these individuals. The demand for the suggested segment was confirmed and the specific questionnaire questions were made related to comfort, comfort perception, product profile, style, fashion, performance, and other specificities that gave rise to the final content were formulated. Specific comfort, performance and aesthetics were the essential focus addressed in the article, although the other items correlated with them helping their understanding. The analysis sought to define the aspects to be observed to compose the proposal of sportswear products, offered by the retail and sportswear market to the age group from 45 years, considering the perception of comfort, well-being, performance, and style. The prerogative was to identify the specificities and the class of products that meet the real needs and expectations of these age groups.

Due to changes and declines in physical strength and tone, the profile of users, of both genders, may be more conservative, accommodating and much more demanding. The attainment of longevity involves complex issues related to well-being, safety, prevention, preservation, guarantees acquired with healthy habits, which will not be addressed in this article. Therefore, aspects such as comfort and perception of comfort of the products have become fundamental within the expectations of the users for the profile of security, prevention and guarantees.

The analysis presented in this article was restricted to identifying the expectations, satisfaction, or absence of this, of the segment of this age group with the sportswear products made available by the market and list the characteristics and specificities desired or predominant preference.

## 5   Presentation and Analysis of Results

The evaluation was restricted to researching the Brazilian population over 45 years old, since the main geographic area of research in the region of the state of São Paulo, profile and determine the demand of mature users over 45 years of age, the specific questionnaire aimed at users to discriminate aspects that are desired by this target audience, which are based on available product offerings in the market, and identify what is not being offered. The form was submitted online, and was answered by a sample of 77 people, respecting the age group between 45 and 80 years. The sample shows 65.5% female subjects and 35.5% male subjects. Relatively, 70% are married, 12% are divorced, 6.8% are single or in non-formal unions, and 4.5% are widowers. It was verified that 94.8% of the sample performed physical activities.

As for the socioeconomic profile of the sample group, it is formed by financially stabilized individuals who are still an active part of the population or retirees with personal income, who make up the portion of the population that enters the third age, and with a certain financial reserve. In this way, the profile of users analyzed in this study corresponds to a middle-class public.

The survey questions prioritized the aspects and motivation of leisure time leisure practices, and the diagnostic descriptions about the perception and need for comfort, style and performance that are part of their expectations. By the qualitative character associated to the quantitative, several questions allowed more of an alternative of answer, selecting all the options that helped to define in a wide form the diverse practices of exercises in the leisure and all the possible choices between the expectations of the users. The results and details of the profile obtained will be described below.

The research revealed that in Brazil the main reasons for the practice of free time activities occur for 70% of people analyzed for prevention (self-prevention), followed by leisure or hobby with 25%. Only 15% practice exercises to socialize and interact socially. About 30% exercise because of medical advice. It is important to point out that the same person can exercise for more than one reason, as shown by the analysis of the answers obtained.

Walking was the predominant activity for 71% of those who participated in the research, confirming previous data of Fig. 1, as well as gymnastics/Fitness Center was the second most common activity for the group analyzed, with 40% of the answers followed of cycling, which positioned itself in third place, as a mobility and leisure activity, in addition to preventive and beneficial exercise, with 28% of the answers. In these cases there was also the possibility that more than one item could be indicated by the respondents. Recalling that the analysis presented here focuses specifically on the evaluation of the clothing used in physical activities performed during the individuals' free time, in order to obtain quality of life. The perception of comfort is confirmed as the most important feature, and in an essential aspect, for the selection of clothing aimed at the practice of physical activity, among users in the age group from 45 to 80 years. Its relevance is absolute, being the option chosen by the majority of the respondents, in all the questions that indicate aspects, such as: physiological, sensorial, psycho-aesthetic, ergonomic. Products intended for these users are characterized by choices that preserve comfort and essential aspects that promote physical and emotional well-being, and which reflect the preservation of the health status and the life-style achieved.

The scale of importance of the aspects that this public considers essential in the decision about the expectation and adequacy of clothing characteristics for this purpose. "Comfort" is considered to be an essential aspect for about 30% of respondents, comfort associated with well-being, followed by aesthetic and beauty aspects in 26% of responses. This tendency becomes much more evident when specifically asked about the importance of comfort compared to "aesthetic/beauty aspects" and other aspects as options to be considered in choosing a specific product to be acquired for the purpose of physical activity here. Comfort accounted for 91.7% of respondents' preference. "Aesthetic aspects and beauty" reached 6,9%. "Comfort and well-being" come first as a fundamental aspect of sportswear.

The graphics indicate a great importance for the perception of comfort and the specific comfort by this class of users. The numbers for comfort, within the question directed between comfort and beauty, far outweigh the need for aesthetic and/or fashion attributes within the individual's social posture in choosing the sport/fitness product for the purpose of physical exercise in time free. The numbers show that the physical and physiological well-being ensured that the emotional and psychological sensation of physical and psychic security within the limitations of the ages is enhanced. This is confirmed in the three questions represented by three images, Figs. 2, 3 and 4.

In another question, several specificities were delineated, and the determinants for the users in the choice of sports fashion apparel again emphasized comfort and well-being - now associated with the sensorial perception of softness of the fabric - thermal control of the fabric, control of sweat and odor, practicality of use and washing, and tissue technology in favor of performance in the exercises. Importance selection

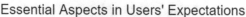

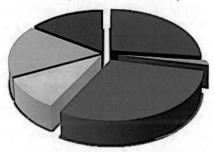

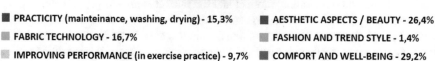

■ PRACTICITY (mainteinance, washing, drying) - 15,3%    ■ AESTHETIC ASPECTS / BEAUTY - 26,4%

■ FABRIC TECHNOLOGY - 16,7%    ■ FASHION AND TREND STYLE - 1,4%

■ IMPROVING PERFORMANCE (in exercise practice) - 9,7%    ■ COMFORT AND WELL-BEING - 29,2%

**Fig. 2.** Essential aspects in the selection of clothes for the practice of physical activity. Author's chart (2018).

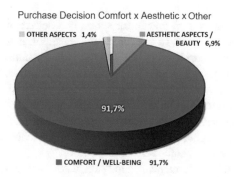

**Fig. 3.** Expectation in the purchase decision between comfort × aesthetic aspect/beauty × other aspects. Authors Charts, 2018.

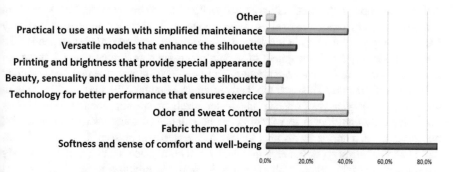

**Fig. 4.** Specificities for the mature user in sportswear/fitness clothing. Author's chart, 2018.

demonstrates that aspects of "fashion", trends, prints, or fashion-style modeling for these products are unwanted or relevant, as well as sensuality and necklines. It is important to define that the "aspects of aesthetics and beauty", as previously shown in Fig. 3, are distinct from "aspects of fashion" or "fashion trends". Therefore, a contemporary and balanced design with elegant modeling and aesthetic beauty is desired among the complementary features. Conclusively, the sensorial aspects stand out in the choices of this public as "softness", "comfort feeling" and "well-being", "thermal control" of the fabric, "sweat control", "technological aspects" and those that add better performance and practicality.

People can convey their image through the clothing they wear is essential for the decision to purchase a clothing product and the market is able to provide clothing that meets these expectations becomes essential in a market with great sales potential. About 24% of people indicated they did not like the clothes they found to get at the outlets, or those they observe in other physical activity practitioners. That is, it is identified that the expectations of individuals over the age of 45 years are not being met.

## 6  Final Considerations

The perception of comfort in garments for sports is a determining factor for the vast majority of users over 45 years of age, as shown by the research presented, and this public cannot fail to be considered by the apparel industry under penalty of losing an enormous consumer market that only tends to grow. This group, which presents itself as actively productive, values the well-being and the quality of life, provided by the practice of physical exercise and a healthier life, but also value the comfort and safety of the clothing during these practices. Contrary to expectations, for this public, interest in fashion was not the highest priority requirement in the choice of clothing when it comes to practicing physical activities.

"Specific comfort," "performance," and "satisfactory aesthetics/aesthetic balance," are considered to be complementary factors of interest that must maintain the essence of the purpose of improving and facilitating physical, sensory, and physical exercise and well-being. Thermal, resulting in pleasant and comforting sensations. For this group, technological features add value to the products and are welcomed as well as user interest. Aspects of softness, softness, adequate temperature management, odor and perspiration reduction, all welfare technology were also highly valued in sportswear/fitness products. Exercise practitioners and athletes demonstrate that they are increasingly demanding in this regard, regardless of their age group and gender. To create the identity for this segment of people, items such as lightness, good sweating, flexibility, odor control and perspiration, and compression are essential because they enhance performance. This was another highlight, obtaining the best performance in the exercises, higher performance and better reach of specific comfort levels. New fibers certainly contributed to widening the boundaries of using sportswear products, but the main demand is to respond clearly to the needs expressed. Concepts of simplified and balanced style, but technological, good color selection and modeling satisfy the segment over 45 years. In short, a specific range of products to meet the specific, physical or physiological specificities of belonging and social identity of this mature, ageless, urban and long-lived society.

**Acknowledgments.** The authors thank the Foundation for the Support of the Research of the State of São Paulo – FAPESP, through Process N° 11169-4 FAPESP, for the support provided to carry out this research.

# References

1. Soares, C.L.: As roupas nas práticas corporais e esportivas: a educação do corpo entre o conforto, a elegância e a eficiência (1920–1940). Autores Associados, Campinas (2011)
2. Soares, C.L.: Elegantemente vestida: A Educação do Corpo Feminino e as Roupas Esportivas (1920–1940). Labrys Êtudes fêministes. https://www.labrys.net.br/labrys20/brasil/carmen. htm (2012)
3. Guiselini, M.: Aptidão Física, Saúde, Bem-Estar: Fundamentos Teóricos e Exercícios Práticos, 2a edn. Phorte Editora, São Paulo (2006)
4. Eu Atleta. In: Globo.com. Globo Esporte Saúde. Criador do método Cooper diz que só exercício físico não garante a saúde, 27 October 2015 (2015). http://globoesporte.globo.com/eu-atleta/saude/noticia/2015/10/criador-do-metodo-cooper-diz-que-so-exercicio-físico-não-garante-saude.html
5. Exame: Revista Exame. Um Mundo Mais Velho e Melhor- Edição Especial Longevidade. novembro 2013, Ed. 1053, Ano 47, N° 21 (2013). http://exame.abril.com.br/revista-exame/um-mundo-mais-velho-e-mais-forte/
6. Sebrae: Portal Sebrae. Potencialidades da Moda Fitness (2015). http://www.sebrae.com.br/sites/PortalSebrae/artigos/potencialidades-da-moda-fitness.cfe06b9049e3f410VgnVCM1000004c00210aRCRD
7. Ministério Do Esporte: A prática de esporte no Brasil. Diagnóstico Nacional do Esporte (2015). http://www.esporte.gov.br/diesporte/2.html
8. Broega, A.C., Silva, M.E.C.: O Conforto Total do Vestuário: Design para os Cinco Sent dos. Universidade do Minho, Guimarães, Portugal (2009)
9. Crane, D.: A Moda e seu Papel Social – Classe. Gênero e Identidade das Roupas, Editora Senac (2006)
10. Gardenal, Isabel: Quando a roupa educa o corpo. Docente conta a história da introdução do vestuário para a prática esportiva, 8 a 14 de nov. – Ano XXIV – No 480. Jornal da Unicamp: Campinas (2010)
11. Moore, S.C., et al.: Leisure time physical activity of moderate to vigorous intensity and mortality: a large pooled cohort analysis. PLoS Med. **9**(11), e1001335 (2012) 6 November 2012. United Kingdom: University of Cambridge, http://dx.doi.org/10.1371/journal.pmed.1001335
12. Vigetel Brasil 2016 - Vigilância de Fatores de Risco e Proteção de Doenças Crônicas Por inquérito telefônico. Ministério da Saúde (2016). http://portalarquivos.saude.gov.br/images/pdf/2017/junho/07/vigitel_2016_jun17.pdf
13. PNUD 2017- Programa das Nações Unidas para o Desenvolvimento - Relatório Nacional de Desenvolvimento Humano do Brasil 2017 - Cap. 4. (United Nations Development Program – Brazil's National Human Development Report 2017- Movement is life! Physical and Sports Activities for all people (2017). http://movimentoevida.org/

14. Sebrae Mercados. Portal Sebrae. Moda Fitness Mercado em Ascenção no Brasil (2014). http://www.sebraemercados.com.br/wp-content/uploads/2015/10/2014_08_04_BO_Maio_ Moda_ModaFitness_pdf.pdf
15. Simmel, G.: Filosofia da Moda e outros Escritos. Ed. Texto & Grafia Lda, Lisboa (2008)
16. Schmid, A.L.: A Ideia de Conforto: Reflexões sobre o ambiente construído. Pacto Ambiental, Curitiba (2005)
17. Barcellos, E.E.I., Mercaldi, M., Landim, P.C., Botura Jr., G.: De Redig ao P&D: A Trajetória da Abordagem da Antropologia no Design. In: Proceedings of the IV International Conference on Design, Engineering, Management for Innovation IDEMI 2015, Florianópolis, pp. 527–540 (2015)
18. Weil, P., Tompakow, R.: O Corpo Fala: a linguagem silenciosa da comunicação não verbal. Ed. Vozes, (2001)
19. Slater, K.: The assessment of comfort. J. Text. Instit. **77**(3), 157–171 (1986)

# Design and Research of Health Aids Based on App in the Elderly

Yu Zhao[(⊠)], Xiaoping Hu, and Delai Men

South China University of Technology,
Guangzhou University City, Panyu District, Guangzhou, China
40280919@qq.com, mendelai@scut.edu.cn

**Abstract.** As the current demographic structure changes and the world's aging population gradually increases, the elderly population has a higher risk of being ill and the health problems of the elderly should draw wide public concern. Older people are groups that need special attention from people. Nowadays, the rapid development of medical science and technology is not a problem. However, elderly people have begun to degrade their memory and memory. Elderly people can not take medicine on time and forget the doctor's advice, thus failing to achieve the desired recovery effect. Therefore, how to make the elderly better self-rehab and maintain their health remains to be studied. In the era of mobile information, medical, diet, tourism and other application terminals come into being, providing more platforms for the health of the elderly. However, the target group for the design of health-care apps for the elderly is the elderly, which requires that the products The function and form should be different from the general app, so how to design health-care app for the elderly is of great significance to the entire elderly population. This article combines the experience of the elderly to design a specific analysis of how to make the elderly healthy living and maintaining a healthy app. The purpose is to remind the elderly to urge medicine on time, rest on time, eat rationally and help plan and do a healthy lifestyle. This article begins with a discussion of the health needs of the elderly. Based on the status quo of health-care apps in the elderly, this article discusses in depth the design of a health-care app that meets the cognitive characteristics of the elderly. To study the influencing factors such as the physiological characteristics, psychological characteristics and cultural characteristics of the elderly, to find out the difficulties in designing the app for the elderly, and finally to discuss the cognitive behavior of the elderly using the mobile phone. The overall design combined with the elderly physiology, psychology, cultural factors for design. Awareness of the elderly aspects of degradation The problem of providing more systematic and targeted design principles and methods from the aspects of icons, text, keys, colors, interface typesetting and interaction processes. According to the above points to seek reasonable and effective app to promote the health of older adults to restore the design.

**Keywords:** Elderly · Health supplementary · App design

© Springer International Publishing AG, part of Springer Nature 2019
N. J. Lightner (Ed.): AHFE 2018, AISC 779, pp. 367–372, 2019.
https://doi.org/10.1007/978-3-319-94373-2_40

# 1   Introduction

## 1.1   The Analysis of the Status Quo of Elderly Health Assistance App

With the development of society, new changes have taken place in the population structure and the trend of population aging has become increasingly evident. The aging population has brought many new problems and challenges to society. With the increase of the elderly population, the prevalence of the elderly population is also on the rise. The medical care in the community is also constantly improving. Elderly people's medical care is guaranteed. However, due to their own functions and psychology, memory and the surrounding environment The factors that affect their health and life will still be affected.

As the population ages, science and technology are also evolving. In particular, the rapid development of the Internet has led to many kinds of terminals in the areas of medical care, health, and life. Various kinds of app have infiltrated all aspects of people's lives In today's information society, the elderly should also enjoy better the fruits of scientific and technological progress, linking the mobile Internet with the elderly so that they can better serve the elderly, especially the elderly who are sick They are in a slow recovery period after their illness or treatment. It is a common phenomenon that memory loss is a common phenomenon. Many things require the reminder of others, and their children are too busy with work to take care of the full scale and thus affect their normal recovery. In this context, the design and study of a app for the elderly health aids is an important issue.

As a new industry, app has broken through the traditional single communication function of mobile phones and brought artificial intelligence closer to life. This has brought us a new approach to solving problems that can help to develop smarter seniors' health through big data processing solutions Auxiliary app, a broader aspect of participation in the elderly service system. However, at present, the research field of app for health care for the elderly is still at an initial stage. Currently, such app operations are too complicated or too single in function to be acceptable to young people. However, the elderly in general can not adapt to such changes in mobile phone products Sexual development. Some of the current research and design have not yet taken full account of the mental health of senior citizens, psychological needs and cognitive behavior.

## 1.2   The Significance of Design and Purpose

Based on the current status of app, this study intends to explore its content based on the cognitive behavior, psychological needs and physical function of the elderly. By analyzing and studying such existing app on the market, Deficiencies in this area, to supplement them, aims to provide a good user experience environment for the elderly, as well as to better promote the physical and mental health of the elderly and promote more people involved in the activities of caring for the elderly, At the same time, it also provides a theoretical basis for app for health care for the elderly to promote the development of the whole field.

The purpose of this study is to investigate the elderly's expectations and goals, to find out their specific needs by actually investigating the elderly's understanding of the status of this type of app and the actual use of the disease and elderly patients, and then by analyzing the existing app Interface design, combined with the elderly psychological needs and physiological needs, provide a clear idea.

## 2  The Concept and Type of Health Aids App

Now people-oriented concept has been involved in all aspects of life, of course, the design field is even more so, the purpose of design to facilitate more conducive to human beings, human needs must be the ultimate goal of design, so that human beings experience a more warm care. With the continuous improvement of the times and the rapid development of science and technology, smartphones and networks have become commonplace. The general improvement of people's living standard makes people more desire for health knowledge. Meanwhile, the information age, the development of mobile terminals such as smart phones increase the transmission of health knowledge. In this environment, smart phones and mobile networks Combining the health apps produced has the potential to grow. Although healthy app is rapidly developing, apps for the elderly are few and far between.

Health Aids apps are third-party applications for smartphones or wearables that help users document features such as analyzing health data, guiding a healthy exercise diet, and leading a healthy lifestyle. This shows that the classification of such app is varied. Generally divided into a few: First, the data recording app, app relatively simple function, based on the user's exercise to form a data analysis, the final feedback to the user, which users can see their daily exercise. The second is the information consulting app, the function of such app is: After the user input data and related information will appear the corresponding answer, after entering their own health problems can self-diagnosis, you can also ask the experts, or to recommend appropriate Hospital or medicine. The third is the health plan app. The main function of such app is to formulate a reasonable sport plan and diet plan for the data input by the experience groups. Fourth is the diagnostic app, such app is equivalent to an online hospital, but generally charge a fee, so the usage is not high.

At present, there are mainly four kinds of health aids in China. Although these four kinds of app are relatively complete in function, their applicable population is mainly young and middle-aged people. Many elderly people have difficulties in their operation. What kind of app Health Supplement app Suitable for the elderly remains to be studied.

## 3  The Elderly Health Assistance App Problems

The rapid development of the current app, a wide range of app research and development although considering the user groups, but to be exhaustive or there is a certain gap. Some needs of the user groups are still not met, and there are still some problems in the AHA for app: 1, Homogenization of Content Function: The ever-increasing content of app has caused many developers to borrow or copy existing apps, Their own characteristics, there is no fresh features, users experience different products to obtain what is no difference; 2, the health data is not accurate: due to the phone hardware problems, or the phone is not around or app own problems and app record data and The fact does not match and thus can not be resolved accordingly; 3, the credibility of information content is low: Now many of the app developers for profit for the purpose, in the context of health knowledge does not have developed the product, many of the content is online 4, the function is relatively simple: the user experience the product is to solve the practical problems, and some app's function can only system record, the mechanical feedback user's Problems, different ways to get the same answer is that users do not get a better experience.

## 4   The Elderly Health Supplement App Need to Have What Functions

Currently there are many health apps on the market, but very few for the elderly, and those for the elderly health app function is too simple, content is similar, or deliberately guide the behavior of consumer spending, then a good old age health care app should have what function?

The first is the most basic answer function: to help users find a solution to the user input problems. Then such app should be a specific hospital as the background, to link the field hospital is the focus, so you can increase the user's identity. At the same time, for the elderly to reduce the physiological function designed to remind users to rest on time, taking medicine, exercise and other functions; according to the user's body to develop their own diet and health campaign. There will be a simple self-testing system, push health tips and other content, as well as prevention of disease teaching, appointment doctor's functional design. In order to reduce the logical thinking ability of the elderly, the design should be properly guided by the steps that are likely to make the elderly understand the obstacles in the design, such as the information prompts for the operation mode and the operation purpose; the operational feedback and the like to help the elderly to improve the operation The purpose of forming a sense of identity, can have a clear understanding of their physical condition.

## 5   Design and Analysis of Aged Health Aid App Interface

Elderly people may experience fear when encountering unexpected situations or encountering difficulties. Therefore, they should be given feedback in every aspect of their interface operations, such as visual, tactile and audible, so that they can understand clearly what they are doing Whether they are correct and effective can reduce their psychological burden when using the product.

### 5.1   Physiological Level Analysis

As we grow older, there will be a series of changes in the human body. Citizens over the age of 60 in China are collectively referred to as the elderly, and the physiological function of such people has already begun to degenerate, so the special physiological conditions of the elderly also affect the entire app interface design. First of all, the vision, the elderly will be a serious decline in visual acuity, and may also be accompanied by some diseases such as presbyopia, cataracts, etc. app interface design is mainly to convey information in visual language, which requires the elderly for health supplements app interface design should take full account of the layout of the interface, color, font size and other issues on the elderly impact; followed by the auditory sense, the sensitivity of the elderly decreased hearing, there will be physiological hearing impairment is a normal phenomenon, Consideration should be given to the size, comfort and identification of the app sounds; in the tactile sense, the skin of the elderly also changes, the sensitivity decreases, and the response becomes sluggish, so designing the app interface must also be considered The complexity of the interface operation, the operation of the reminder function.

## 5.2 Psychological Level Analysis

After entering the senile age with the changes in the human body have a psychological change, which also has an important impact on the app interface design. Forgetfulness is a common phenomenon in the elderly. It is closely related to the psychological factors. This phenomenon often causes the inferior groups to feel inferiority and self-confidence. In the meantime, with aging and recession of the brain tissue, anxiety, mood changes, depression, Paranoid and other psychological characteristics of the elderly are also often manifested as emptiness, excitement, the lack of a proactive approach to things. A survey shows that 48% of elderly outpatients with poor financial conditions have depression, while those with good health and economic conditions have depressive symptoms, 44%, and many people have monthly attacks once. Lasts for several hours or days, manifested as depression, worry, depression and anxiety, and more memories of the past have a sense of responsibility. Therefore, in the design of the app interface to take full account of the emotional needs of the user groups, appropriate to add some encouraging words, and to give users more sense of security.

## 5.3 Cultural Analysis

Elderly groups as a special group of their cultural factors can also cause different degrees of diversity. First of all, the concept is that seniors generally tend to be conservative and temporarily unacceptable to new things. In terms of cultural background, the elderly and young people are also different. In terms of health care, most elderly people would like traditional health regimens. For the traditional Chinese medicine Treatment and Western medicine treatment, the elderly groups will be more biased toward traditional Chinese medicine, which is inseparable from the growing environment and the accepted culture of the Chinese elderly. Therefore, the design of the app interface should pay attention to match the cultural background of the user experience, the language should be easy to understand, as much as possible to meet the needs of users.

# 6    Elderly Health Assistant App Interactive Design Analysis

The evaluation of an app interaction design is based on the content of the product and does not have a very accurate standard and method. The Elderly Health Assistants app user community is the elderly, and the interactive design of such apps has a significant impact on the user community.

Simplicity: The interaction process for the elderly should be as simple as possible, to be able to easily identify the operation, such as a simple click and slide is the most easy to grasp and operate the elderly.

Visualization: To achieve the interface is not only visible to the user content but also changes can be seen that many of the app's jump page in the process of opening or opening a blank, it is easy to cause the user's operating errors.

A key: the elderly will have unexpected situations too late to operate, a key for help, a key positioning can effectively handle such incidents.

Foolproof, Foolproof: As much as possible to remind and design under the conditions to ensure simplicity, users in the contact with new products and unfamiliar objects easily lead to fear of dare not to operate, so to help guide the user to avoid Wrong and confused.

Rectification: User error operation is normal, in the event of error operation, to promptly make reminders and guidance, error handling steps, the more the way to remind.

Assist Memory: Due to the memory loss in the elderly, such app should have the function of assisting memory. When the user inputs the information, it helps the user to record the information for marking or tagging so as to prevent users from having similar needs.

# 7    Conclusion

The aging of the world's population has become a hot topic, an inevitable phase of social development and a phase we are going through. Elderly groups are a special group to be concerned about. They should also enjoy the social changes brought about by the development of science and technology. Design is an important way to change the way they live. This article aims to analyze the current situation and problems of elderly health-care apps.

# References

1. Liu, L.: Status Analysis and Research of Health app. Technology world (2016)
2. Guo, X., Gong, M., Shu, H.: Mobile Health app Design Strategy for Elderly Patients with Chronic Diseases. Design (2017)
3. Zhang, X., Gu, L.: Medical app Information Architecture and Interface Design for the Elderly. Design (2015)

# Improving Mobile Interfaces for the Elderly

Ana Rebeca Araujo[✉], Eveline Sá, Ivana Maia, Karla Fook,
and Luíza Rosa

Federal Institute of Education, Science and Technology of Maranhão,
São Luís, Brazil
anarebeca.ar@gmail.com,
{Eveline,Ivana.Maia,Karladf}@ifma.edu.br,
lulibeatriz@hotmail.com

**Abstract.** The purpose of this research is to investigate how to improve accessibility in mobile interfaces for the elderly, considering the disabilities commonly acquired with age, such as reduced mobility and visual impairments. In this study, touch gestures, such as double tap and tap and hold, were analyzed to determine which gestures are recommended for applications aimed at elderly, and how written descriptions can improve their performances. Trials with a group of elders showed that this group performed better in interactions that used written descriptions instead of icons, and required longer touch gestures. The results suggest that implementing these factors in interfaces can make them more accessible to older users.

**Keywords:** Elderly · Human-computer interaction · Mobile interfaces

## 1 Introduction

In Brazil, as well as in other developing countries, people who are 60 years old or above are considered elders [10]. Worldwide, research indicates that the elderly population is increasing constantly [3, 14]. It is a diverse population, with different educational backgrounds, and sometimes contributing to the household income, or even retired and readapting to the domestic life [7].

Research also indicates that the social support received by elders, such as contact with friends and satisfaction with that contact, tend to decrease as they age, as well as the number of social relations [8]. Additionally, elders tend to feel isolated and socially excluded, and their social circles tend to be even smaller if they have low income [4, 8].

In addition, there are complications that result from the natural aging process, and may cause cognitive problems and affect the senses of the elderly. The first most common problem found in older people is vision impairments. This includes needing more light to distinguish objects clearly [5]. There are also changes in perception of touch, pressure and vibration, especially in the hands and feet because these parts slowly lose the sensitivity as the years go by [5]. Other problems include gradual hearing and motor coordination loss [8].

Despite their disabilities, research not only shows that elders are interested in interacting with technology, but are also active online [2, 4, 7]. Besides, the Internet

N. J. Lightner (Ed.): AHFE 2018, AISC 779, pp. 373–382, 2019.
https://doi.org/10.1007/978-3-319-94373-2_41

and technology can bring benefits to the elderly. These benefits include improving social life and contact with friends and family, and therefore decreasing feelings of loneliness [4, 8].

However, the elderly are usually overlooked as a target audience by developers because applications are generally aimed at mass populations and do not consider the individual needs of older users [1]. The lack of appropriate design forces older users to use technological products that are not specific for them, and can impact how they maintain their independency [1]. For that reason, it is important to consider the elderly when designing applications, and more specifically, mobile interfaces, in order to meet the needs of this population.

This research was structured to analyze how to improve mobile interfaces to elderly users, considering their special needs. The main aspects of interfaces considered were interface layout, and touch gestures supported by Android mobile phones. Additionally, trials were conducted with older users to evaluate the interface of two popular applications, Whatsapp and Telegram. Lastly, the results of the trials were used to propose orientations to the design of interfaces aimed at older populations.

## 2   Designing Interfaces for Older Users

The design of interfaces for older users must consider the fast evolution of mobile technology, and the new interactions methods that it supports. For example, in mobile phones, there are many touch gestures supported by different applications, such as tap, tap and hold, double tap and many more.

Research suggests that the touch gestures required to perform tasks must be as simple as possible, such as tapping and swipe [1, 6, 12]. However, by analyzing the touch gestures factor combined with other aspects of the interface, this research aimed to suggest additional approaches to designing interfaces of mobile applications for the elderly.

To study this interaction, the applications Whatsapp and Telegram were selected for experiments with elders. These two free applications have very similar interfaces in the Android platform (Fig. 1), and similar functions, which include sending images, text and voice messages [11, 13].

Another factor that lead to the choice of these applications is the design approach to certain functionalities. For example, to access the icon menu of delete, copy, and forward text in Whatsapp, it requires long pressing a message (Fig. 2). On the other hand, Telegram offers two ways of accessing a similar menu. One way is by long pressing a message, similarly to Whatsapp, and the second is through a quick tap on a message that will show a menu with written options instead of icons (Fig. 2). In the example shown in Fig. 2 the options displayed are reply, save to gallery, forward, edit and delete.

This particular difference between the two applications combines the aspects that were tested in the experiments, since not only the touch gestures could be evaluated, but also the use of words instead of icons in the menu. Furthermore, the experiments were elaborated to investigate if elders have any struggles regarding the touch gestures, also if writing the options in a special menu instead of using icons can improve their performances, and finally if the elders are comfortable with the layout of the applications.

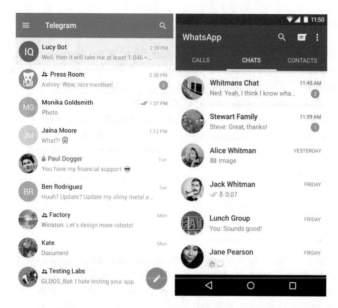

**Fig. 1.** Mobile interfaces of Telegram (*left*) and Whatsapp (*right*).

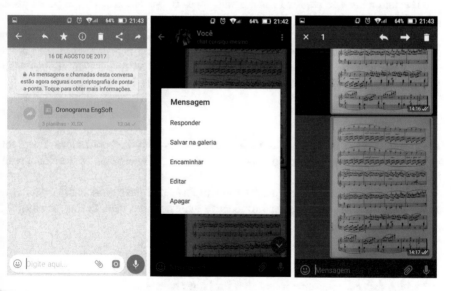

**Fig. 2.** Whatsapp icon menu (*left*), Telegram written menu (*center*) and Telegram icon menu (*right*).

# 3   Materials and Methods

One of the techniques available to evaluate interfaces is the data collection. Among the various approaches of this technique, we can highlight observation of users, interviews and questionnaires. Usually, questionnaires and interviews are used to gather the opinion of users, in either small or larger groups [9]. In the observation, the examiners can observe not only the problems that users face when using the application, but also the positive aspects of said application. In environments similar to laboratories, the examiner can have more control over the variables of the experiment, such as tasks performed, user's focus, and duration [9].

For this research, it was used a combination of these techniques. The events of the experiment are described below.

## 3.1   Participants

The participants of the trials were attending sessions at the Grupo de Pesquisa Velhice, Cultura e Sociedade (Research Group Aging, Culture and Society), which is a group that does volunteer work with elders, such as group therapy, choir practice, and other activities. The volunteers were selected for the study after one of their regular meetings. All of the participants live in, or close to, downtown in São Luís do Maranhão, near the place where the volunteer work happens.

The minimum age required for the study was 60 years olds, but the participants were all 65 and above. A total of 8 (eight) women volunteered for the study.

The educational background of the participants varied, some of them were able to read and write but others were illiterate. The technological background of the participants was more homogenous; even if some of them had had casual contact with smartphones before, they were unfamiliar with how to use it.

## 3.2   Materials

The materials used in the trials were Android phones with the applications Telegram and Whatsapp, and written questionnaires to evaluate the interaction of the elders with the interface.

Participants also signed a consent form to state that their participation was voluntary, and no data would be used to identify their personal identities in the study.

## 3.3   Design

The trials were structured to observe the interaction of elders with mobile interfaces, and which aspects affect that interaction for better or worse.

The aspects of the interfaces evaluated were icons, gesture interaction and button placement of the applications Whatsapp, version 2.17.323, and Telegram, version 4.3.0, in the default settings. The tasks performed by the participants were sending a voice message, answering texts individually, and deleting texts.

The evaluation of the interaction was measured by observation and application of questionnaires. The participants either handwritten their answers, or recorded them.

The experiment took place in the meeting room of the group, and the physical aspects of the environment did not impact the results of the experiment.

There were three examiners to perform the experiment individually with the volunteers. Each examiner had one set of the materials needed for the experiment.

## 3.4    Procedure

The examiners arrived at the meeting room where the group of elders was waiting. The examiners explained the purpose of the research, the consent form, and a brief overview of the experiment. Each examiner watched one participant at a time during the trial sessions that lasted between 25 and 35 min each. The examiners told the participants that they would be asked to perform three tasks on the phone, and then they would be asked some questions about their interaction. Participants also signed a consent form to state that their participation was voluntary, and no data from the study would be used to identify their personal identities.

Before asking the participants to begin the experiment, they were introduced to the applications that they would use. Briefly, it was explained how the applications work because most of the participants were unfamiliar with the applications. Then, the trials proceeded by having the participants perform the tasks, firstly on Whatsapp, then on Telegram. After performing the tasks, the participants answered the two questionnaires (Appendix A and B).

The participants were closely watched during the experiment and the examiners also took notes about the interaction.

## 4    Results

The results of the general questions questionnaire (Appendix B) show that the majority of the participants finds it difficult to recognize the shape of the icons, and consequently guess its meaning and/or function. They also reported that the interface does not give any visual clues about how to start using the application. Moreover, the tasks considered the most difficult ones required users to quickly tap the interface (typing, selecting texts, etc.), contrary to the tasks that required pressing the buttons for longer (sending a voice message. Below are the detailed findings (Figs. 3, 4, 5, 6 and 7) of the Questions per task questionnaire (Appendix A).

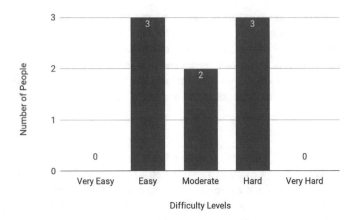

**Fig. 3.** Difficulty levels when performing the task. (Source: Authors' collection)

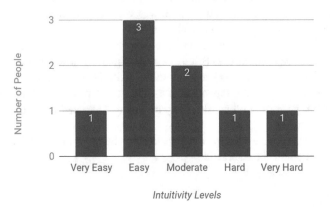

**Fig. 4.** Intuitiveness of the task. It was explained to the participants that the intuitiveness asked here was regarding the actions needed to perform the task, and if they considered the actions easy to identify and perform. (Source: Authors' collection)

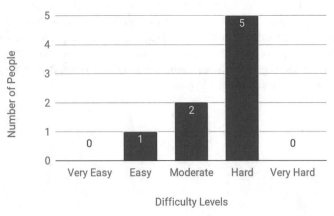

**Fig. 5.** Buttons' layout. The characteristics of the layout that the participants were asked about were size and position in the screen, which they considered difficult to interact with. (Source: Authors' collection)

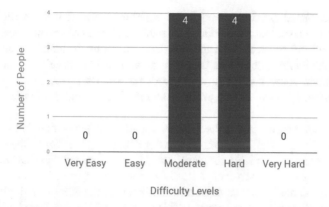

**Fig. 6.** Meaning of icons. It was observed in the experiment that the participants found the buttons confusing and could not easily memorize the function of the buttons. (Source: Authors' collection)

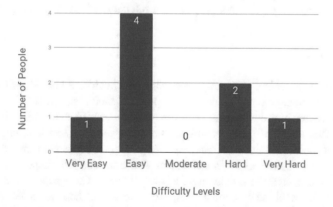

**Fig. 7.** Writing X Icons. 62.5% of the participants said that the tasks were easier to perform in the application that provided the written description of the functions (Telegram), instead of using only icons (Whatsapp). (Source: Authors' collection)

## 5 Discussion

As expected, the participants had trouble identifying the functions of the buttons through the icons. This is most likely due to their unfamiliarity with mobile phones. Although the study was originally designed to participants with some technological background, the people who volunteered did not have regular contact with Android phones. This could indicate that interfaces are not designed to "new older users", and therefore could potentially prevent them from trying to interact with technology. To add to that hypothesis, in informal conversations with the participants, they said that most of the family members who lived with them had smartphones, but they were averse to using the phones due to fear of breaking the device or not learning how to use it.

One unexpected trend observed in the experiment was that the participants performed better in tasks that required long pressing an element of the interface. This trend appeared as a surprise because the authors consulted during the literature review did not mention it. Additionally, based on the observation, it can be speculated that users were trying to obtain some kind of physical feedback similar to the feeling of pressing physical button, but were unable to since the interface has buttons drawn all over the screen.

An interesting outcome was the fact that not all participants thought the interaction with the written menu of Telegram was easier than using the icons. Since the participants did not find recognizing the icons easy, it was expected that they would prefer reading the function of each icon instead of trying to guess it. However, a possible reason for this could be that some users were illiterate, therefore would not be able to identify the options in the written menu. This aspect would benefit from being analyzed again, with a group of literate participants.

Lastly, it was observed that the participants were very interested in learning about the smartphones once the examiner helped them overcome their fear of damaging the device. It shows that this population wants to enjoy the benefits of technology, but the its newness creates a barrier that prevents the interaction from happening.

## 6  Conclusion

The population of elders is rapidly increasing worldwide. Although willing to use technology and being already active online, physical factors prevents older users from fully experiencing the advantages of using smartphones in their daily life, such as improving their social life and becoming more independent. Therefore, improving the interfaces of mobile applications can help elders interact better with mobile phones.

Two positive aspects of the interfaces of Telegram and Whatsapp noticed in this study are the long pressing gesture and the written menu. These aspects can be used to improve interfaces of other applications, either to adapt them to older users, or to develop new applications aimed at this audience. By implementing these aspects, developers help the elderly population improve their performances on mobile phones and decrease the frustration of not being able to interact with technology that can significantly enhance their quality of life.

Future research on this topic can explore how to make icons more understandable for the elderly, especially those with limited educational background.

To conclude, implementing written menus in applications, and adapting interfaces to require more long pressing gestures are simple ways of improving mobiles interfaces for the elderly.

**Acknowledgments.** To Federal Institute of Education, Science and Technology of Maranhão, and FAPEMA, for supporting this research.

## Appendix A: Questions Per Task

1. About the method required to perform the task (long pressing while speaking), how would you describe the task?
   ( ) Very easy ( ) Easy ( ) Moderate ( ) Hard ( ) Very Hard
2. About the task itself, how difficult was figuring out how to do it?
   ( ) Very easy ( ) Easy ( ) Moderate ( ) Hard ( ) Very Hard
3. About the positions of the buttons regarding the task, how difficult was finding them?
   ( ) Very easy ( ) Easy ( ) Moderate ( ) Hard ( ) Very Hard
4. About the meaning of the icons in the interface, how difficult is understanding their functions?
   ( ) Very easy ( ) Easy ( ) Moderate ( ) Hard ( ) Very Hard
5. About the written descriptions used instead of the icons, how difficult is using that option?
   ( ) Very easy ( ) Easy ( ) Moderate ( ) Hard ( ) Very Hard

## Appendix B: General Questions

1. What's your opinion about the application's icons?
2. Would you call this app "easy to use"?
3. How would you change the icon to make it easier to use?
4. Which task was the most difficult to do?
5. Is there any aspect of the interface (color, font, icons, button size, etc.) that bothers you?

## References

1. Abrahão, A.L.B.: Estudo de Acessibilidade e Interação Multitouch com utilizadores seniores. Master Thesis. Faculty of Science and Technology of Coimbra, Coimbra, Portugal (2013)
2. Alban, A., Marchi, A.C.B., Scortegagna, S.A., Leguisamo, C.P.: Ampliando a usabilidade de interfaces web para idosos em dispositivos móveis: uma proposta utilizando design responsivo. Novas Tecnologias na Educação 10, 1–10 (2012)
3. Business Wire. https://www.businesswire.com/news/home/20180223005691/en/Global-Bidets-Market—Smart-Bidets-Rise
4. Cardoso, R.G.S., Stefanello, D.R., Castro Soares, K.V.B., Almeida, W.R.M.: Os benefícios da informática na vida do idoso. In: Computer on the Beach 2014, Florianopolis, Brasil, pp. 340–350 (2014)
5. Farage, M.A., Miller, K.W., Ajayi, F., Hutchins, D.: Design principles to accommodate older adults. Glob. J. Health Sci. 4(2), 2–25 (2012)
6. Google. Usability: Accessibility. https://material.io/guidelines/usability/accessibility.html
7. Macedo, M.K.B., Pereira, A.T.C; Ambiente Virtual De Aprendizagem – Moodle: Voltado Ao Usuário Idoso. Conahpa, pp. 1–13 (2009)

8. Pires, A.C.S.T.: Efeitos dos videojogos nas funções cognitivas da pessoa idosa. Mater's thesis, Faculdade de Medicina da Universidade do Porto, Porto, Portugal (2008)
9. Prates, R.O., Barbosa, S.D.J.: Avaliação de Interfaces de Usuário - Conceitos e Métodos. In: Anais do XXIII Congresso Nacional da Sociedade Brasileira de Computação. XXII Jornadas de Atualização em Informática (JAI). SBC 2003(2003)
10. Santos, S.S.C.: Concepções teórico Concepções teórico-filosóficas sobre -filosóficas sobre envelhecimento, velhice, idoso e enfermagem ger envelhecimento, velhice, idoso e enfermagem gerontogeriátrica ontogeriátrica. Revista Brasileira de Enfermagem Reben **6,** 1035–1039 (2010)
11. Telegram, https://telegram.org/faq
12. W3C, https://www.w3.org/TR/mobile-accessibility-mapping/
13. Whatsapp Inc, https://www.whatsapp.com/about/
14. The Wall Street Journal. https://www.14.com/articles/elderly-in-u-s-are-projected-to-outnumber-its-children-for-first-time-1520967362

# Study on the Visual Experience of Senior People Shopping Website Interface

Xueying Mei[(⊠)] and Delai Men

South China University of Technology,
Guangzhou University City, Panyu District, Guangzhou, China
912378651@qq.com, mendelai@scut.edu.cn

**Abstract.** Based on the senses of seniors' visual experience, this study analyzes the relationship between visual effects, interaction effects and experience effects produced by shopping website interfaces which are arranged by different layouts and different colors. Summed up the elderly shopping site design system theory. With the help of relevant experiments, questionnaires and data statistics, this study combines the cognitive psychology of the elderly with ergonomics and other disciplines to systematically sort out the design principles of the shopping sites for the elderly and conclude a set of complete Senior shopping website interface design.

**Keywords:** Elderly · Interactive interface · Shopping website
Visual design

## 1 Introduction

### 1.1 Research Significance

The article takes the visual design of the interface as the starting point, combines the layout design of color and interface, and sums up the system theory of the visual design of the shopping interface of senior citizens through experimental analysis. And papers in the research project will ergonomics, cognitive psychology and other disciplines blend with each other in the study of the topic, on the one hand for the interface of the website provides a more careful design ideas and theoretical support, and such research for the design Advocated "human design concept" also provides some theoretical support. On the other hand, such a research method can make the design of this science and art more interdisciplinary more rational, for interdisciplinary design and research integration has a certain theoretical reference value.

Designing a website that better matches the visual experience of older people also increases the motivation of older people to use the internet. To enable the elderly better access to online counseling, more use of the network, you can add more fun to the elderly in their later years. More and more attention has been paid to the applicable design of the elderly, which has become an urgent task for improving the quality of life and quality of the elderly. In the face of the ever-increasing number of elderly users, shopping websites that are able to get satisfied and recognized by the elderly can bring

© Springer International Publishing AG, part of Springer Nature 2019
N. J. Lightner (Ed.): AHFE 2018, AISC 779, pp. 383–388, 2019.
https://doi.org/10.1007/978-3-319-94373-2_42

high returns to the network platform, get a better experience and better enable the elderly to improve their status.

## 1.2    Research Significance

**Social Status Quo.** Nowadays, there are an endless number of online platforms, and major online brands are also making their websites more detailed and diverse. However, most brands neglect the use of seniors, especially shopping sites. Older people do not want to use it is not convenient to use, the font is too small, too young products are the problem. Also need to distinguish font size, font. Most of the time spent on the Internet to learn and search on the Internet to experience the real convenience of the time but rarely. Psychologically, older people are more reluctant to accept new things, and thus can not expedite the network more conveniently. There are also some older people, who themselves accept new things, and are accustomed to using the Internet, but with age. Both visual acuity and reverberation have declined, making it difficult for the originally familiar websites to be used, so they have also gradually abandoned their use of the Internet.

**Research Status of Elder Shopping Websites.** In the increasingly serious environment of China's aging, the problem of aging has begun to be emphasized throughout the country. Especially in the design, product design, interactive design are introduced to the elderly as the center of the custom design. However, in the shopping site is still blank, the site search for shopping sites for the elderly, the results obtained only 8 and so on. And the only shopping sites for the elderly did not start from the needs of the elderly, from the overall interface layout to color matching are not very good old sticky shopping site features. There is also more to explore in the display and layout of merchandise. At the academic level, there are only about 10 papers on the shopping websites for the elderly as of 2015, which proves the extent to which this topic is to be developed. Overall, these essays are merely about the availability of shopping sites for seniors, and there is little practical guidance on a research level. Most stay at the forward-looking level

## 2    The Need for the Elderly Shopping Sites

### 2.1    The Current Situation of the Needs of the Elderly Website

From the characteristics of the elderly themselves, they learn the computer, surfing the Internet also has many advantages. Including the elderly retired at home, time is abundant, enough time to learn online access Seniors mental life is relatively monotonous, access to various services can be enjoyed after the Internet, greatly enriching life in old age Longing to understand the outside world and communicate the expression, the network provides access to Information window and online platform for the exchange of knowledge of the elderly quality and physical quality continues to increase, basic learning computer and Internet population large base of strong determination of the elderly, once there is a strong interest, can be more dedicated, devoted to learning, enthusiasm is high. In addition, surfing the Internet to enjoy the fun, online shopping, chat, send and receive e-mail, is conducive to physical and mental health, maintain a young mind.

## 2.2    The Need for the Elderly Shopping Sites

I analyzed several major shopping websites. In the board design, the traditional website to maximize the seasonal new products and discounted products to maximize the visual, so that users can see at a glance preferential goods. In the text editor, the main push product uses a larger font size and advertising fonts to highlight the product. Traditional bold characters are used in navigation and non-main items. In color matching, the main red, yellow, high-based pure, with white form the primary and secondary visual effects. In the navigation, some websites will recommend the navigation position of the commodity according to the user search volume, and will also arrange the classification according to the commodity purchase volume.

But their shortcomings are also obvious. Traditional shopping sites in the text editor, the use of font size, more consideration of young people's needs, with stylish font style to attract the eye. But older users find it hard to distinguish these words. In operation, the traditional shopping process is complex, but also in the selected goods on the basis of 4–5 steps in the operation, and there is no obvious reminder to prevent fraud and other signs, the elderly did not experience the shopping experience the actual protection.

## 2.3    The Advantages and Disadvantages of Traditional Shopping Website Interface Design

The increasing popularity of the Internet, the elderly learning and the use of the network is an inevitable requirement and trend, the elderly also want to be closer to the lives of young people. While meeting younger users, the Internet also needs to consider the needs of older users. The respect and care for the young are the traditional virtues of the Chinese nation. In addition to providing rich and substantial material security for the elderly, they should also enhance their spiritual life. The elderly should have access to appropriate education, culture, religion, entertainment and social resources to enhance their life satisfaction. The elderly population have special needs on the Internet. For example, they are not as quick and agile as they are when they are young. Therefore, they need to communicate with their relatives and friends through online shopping to understand the society. They are prone to feeling lonely. They also need to make friends in the online world and participate in the online community; They need to learn new knowledge, need to find all kinds of knowledge needed online, and participate in study and so on.

## 2.4    The Visual Focus of Older People Using the Internet

The visual ability of the elderly is weakened. Their visual receptivity is reduced; their basic functions include vision and depth of vision are also worse than those of young people; and their ability to recognize small objects is greater than that of large objects.

In addition, the processing speed of visual information has also been greatly reduced. visual attention has also been reduced to a considerable extent, and the visual attention of the elderly are more vulnerable to irrelevant stimuli. Increasing the illuminance of an object or improving the contrast between the object and its background can, to some extent, improve the visual acuity of the elderly.

Light color selection Scientific research shows that the elderly feel less on the color, for example, 60–70 years old color discrimination ability of young people is 76%. Elderly people often see colored objects as faded, experiments show that blue and green fade up, red fade at least. Relatively speaking, older people are more sensitive to warm light of longer wavelength, so the design is best to use warm yellow, warm white color. The use of such colors not only makes the elderly feel visually comfortable, but also because of warm colors, soft, so that the elderly psychologically produce a warm, pleasant feeling.

## 3   The Elderly Shopping Website Interface Design

### 3.1   The Elderly Shopping Website Interface Layout Design

In the overall layout and visual effects: to maintain the interface layout is concise, clear and consistent, so that older users can find the information they need more easily and not easily distracted. The visual area of older people becomes smaller, so the most important content should be placed near the center of the window in a conspicuous manner, such as larger fonts and prominent colors, avoiding placing important content on the right and the bottom; avoiding The use of floating windows and frequent flashing dazzling dynamic content, to avoid bouncing windows and multiple windows, otherwise it will seriously distract elderly users. Interface font size to be reasonable, too large fonts and relatively large line spacing is more appropriate. The need for important display of interface information, to highlight the way to performance, such as on the page center area or highlight the color, easy for elderly users to identify.

### 3.2   The Elderly Shopping Web Interface Text Editing

In the use of text: reduce the interface information density, give accurate information input prompts to improve the interface response speed and feedback capabilities. Must take into account the overall appeal of the text effect, space for different categories of text to be properly concentrated, and the use of blank to distinguish, older users with a clear visual impression; for ease of reading, text layout should be as simple as possible, similar to the magazine page Of the typesetting; To meet the visual characteristics of the elderly, should increase the color contrast of the text and background, and reduce the screen glare; text to 12–14 level appropriate, the title bolded; words should be used by the average user is familiar Words, and use easy language to avoid using unnecessary complex and abstract language; the text suggestions are expressed in a positive way and simple sentences are used.

### 3.3    The Elderly Shopping Site Image Editing Interface

In the use of images: the use of simple, symbolic or strong relevance icon, button design, reduce the memory burden on elderly users. The use of symbolic images can speed up the information retrieval of the elderly users. The use of images instead of words can reduce the memory burden of the elderly users. The images should be intuitively associated with the images and should pay attention to the consistency of the website images. The pixels of the image buttons should not be too small, Should be at least 25 pixels; important information can be emphasized with the help of the image; to design the right amount of dynamic images in the webpage can effectively attract the attention of the elderly users. However, to avoid the animation movement frequency should not be too large, otherwise it will reduce the elderly users Recognition ability. Design images, vivid images, pictures, improve the attractiveness of the interface information for the elderly.

### 3.4    The Elderly Shopping Site Interface with Color

In the use of color: the use of color should follow a uniform standard, to avoid the use of low contrast color and blue-green range of colors, to avoid small blue information; a large number of text content should not be brightly colored, should use more bright tones, To reduce the visual search time; the title suitabl.

### 3.5    The Elderly Shopping Site Design Interface Operation

In terms of ease of use: Fixed interface search box and navigation bar location, unified search box and navigation bar design and logic to reduce cognitive burden on older users. Window to avoid the use of scroll bars; drop-down menu does not meet the visual requirements of the elderly users, it is not suitable for older sites drop-down menu; radio button with the use of images, it is more easy for elderly users. In addition, the use of multi-list and list of expressions, so that elderly users can bring convenience. In the hyperlinks: to express the hyperlinks on the page clearly; the use of images instead of text hyperlinks, the image should be properly visual processing, to avoid making users think it is a general image and is ignored; in order to allow older users more easily identify the hyperlink, Before the hyperlink with a small image to emphasize the function of the link. To ensure the effectiveness of the link, the distinction between access and can not access the link, to reduce the elderly users do not expect the operation.

### 3.6    The Elderly Shopping Site Link Interface Design Needs

In the language expression of the usability evaluation of the shopping website interface, expressions that are valid include: timely response of the interface, accurate classification of the interface information, effective interface linking, prompt information or fuzzy matching information when the interface text is input. Therefore, when considering the design of the effectiveness of the shopping interface for the elderly, we should pay attention to the density and accuracy of the interface information, the usefulness of the interface interaction function elements and the input prompt information, and the changes and feedbacks of text, pictures and icons when interacting with the interface Timeliness and so on.

# 4 Conclusion

This article systematically summarizes the framework of the shopping website for the elderly by means of experiment and observation. Based on the use of online shopping, the article pays more attention to the experience of the elderly and gives the elderly more chances to enjoy and accept the internet.

The summary of the elderly shopping site design principles once applied to the specific practice of the project, I believe will provide useful theoretical guidance for the existing shopping site, so as to design more and better user experience. So that the elderly in the use of shopping site interaction more natural and more humane. It is expected that the design principles summarized in the text will also provide some guidance to other elderly website designs.

# References

1. Chattaraman, V., Kwon, W.-S., Gilbert, J.E., Soo, S.I.: Virtual agents in e-commerce representational characteristics for seniors. J. Res. Interact. Market. **5**(4), 276–297 (2011)
2. Hande, T., Altin, G.C., Elvan, B.A., Fethi, C.: The relative importance of usability and functionality factors for e-health web sites. Hum. Fact. Ergon. Manuf. Serv. Ind. (2013)
3. Bentler, P.M., Chou, C.P.: Practical issues in structural modeling. Sociol. Methods Res. (1987)
4. Cerella, J.: Information processing rates in the elderly. Psychol. Bull. (1985)
5. Kirakowski, J., Cierlik, B.: Measuring the usability of web sites. In: Proceedings of the Human Factors and Ergonomics Society Annual Meeting (1998)
6. Jeng, J.: What is usability in the context of the digital library and how can it be measured? Inf. Technol. Libr. (2005)

# The Study of O2O Urban Community Service Platform Design Based on the Elderly Demands

Yi Zhang[(✉)] and Delai Men

Guangzhou Higher Education Mega Centre,
South China University of Technology,
382 Zhonghuan Road East, Panyu District, Guangzhou 510006,
Guangdong, People's Republic of China
326087534@qq.com

**Abstract.** The aging trend with large-scale rapid growth,heightening the risk of the world's most populous country "getting old before getting rich". At the present stage, Elderly people live in residential communities are in the majority. Some old Neighborhood Communities due to have a large number of aged people, community activities become less, even community services and the infrastructure are also gradually decline. Most of the community service system is not perfect, and the existing system is only attached to the youth groups. What's worse, concerned about the design of the elderly are very few. Traditional communities due to lack of big data information, single service facilities, and low intellectualization, led to relatively orderless community management, and more and more elderly with negative interaction. Therefore, for the elderly who live in vacant rooms for prolonged periods of time, they have less social activity even do not exercise often. It's possible that the spirit is willing but the flesh is weak. Persist in so doing, their physical and mental health will be endangered gradually. The paper aims to explore the characteristics and needs of the elderly by combining the Maslow hierarchy of needs and propose a O2O community service system suitable for the elderly as well as a multi-directional vertical format combination mode, which benefits the elderly community in urban communities. Put forward an innovative community service system focused on the elderly, set up the online to offline smart community platform framework, and initially complete the online community service platform interface design. Insist on the people-oriented, improve the life happiness index of the elderly.

**Keywords:** The elderly demands · Urban community service platform
O2O · Innovative design

## 1 Introduction

According to statistics, in 2015, the population aged 60 and above reached 222 million, accounting for 16.15% of the total population. It is estimated that by 2020, the population of the elderly will reach 248 million, and the level of aging will reach 17.17%,

© Springer International Publishing AG, part of Springer Nature 2019
N. J. Lightner (Ed.): AHFE 2018, AISC 779, pp. 389–396, 2019.
https://doi.org/10.1007/978-3-319-94373-2_43

of which 30.67 million will reach the age of 80 or over; in 2025, the population over the age of 60 will reach 300 million and China will become super-aged countries [1].

On the one hand, with the aging development, the demands of social services for the elderly is on the rise; On the other hand, due to the increase of the only child, family model is getting smaller, empty-nest or living alone elderly are also increasing, gradually the traditional family pension function getting weakened. Therefore, to explore a sustainable development system that is multi-disciplined and participatory and compatible with the current economic level of our country is crucial to cope with the issue of aging.

In countries with a developed market economy, pay great attention to the community pension function, and community organizations and mass organizations have been organized and implemented in a concrete way. They proposed the "solar system" architectural pattern in residential design. To the elder house as the center, in the surrounding construction of medical services for the elderly, entertainment, learning, fitness facilities. Some countries have also set up "day care centers," sending the elderly to the center during the day and reuniting with their children at night. It not only solves the difficulties of children taking care of the elderly during their daytime work but also meets the spiritual needs of the elderly and their children. The unique advantages of community-based care meet the requirements of a market economy, also supplement the deficiencies of family pensions after changes in family structure.

Since the 1980s, the developed countries in Europe and the United States have started to implement the community care model and implemented the old-age pension policy by integrating various community resources in order to reduce the cost of supporting the elderly, improve the service quality and enhance the welfare of the elderly, so as to achieve the goal of active aging. In the late 1980s, the Chinese government promoted the development of community service through the introduction of various policies and pilot projects for socializing social welfare across the country. In 2010, there were 153,000 community service facilities nationwide, including 12,720 community service centers, 539,000 convenience and profit-making outlets, community service facilities coverage rate reached 22.4% [2].

Community-based pension model is imperative. With its unique advantages to help the elderly in community make a more convenient and healthy life. Today in the smart era, O2O community service platform can able to more in-depth services to the elderly.

## 2  Methods

### 2.1  Field Study

In order to have a range of targeted surveys, an old community in Luoyang, Henan Province which lived in many old people was to be visited. It is located in urban area, and there is a supermarket, many shops surrounding. Discover through field visits, this community has an independent neighborhood office and convenience center. That provides the basis for the study of this topic.

## 2.2    Questionnaire

This Study was to determine the urban Community Residents needs, demands and the daily behavior hobby of people older than 60 years; So, this questionnaire was prepared for the purpose.

A total of 50 elderly people over the age of 60 were randomly selected as the survey subjects. Interview with them through the survey, get some information about their needs for community-based services and the actual status of community services. Due to the age-specific interviewees, the questionnaire design is relatively easy to understand and conform to elderly.

## 2.3    Analysis

The collected data information was used for SPSS software analysis. Purpose to figure out the link through data.

# 3    Results

Statistics from the results of 51 valid questionnaires, there are 18 male investigators, 56% of the total; And there are 33 female investigators, 64.71% of the total. In order to facilitate the finishing analysis, the three age groups are divided. The elderly aged 60–70 accounted for 33.3%, aged 71–80 accounted for 37.25%, aged above 80 accounted for 29.41%. The data show that the elderly in this community have a high degree of aging.

## 3.1    Demographic

As shown in Table 1, the interviewed urban elders have a good level in education and personal income, which can improve their quality of life. From the survey situation, the vast majority of older people's monthly income is still relatively high, mostly in the 2000–3000 yuan. This may be related to the occupations that the old people were worked in before. According to the interviewed elders, they learned that their occupation is mainly divided into five types: worker, farmer, Government agency, Enterprise staff and Individual private. Among them, 45.1% of the total choose the Enterprise staff.

From the way of living, most elderly people choose home-based care, and only 3.9% of the elderly choose to live in community nursing home. Live with spouse accounted for 47.1%, on the one hand, it shows that the old couple live together and take care of each other more; On the other hand, also reflects the growing number of empty nesters. According to the statistics of Luoyang Aging Committee, among the 170,000 elderly over 60 in Luoyang City, the proportion of "empty nest" elderly people is nearly 40%.

More and more elderly concentrate on their health, according to the collected information, 82.1% of the elderly in good health, which pay more attention to medical and spiritual needs.

**Table 1.** The basic information of the subjects

| Characteristic | Categories | f | % |
|---|---|---|---|
| Education | Illiterate or rarely literate | 5 | 9.8 |
| | Primary to junior high school | 17 | 33.4 |
| | High school | 4 | 7.8 |
| | Secondary school | 18 | 35.3 |
| | College and undergraduate | 7 | 13.7 |
| | Total | 51 | 100 |
| Personal income | <RMB1000 | 4 | 7.8 |
| | 1000–2000 | 11 | 21.6 |
| | 2000–3000 | 15 | 29.4 |
| | >RMB 3000 | 21 | 41.2 |
| | Total | 51 | 100 |
| Career before retirement | Worker | 6 | 11.8 |
| | Farmer | 6 | 11.8 |
| | Government agency | 6 | 11.8 |
| | Enterprise staff | 23 | 45.1 |
| | Individual private | 5 | 9.8 |
| | Others | 5 | 9.8 |
| | Total | 51 | 100 |
| Way of living | Live alone | 12 | 23.5 |
| | Live with spouse | 24 | 47.1 |
| | Live with children | 13 | 25.5 |
| | Community Nursing home | 2 | 3.9 |
| | Total | 51 | 100 |
| Number of children | Only one | 6 | 11.8 |
| | Two or three | 36 | 70.6 |
| | Four and above | 9 | 17.6 |
| | Total | 51 | 100 |
| Physical health | Poor (need someone to take care) | 9 | 17.6 |
| | General (able to take care of themselves) | 28 | 54.6 |
| | Good (able to freely arrange life, entertainment, etc.) | 14 | 27.5 |
| | Total | 51 | 100 |
| Community service needs | Living needs | 11 | 21.6 |
| | Health care needs | 20 | 39.2 |
| | Cultural needs | 20 | 39.2 |
| | Total | 51 | 100 |

## 3.2   Elderly Demands

Correlation analysis was used to analyze the relationship between the health status of the elderly and their community service needs.

Correlation analysis is used to study the relationship between quantitative data, whether there is a relationship, the relationship between the degree of closeness.

The Pearson correlation coefficient is used to indicate the strength of the correlation. From the Table 2 shows that results the living needs and the Physical health which difference was significant ($p < 0.01$). This also shows that there is a negative relationship between the state of physical health and the living needs of the elderly. The worse the physical condition is, the higher the demands for community service of living. Also, there is a positive correlation between the state of physical health and the Cultural needs of the elderly. The better the body condition is, the higher the demands for community service of living.

**Table 2.** The study on correlation between elderly demands and Personal situation

| Characteristic | Categories | Value (p) | | |
|---|---|---|---|---|
| | | Physical health | Way of living | Personal income |
| Living needs | Housekeeping services | −0.545** | 0.245 | −0.262 |
| | Support home delivery supermarket | −0.576** | 0.236 | −0.268 |
| | Elderly canteen party | −0.561** | 0.234 | −0.281** |
| | Day-care nursery | −0.596** | 0.219 | −0.254 |
| | Daily life care | −0.576** | 0.236 | −0.268 |
| Health care needs | Home medical care | −0.028 | 0.080 | 0.114 |
| | Regular health care speech | −0.004 | 0.064 | 0.123 |
| | Accompanied by see the doctor | −0.005 | 0.042 | 0.121 |
| | Counseling | −0.003 | 0.045 | 0.163 |
| | Health care | −0.008 | 0.098 | 0.104 |
| Cultural needs | Entertainment (chess or painting class) | 0.495** | −0.272 | 0.100 |
| | Travel (regular group travel) | 0.496** | −0.262 | 0.079 |
| | Physical exercise (Health Consciousness) | 0.478** | −0.210 | 0.073 |
| | Legal Aid (lecture or meeting) | 0.460** | −0.202 | 0.055 |
| | Reading (communication) | 0.461** | −0.253 | 0.084 |

*$p < 0.05$ ** $p < 0.01$

# 4  Discussion

## 4.1  Demographic

From the information collected is not difficult to find that the elderly who lived in this community have a strong sense of health care because of the comfortable living standards they have had. And due to their generally higher literacy levels, there is also a high willingness to accept new things. The growing trend of empty-nesters has made them more in need of convenient living mode and mental care and attention. Therefore, a O2O community service system suitable for the elderly as well as a multi-directional vertical format combination mode, which benefits the elderly in urban communities.

## 4.2   Elderly Demands

The American psychologist Maslow first proposed the theory of the level of human needs in The Human Motivation Theory in 1943. Based on the hierarchy of needs of animals and human beings, Maslow divides the level of human needs from low to high into five levels: physiological needs, needs for safety, love or belonging needs, needs for respect, Self-actualization needs [3].

Economic income is the basis to meet the physiological needs, the degree of satisfaction of physiological needs depends on the level of economic income of the elderly. The main sources of life for Chinese elderly are retirement pensions and the support from other family members such as their children. It can clearly be seen that the level of economic income of the elderly, thus affecting the physical needs of the elderly to meet.

To ensure the safety of life and health are the most pressing needs of the elderly in terms of security needs. Closely related to this two areas are medical needs and health care needs of the elderly.

The advent of the silver age forced the number of empty nesters increased sharply, there are many problems with the emotional aspects of the elderly in our country. So, taking community as a platform, we should pay attention to the mental health of the elderly.

Similarly, older people also want recognition and respect, access to higher social status and self-respect. The simple wish of the elderly is that have a stable old life and maintain their prestige in the family. Make sure that they have the retirement pension, the medical care, the education chance and their own accomplishment and enjoyment.

The theory of social emotion selection suggests that the reduction of social network and social participation of the elderly should be regarded as the redistribution of resources by the elderly. Therefore, the construction of a community platform that can provide more entertainment activities, organize parties, home visits and other services for elderly is particularly important.

## 5   Design

### 5.1   App Function

In this paper, the interactive mobile platform design aim to meet the daily needs of the elderly, the community can integration all peripheral public resources. Integrate the vertical business resources available in the surrounding area and open up new online to offline community services. Put forward an innovative community service system focused on the elderly. Through the network platform to establish real-time contact, so that if the elderly need service, they can apply on the platform, then the service side can response timely.

The application set the main terminal has seven, User terminal (mainly for the elderly, children can also be used), community supermarket terminal, community hospital terminal, community housekeeping service terminal, neighborhood committees' terminal, elderly Activity Center terminal, and community volunteer terminal.

To meet the needs of living is the supermarket terminal, housekeeping service terminal and volunteer terminal to work together to complete. Community supermarkets and surrounding shops can send their products to homes for the elderly who cannot go out; housekeeping service centers provide on-site housekeeping services; and community volunteers can learn about the needs and help for the elderly through service systems.

The realization of the health requirement is the basis for the connection between the elderly terminal and the community hospital terminal. The services that community hospitals can provide to the elderly through service systems are regular reminders of elderly medical examinations, home-based treatment and psychological counseling services, as well as elderly people in distress and timely assistance.

The community should organize activities and provide opportunities for learning to enrich the lives of the elderly and timely send the latest activities information through the community service system to the elderly terminals. In addition, community volunteers can learn from the platform which elderly need to accompany, booking online and real-time implementation.

Different from the other, the highlight of this App features design is audiences are elderly, but elderly and their children both can be users. That will relief empty-nesters the sense of lonely, furthermore, make their children more concerned about their old parents.

## 5.2  Visual Interface Design

The design of the interactive interface used by the elderly should follow the design principles of barrier-free, including high contrast, consistent page layout, short text, large size and so on.

Taking into account the cultural level and operational ability of the elderly, the information input method avoids the typing as much as possible. More comprehensive option for the elderly to choose will be great, which corresponds to the option of merchandise with pictures, reducing the probability of error selection.

Last but not least, the elderly are having the problem with the motor impair, so their process of cognition is slower than the young people. This is important for the pictures lighting on screen do not fade too quickly. As far as possible to keep the picture still, and have a simple operation.

# 6  Conclusion

The aging issues arouse public concern, making the situation better needs the Multipart supporting. Only find the fundamental solution to solve the problem can get a good result. The O2O Urban Community Service Platform has a good future in China. The government pay more attention on and provides policy support will make the platform run better, serve for the elderly further.

# References

1. China Industrial Information. http://www.chyxx.com
2. National Bureau of Statistics of People's Republic of China: China Statistical Yearbook. China Statistics Press, Beijing (2011)
3. Liqiang, Z.: Probe into the needs of the elderly from Maslow's theory of demand. Nanjing, Jiangsu (2010)

# Postural Balance and Vitamin D Receptor Gene Polymorphism in Physically Independent Older Adults

Regina Poli-Frederico[1](✉), Marcos Fernandes[1],
Rubens A. da Silva[1,2], and Karen Fernandes[1]

[1] Master Program Rehabilitation Sciences UEL-UNOPAR,
Av. Paris 675, Jd. Piza, Cx. P. 401, Londrina, PR 86041-140, Brazil
reginafrederico@yahoo.com.br

[2] Département des Sciences de la Sante, Programme de physiothérapie
de Université McGill offert en extension to the Université du Québec
à Chicoutimi (UQAC), et Laboratoire de recherche Biomécanique
& neurophysiologique en réadaptation neuro-muscle-Squelettique – Lab BioNR,
Saguenay, QC, Canada

**Abstract.** This study aimed to assess the association between VDR polymorphisms and postural balance in physically independent elderly. 142 elderly persons were enrolled at this case-control study. In order to assess the balance, the individuals performed three 30-s trials of one-legged stance balance test on a BIOMEC400 force-platform (EMG System of Brazil, SP Ltda.), following a standardized protocol (with 30 s of rest between each trial). The main balance parameters used for analysis were: center of pressure area (COP), sway velocity (cm/s) and frequency (s) in both the antero-posterior (A/P) and the medio-lateral (M/L) axes. The VDR TaqI polymorphism analysis was by PCR-RFLP. The case group showed lower values of COP, sway velocity in A/P and M/L axes (p = 0.0007). Similar data were observed regarding frequency in A/P (p = 0.04) and M/L axes (p = 0.03). Therefore, carriers of the "C" allele have a better postural balance when compared to individuals with "T" allele.

**Keywords:** Falls · Postural balance · Vitamin D receptor · Elderly

## 1 Introduction

The most important physiological changes age-related [1] regarding physical performance are the decline in muscle strength, aerobic capacity and falls. Balance is another function that often becomes impaired with aging [2–4]. Balance involves several control systems, including motor control mechanisms and sensory integrative processes (visual, vestibular, and proprioception), which undergo significant changes with age [5, 6]. The role of genetic factors, such as the genetic polymorphisms of BsmI, TaqI, ApaI and FokI in the vitamin D receptor (VDR) gene in fracture risk has been extensively reported [7–13]. But, the exact association has failed to be well defined and still remains to be further evaluated.

© Springer International Publishing AG, part of Springer Nature 2019
N. J. Lightner (Ed.): AHFE 2018, AISC 779, pp. 397–404, 2019.
https://doi.org/10.1007/978-3-319-94373-2_44

Both active forms of vitamin D and standard supplemental vitamin D have been suggested to prevent falls among older individuals. The benefit of vitamin D in falls/fractures extends beyond improved bone health. Vitamin D can strengthen muscle and hence reduce falls. Meta-analysis has shown that supplemental vitamin D at a dose of 700 IU to 1000 IU a day reduces the risk of falling among older individuals by 19% [14]. The current opinion is that in community-dwelling elderly, vitamin D supplementation reduces the rate of falls or risk of falling in a subgroup of people with low vitamin D levels but its benefit is absent in people without deficiency [15].

Vitamin D Receptor (VDR) is a nuclear hormone receptor which was the first to be implicated in osteoporosis and it has been targeted in the research of genetic determinants influencing bone status, once the activity of vitamin D is mediated by VDR activation. However, despite there are some evidence concerning VDR polymorphisms and falls, a relation between VDR polymorphisms and balance has not been properly addressed. Thus, this study aimed to assess the association between VDR polymorphisms and postural balance in physically independent elderly.

## 2    Materials and Methods

**Subjects.** In the present cross-sectional study, initially 483 physically independent elderly individuals registered with basic health units from the local population were screened for the evaluation of the risk of osteoporosis. Detailed information on age, medical history and life style was obtained from these subjects. A total of 142 elderly individuals were found to be eligible (mean age 68 ± 6.0) and were enrolled at this case-control study.

**Postural Balance.** Postural balance assessment was performed during one-legged stance test [16, 17] using a force-platform (400 BIOMEC, EMG System of Brazil Ltda, Brazil). Reaction force signals were recorded and filtered (low pass filter of second order, Butterworth, 35 Hz, with sampling of 100 Hz) and processed by routine stabilographic analysis on its own software's system. Subjects were familiarized with both the equipment and experimental protocol before the test. Balance test consisted in remaining barefoot on one leg with the limb of choice; the contralateral limb was flexed approximately 90° with arms along the body. The subject stood with eyes opened, looking at a target placed in front at eye level, two feet away (Fig. 1).
Participants performed three trials of maximum 30 s, with rest periods of approximately 30 s between each attempt. The main parameters for stabilographic analysis used in the present study were 95% confidence ellipse area of center of pressure (COP area in $cm^2$) and mean velocity sway of COP (MVel in cm/s) for anteroposterior (A/P) and medial-lateral (M/L) direction of movement. The variables were computed across time-series for each trial and the mean was used for analysis.

**Collection of Material for DNA Analysis.** DNA was obtained from 200 μL of peripheral blood leukocytes, collected using EDTA, with the use of a DNA extraction kit (PureLink Genomic DNA Kits - Invitrogen), in compliance with the manufacturer's instructions. The extracted DNA was stored in a freezer at −80 °C until the polymorphism analyses were carried out.

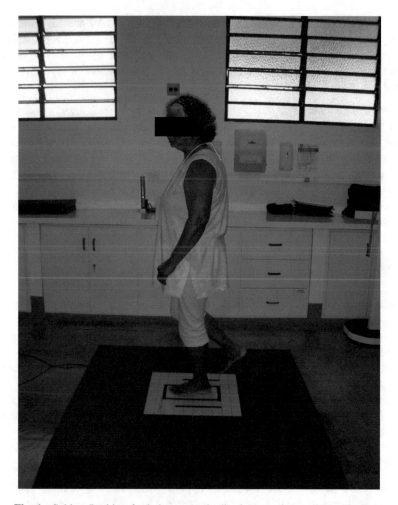

**Fig. 1.** Subject Position for balance standardized protocol on a Force Platform.

The evaluation of DNA quality and quantity was performed through an analysis of absorbance in a spectrophotometer (NanoDrop 2000 – Thermo Scientific) at 260 nm and 280 nm. Dilution of the DNA was subsequently performed with Milli-Q® ultra-pure water for a final concentration of 30 ng/µL.

**Analysis of Polymorphisms in the VDR Gene by Means of the Real-Time Polymerase Chain Reaction (PCR).** In order to analyze the SNPs of the Taq I VDR gene (rs731236), the DNA fragment amplification technique was carried out by means of a real-time polymerase chain reaction (PCR), using the TaqMan® system (Applied Biosystems, Foster City, USA). The standardized reaction used contained 20 µL of final volume, comprising 10 µL of Taqman® Genotyping Master Mix (1x), 0.5 µL of probe (1x) (Applied Biosystems, Foster City, USA), 7.5 µL of Milli-Q® ultrapure water and 2 µL of DNA (30 ng/µL). The thermocycler StepOne Plus™ Real-Time

PCR System (Applied Biosystems, Foster City, USA) was employed, with the fol
lowing cycling: 60 °C for 30 s (pre-denaturation), 95 °C for 10 min for initial denat
uration, 50 cycles of 95 °C for 15 s (denaturation) and 60 °C for 90 s (prime
sequencing) and a final cycle lasting 30 s at 60 °C. The evaluation of the results was
carried out using StepOne Software v2.3.

**Statistical Analysis.** Statistical Package for Social SPSS statistical software (v.18
SPSS Inc., Chicago) was used to analyze the data. Frequencies, means and standard
deviation were calculated for each variable. The $\chi 2$ test was used to test the association
between osteoporosis and the independent variables such as: sex, age, body mass index
and genotype and allele frequencies. The $\chi 2$ test was used for the Hardy-Weinberg
equilibrium analysis. Simple and multiple logistic regression analysis was employed to
test the association between postural balance and the independent variables (sex, age
BMI and genotypes). The level of significance adopted for all the analyses was $p < 0.05$

# 3  Results

**Sample Characterization.** In this case-control study, 142 elderly individuals were
recruited, being 100 women (70.4%) and 42 men (29.6%).

The mean age of this sample was $68.02 \pm 5.9$ (Minimum age: 60 and Maximum
age: 83). No difference was observed between the age of the groups ($p = 0.26$)
according to Unpaired t test. Similarly, no difference was observed in body mass index
when compared the case (G2) and control group (G1, $p = 0.45$).

Regarding gender, the distribution among the groups was also similar according to
Fisher Exact Test ($p = 0.36$). Therefore, it may be assumed that the groups were similar
considering age, gender and body mass index.

Considering genotypes frequencies, it was observed that 62 (43.7%) individuals
harbor TT genotype, while 80 individuals (56.3%) harbor TC and CC genotypes.

**Balance Parameters.** Since all balance parameters had no normal distribution
(Shapiro Wilk test, $p = 0.05$), data were expressed by median and interquartile range
(1st Q.–3rd Q.) and groups were compared using Mann-Whitney's test. The case group
showed lower values of COP [G1 median: 13.8 (8.7–26.1) versus G2 median: 9.9 (7.8–
16.9), $p = 0.009$, Fig. 2], sway velocity in A/P [G1 median: 3.4 (2.9–5.1) versus G2
median: 2.9 (2.4–4.1), $p = 0.01$, Fig. 3] and M/L axes [G1 median: 4.3 (3.3–5.7
versus G2 median: 3.5 (2.8–4.3), $p = 0.0007$, Fig. 3]. Similar data were observed
regarding frequency in A/P [G1 median: 0.9 (0.7–1.1) versus G2 median: 0.8 (0.6–1.0)
$p = 0.04$] and M/L axes [G1 median: 1.0 (0.8–1.3) versus G2 median: 0.9 (0.8–1.1)
$p = 0.03$, Fig. 4]. Therefore, carriers of the "C" allele have a better postural balance
when compared to individuals with "T" allele.

Genetic polymorphisms have been extensively studied in recent years for the early
detection of various diseases with an interest in previous treatment to any harmfu
advance the health of the population [7].

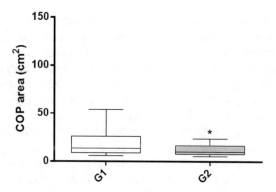

**Fig. 2.** Center of Pressure Area (COP) values for experimental group (EG) and control (CG). * statistical significant differences between the groups, Mann-Whitney test, p < 0.05. Discussion.

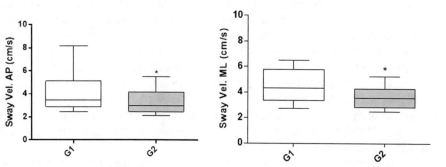

**Fig. 3.** Sway velocity in the anterior-posterior (AP) and Medio-lateral (ML) direction for Case (G2) and Control Group (G1). * Statistical significant differences between the groups, Mann-Whitney test, p < 0.05.

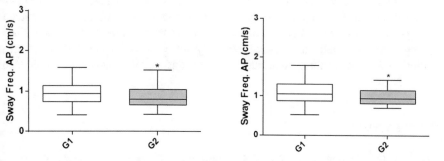

**Fig. 4.** Sway velocity in the anterior-posterior (AP) and Medio-lateral (ML) direction for Case (G2) and Control Group (G1). * Statistical significant differences between the groups, Mann-Whitney test, p < 0.05.

Vitamin D plays an important role in calcium homeostasis and its deficiency has direct effects on bone health, with negative effects on bone remodeling [18]. There is evidence of a beneficial effect of vitamin D for the regulation of various cellular functions and recently the effects of vitamin D on muscle mass and strength have been analyzed [19, 20].

The biological actions of vitamin D in the differentiation of muscle cells, metabolism and function are multiple, acting both directly and indirectly, by genomic and not genomic pathways [18]. The identification of vitamin D receptors in skeletal muscle is direct evidence of the mechanism by which vitamin D acts on the skeletal muscles and its deficiency is associated with muscle loss in the elderly. Furthermore, it was also described a lower expression of vitamin D receptor in skeletal muscles of elderly [14]. However, the association between vitamin D deficiency and balance impairment has not been properly addressed.

At this study, we observed that individuals that carriers of "C" have better balance performance in all variables analyzed. Therefore, the presence of "C" allele may have a protective effect against balance impairment related to ageing process.

The advantage of results from this study is that reliable COP sway parameters were used to contrast balance differences between groups instead of using subjective questionnaires or balance scales such as Berg or Tinneti, similarly from previous work [21]. Functional tests or balance scale can measure balance deficit indirectly, while COP parameters from a force platform can directly analyze balance deficits related to proprioception and postural adjustments [22–24]. In contrast to these previous studies which assessed healthy community-dwelling older adults using double-leg stance tasks the present study included a more challenging balance-control task to shown the impact of vitamin D deficiency, which may be more predictive of balance problems and consequently, a better indicator of falls [25].

The underlying mechanism involved in balance impairment related to vitamin D deficiency is not clearly understood. One possible explanation remains in the fact that low levels of vitamin D have a negative effect in gait speed which may influence indirectly balance. This result has been previously demonstrated by Boersma et al. [26]

This study has potentially implications for public health, once balance may increase falls' risk in elderly. Therefore, it is important to provide valuable knowledge for clinicians and healthcare policymakers concerning the necessity of identify individuals with polymorphism of vitamin D receptor as well as treat vitamin D deficiency. These strategies may help falls' prevention, especially in persons with a high risk of recurrent falling and, consequently, contribute to reductions in fall-related injuries in older adults [27].

# References

1. Fleg, J.L., Morrell, C.H., Bos, A.G., Brant, L.J., Talbot, L.A., Wright, J.G., et al. Accelerated longitudinal decline of aerobic capacity in healthy older adults. Circulation **112** 674–682 (2005)
2. Corriveau, H., Prince, F., Hebert, R., Raiche, M., Tessier, D., Maheux, P., et al.: Evaluation of postural stability in elderly with diabetic neuropathy. Diab. Care. **23**, 1187–1191 (2000)

3. Horak, F.B., Shupert, C.L., Mirka, A.: Components of postural dyscontrol in the elderly: a review. Neurobiol. Aging **10**, 727–738 (1989)
4. Hughes, M.A., Duncan, P.W., Rose, D.K., Chandler, J.M., Studenski, S.A.: The relationship of postural sway to sensorimotor function, functional performance, and disability in the elderly. Arch. Phys. Med. Rehab. **77**, 567–572 (1996)
5. Stelmach, G.E., Teasdale, N., Di Fabio, R.P., Phillips, J.: Age related decline in postural control mechanisms. Int. J. Aging Hum. Dev. **29**, 205–223 (1989)
6. Woollacott, M.H., Shumway-Cook, A.: Changes in posture control across the life span—a systems approach. Phys. Ther. **70**, 799–807 (1990)
7. Ji, G.R., Yao, M., Sun, C.Y., Li, Z.H., Han, Z.: BsmI, TaqI, ApaI and FokI polymorphisms in the vitamin D receptor (VDR) gene and risk of fracture in Caucasians: a meta-analysis. Bone **47**, 681–686 (2010)
8. Fang, Y., Rivadeneira, F., van Meurs, J.B., Pols, H.A., Ioannidis, J.P., Uitterlinden, A.G.: Vitamin D receptor gene BsmI and TaqI polymorphisms and fracture risk: a meta-analysis. Bone **39**, 938–945 (2006)
9. Aerssens, J., Dequeker, J., Peeters, J., Breemans, S., Broos, P., Boonen, S.: Polymorphisms of the VDR, ER and COLIA1 genes and osteoporotic hip fracture in elderly postmenopausal women. Osteoporos. Int. **11**, 583–591 (2000)
10. Alvarez-Hernández, D., Naves, M., Díaz-López, J.B., Gómez, C., Santamaría, I., Cannata-Andía, J.B.: Influence of polymorphisms in VDR and COLIA1 genes on the risk of osteoporotic fractures in aged men. Kidney Int. Suppl. **63**, S14–S18 (2003)
11. Berg, J.P., Falch, J.A., Haug, E.: Fracture rate, pre- and postmenopausal bone mass and early and late postmenopausal bone loss are not associated with vitamin D receptor genotype in a high-endemic area of osteoporosis. Eur. J. Endocrinol. **135**, 96–100 (1996)
12. Chatzipapas, C., Boikos, S., Drosos, G.I., Kazakos, K., Tripsianis, G., Serbis, A., Stergiopoulos, S., Tilkeridis, C., Verettas, D.A., Stratakis, C.A.: Polymorphisms of the vitamin D receptor gene and stress fractures. Horm. Metab. Res. **41**, 635–640 (2009)
13. Feskanich, D., Hunter, D.J., Willett, W.C., Hankinson, S.E., Hollis, B.W., Hough, H.L., Kelsey, K.T., Colditz, G.A.: Vitamin D receptor genotype and the risk of bone fractures in women. Epidemiology **9**, 535–539 (1998)
14. Bischoff-Ferrari, H.A., Dawson-Hughes, B., Staehelin, H.B., et al.: Fall prevention with supplemental and active forms of vitamin D: a meta-analysis of randomised controlled trials. BMJ **339**, b3692 (2009)
15. Gillespie, L.D., Robertson, M.C., Gillespie, W.J., et al.: Interventions for preventing falls in older people living in the community. Cochrane Database Syst. Rev. **9**, CD007146 (2012)
16. Davidson, B.S., Madigan, M.L., Nussbaum, M.A.: Effects of lumbar extensor fatigue and fatigue rate on postural sway. Eur. J. Appl. Physiol. **93**, 183–189 (2004)
17. Gribble, P.A., Hertel, J.: Effect of hip and ankle muscle fatigue on unipedal postural control. J. Electromyog. Kinesiol. **14**, 641–646 (2004)
18. Rizzoli, R., Stevenson, J.C., Bauer, J.M., Van Loon, L.J., Walrand, S., Kanis, J.A., Cooper, C., Brandi, M.L., Diez-Perez, A., Reginster, J.Y.: ESCEO Task Force. The role of dietary protein and vitamin D in maintaining musculoskeletal health in postmenopausal women: a consensus statement from the European Society for Clinical and Economic Aspects of Osteoporosis and Osteoarthritis (ESCEO). Maturitas **79**, 122–132 (2014)
19. Hildebrand, R.A., Miller, B., Warren, A., Hildebrand, D., Smith, B.J.: Compromised vitamin D status negatively affects muscular strength and power of collegiate athletes. Int. J. Sport Nutr. Exerc. Metab. **26**, 558–564 (2016)

20. Gifondorwa, D.J., Thompson, T.D., Wiley, J., Culver, A.E., Shetler, P.K., Rocha, G.V., M Y.L., Krishnan, V., Bryant, H.U.: Vitamin D and/or calcium deficient diets may differentiall affect muscle fiber neuromuscular junction innervation. Muscle Nerve **54**, 1120–1132 (201(

21. Takkouche, B., Montes-Martinez, A., Gill, S.S., Etminan, M.: Psychotropic medications an the risk of fracture: a meta-analysis. Drug Saf. **30**, 171–184 (2007)

22. Holbein, J.M.A., Dermott, M.C.K., Shaw, C., Demchak, J.: Validity of functional stabilit limits as a measure of balance in adults aged 23–73 years. Ergonomics **50**, 631–646 (200'

23. Pollock, A.S., Durward, B.R., Rowe, P.J., Paul, J.P.: What is balance? Clin. Rehabil. **1** 402–406 (2000)

24. Nguyen, D.T., Kiel, D.P., Li, W., Galica, A.M., Kang, H.G., Casey, V.A., et al.: Correlatior of clinical and laboratory measures of balance in older men and women. Arth. Care Res. **6**, 1895–1902 (2012)

25. Hurvitz, E.A., Richardson, J.K., Werner, R.A., Ruhl, A.M., Dixon, M.R.: Unipedal stanc testing as an indicator of fall risk among older outpatients. Arch. Phys. Med. Rehabil. **8**, 587–591 (2000)

26. Boersma, D., Demontiero, O., Mohtasham, A.Z., Hassan, S., Suarez, H., Geisinger, D Suriyaarachchi, P., Sharma, A., Duque, G.: Vitamin D status in relation to postural stabilit in the elderly. J. Nutr. Health Aging. **16**, 270–275 (2012)

27. Haetholt, K.A.: [Cost]effectiveness of withdrawal of fall-risk increasing drugs versu conservative treatment in older fallers: design of a multicenter randomized controlled tria (IMPROveFALL-study). BMC Geriatri. **11**, 48 (2011)

# Author Index

© Springer International Publishing AG, part of Springer Nature 2019
N. J. Lightner (Ed.): AHFE 2018, AISC 779, pp. 405–407, 2019.
https://doi.org/10.1007/978-3-319-94373-2